General Pathology Student Guide

Jessica Claus • Linda Corey Hanley • Joyce Ou
Editors

General Pathology Student Guide

With AMBOSS Shortcuts

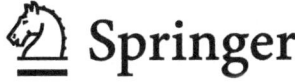

Editors
Jessica Claus
Department of Pathology
and Laboratory Medicine
Brown University
Providence, RI, USA

Joyce Ou
Department of Pathology
and Laboratory Medicine
Brown University
Providence, RI, USA

Linda Corey Hanley
Department of Pathology
and Laboratory Medicine
Brown University
Providence, RI, USA

ISBN 978-3-662-67961-6   ISBN 978-3-662-67962-3   (eBook)
https://doi.org/10.1007/978-3-662-67962-3

© The Editor(s) (if applicable) and The Author(s), under exclusive license to Springer-Verlag GmbH, DE, part of Springer Nature 2024
This work is subject to copyright. All rights are solely and exclusively licensed by the Publisher, whether the whole or part of the material is concerned, specifically the rights of translation, reprinting, reuse of illustrations, recitation, broadcasting, reproduction on microfilms or in any other physical way, and transmission or information storage and retrieval, electronic adaptation, computer software, or by similar or dissimilar methodology now known or hereafter developed.
The use of general descriptive names, registered names, trademarks, service marks, etc. in this publication does not imply, even in the absence of a specific statement, that such names are exempt from the relevant protective laws and regulations and therefore free for general use.
The publisher, the authors, and the editors are safe to assume that the advice and information in this book are believed to be true and accurate at the date of publication. Neither the publisher nor the authors or the editors give a warranty, expressed or implied, with respect to the material contained herein or for any errors or omissions that may have been made. The publisher remains neutral with regard to jurisdictional claims in published maps and institutional affiliations.

Cover illustration: Photo by Dr. Corey Hanley, Providence

This Springer imprint is published by the registered company Springer-Verlag GmbH, DE, part of Springer Nature.
The registered company address is: Heidelberger Platz 3, 14197 Berlin, Germany

Paper in this product is recyclable.

Preface

The present book is based on the German pathology curriculum and was originally developed in a cooperation between two medical students Jessica Claus and Carsten Fechner, medical graduates from Rostock University, Germany.
The redesign and additional production was supported by Doctor Annette Zimpfer and Professor Doctor Andreas Erbersdobler.
All histopathological slides treated in the course are presented in thematic blocks with a focus on macroscopy, histology, etiology and pathogenesis. The clinical pictures are briefly linked with clinical references.
To deepen the course contents, we encourage the students to look up the individual aspects and to reference the bibliography. At the same time, the pathology book contains a barcode, which forwards you to the relevant learning chapter of the AMBOSS learning platform. AMBOSS is a paid program for medical students and doctors. Please check with your medical school to see if it offers free user licenses.

We wish all students a pleasant and successful pathology course.
We ask for feedback on incorrect statements and look forward to your suggestions or suggestions for correction to the course book. We do not guarantee completeness and accept no liability claims.
To prepare for pathology lessons, we recommend the review of histology.

Disclaimer: The cooperation with AMBOSS does exclude financial interests from both parties. None of the editors, authors, Springer Publishing or AMBOSS are receiving financial or other compensation for connecting the chapters to individual parts from the AMBOSS learning platform. The sole intent is to provide readers the opportunity to access further clinical information based on the presented pathology based on an interactive concept.

American Edition by:
Jessica Claus
L. Corey Hanley
Joyce Ou

Acknowledgement

We would like to thank our German collaborators from the department of pathology at Rostock University and the Department of Pathology and Laboratory Medicine at Brown University. Many thanks to all of the faculty, and especially to the trainees and students, who took time to contribute to this effort; and special thanks to Dr. W. Dwayne Lawrence, Professor Emeritus, for his early support of this project, and his continuing encouragement.
- *The Editors* -

Personal Acknowledgments:
Kafka once said: "Paths are made by walking them."
Therefore, I would like to thank the people who paved this path for me. First my family and then my mentors:
Dr. Cornelia Woitek, Dr. Annette Zimpfer, Dr. Andreas Erbersdobler, Dr. Michele Lomme, Dr. Corey Hanley, Dr. Joyce Ou, Dr. William Dwayne Lawrence, Dr. James Sung, Dr. Diana Treaba and Dr. Nina Tatevian.
- *Jessica Claus* -

Editors

Jessica Claus, MD
Resident Physician
Department of Pathology and
Laboratory Medicine,
Warren Alpert Medical School of
Brown University, USA

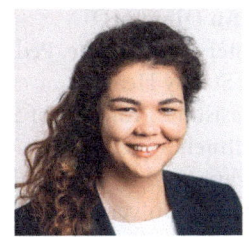

L. Corey Hanley, MD
Associate Professor of Pathology
and Laboratory Medicine
Warren Alpert Medical School of
Brown University, USA

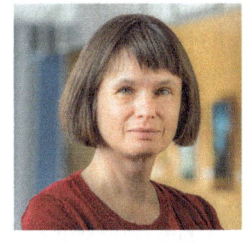

Joyce Ou, MD, PhD
Associate Professor of Pathology
and Laboratory Medicine
Warren Alpert Medical School of
Brown University, USA

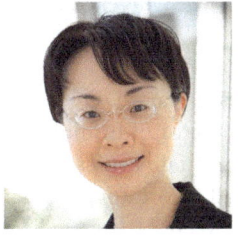

Authors

Carsten Fechner, MD
Resident Physician
Department of Radiology
Kantonsspital Luzern
Luzern, Switzerland

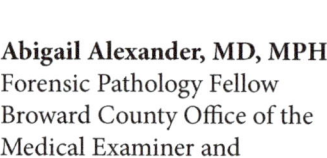

Ann Ding, MD
Internal Medicine, Pediatrics
at Sturdy Health
Assistant Professor of Pediatrics,
Clinician Educator at
Warren Alpert Medical School of
Brown University, USA

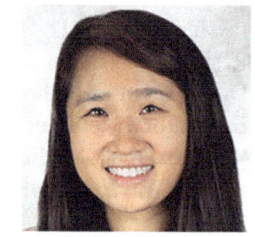

Abigail Alexander, MD, MPH
Forensic Pathology Fellow
Broward County Office of the
Medical Examiner and
Trauma Services, USA

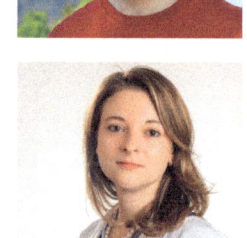

Prof. Dr. Andreas Erbersdobler
Professor and Chief of Pathology
Institute of Pathology
University Medical Center
Rostock, Germany

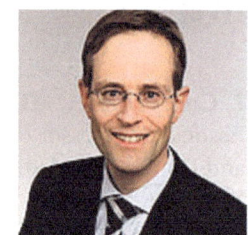

Stephanie Barak, MD
Associate Professor of Pathology
and Laboratory Medicine,
Clinician Educator
Warren Alpert Medical School of
Brown University, USA

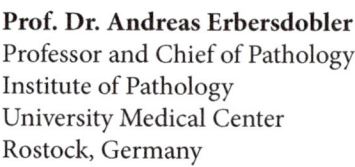

Ricky Grisson, MD, MBA
Associate Professor of Pathology
and Laboratory Medicine
Warren Alpert Medical School of
Brown University, USA

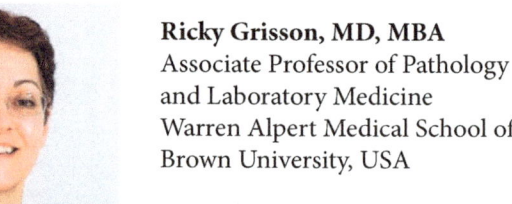

Robert Barno, MD
Resident Physician
Department of Pathology and
Laboratory Medicine,
Warren Alpert Medical School of
Brown University, USA

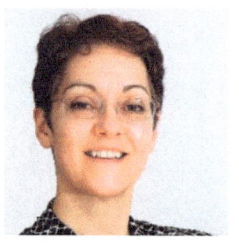

Jesse Hart, DO
Director of Immunohistochemistry
Associate Professor of Pathology
and Laboratory Medicine
Warren Alpert Medical School of
Brown University, USA

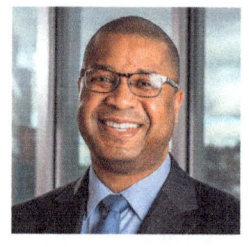

Miguel Carabaño, MD
Resident Physician
Department of Pathology and
Laboratory Medicine,
Warren Alpert Medical School of
Brown University, USA

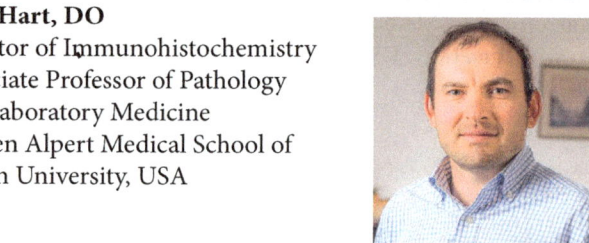

Tao Hong, PhD
Director of Microbiology
Department of Pathology and
Laboratory Medicine,
Rhode Island Hospital
Providence, USA

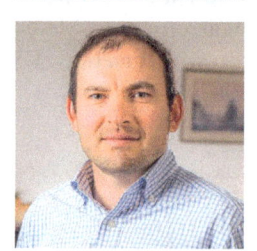

Mariana Canepa, MD
Cyto-/Surgical Pathologist
Associate Professor of Pathology
and Laboratory Medicine
Warren Alpert Medical School of
Brown University, USA

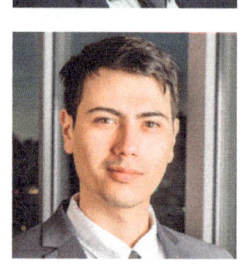

Dr. med. Nora Lamp
Gynecologic Pathologist
Practice of Pathology
Northeast Pathology Network
Rostock, Germany

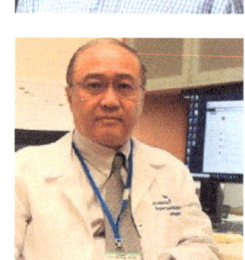

Katelyn Dannheim, MD
Pediatric/Perinatal Pathologist
and Hematopathologist
Massachusetts General Hospital,
Harvard Medical School, USA

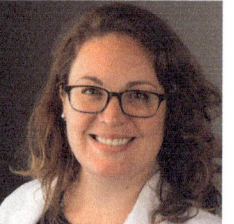

Shaolei Lu, MD
Associate Professor of Pathology
and Laboratory Medicine
Warren Alpert Medical School of
Brown University, USA

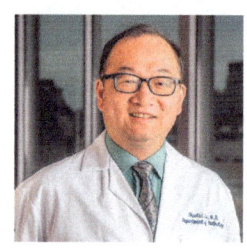

Shivali Marketkar, MD
Assistant Professor of Pathology
and Laboratory Medicine
Warren Alpert Medical School of
Brown University, USA

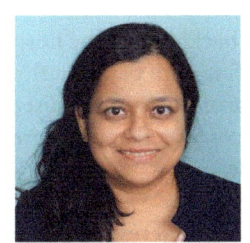

Senior Reviewer

William D Lawrence, MD, MSc
Professor Emeritus of Pathology
and Laboratory Medicine
Warren Alpert Medical School of
Brown University, USA

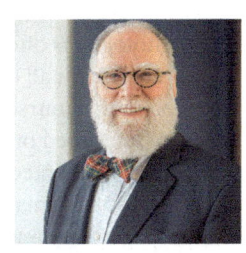

Jao Ou, MD, PhD
Assistant Professor, Radiology
Wake Forest University
School of Medicine, USA

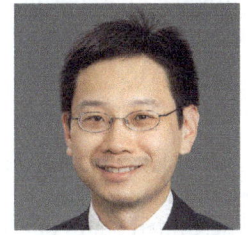

Dr. James Sung, MD
Professor of Pathology
and Laboratory Medicine
Warren Alpert Medical School of
Brown University, USA

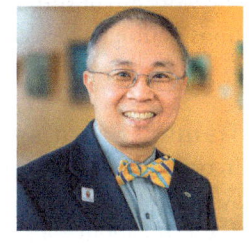

Scetta Samantha, BA
Medical Student
The University of New England
College of Osteopathic Medicine
Maine, USA

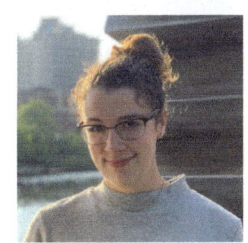

Diana Treaba, MD
Director of Hematopathology
Associate Professor of Pathology
and Laboratory Medicine
Warren Alpert Medical School of
Brown University, USA

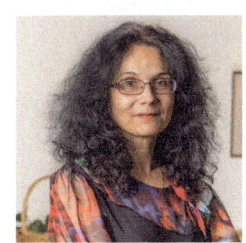

Heejae Yang, BSc, MAT
Brown University Alumni
Providence, USA

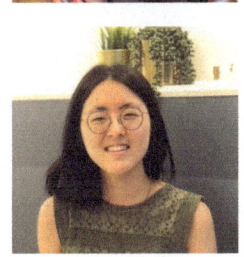

Dr. med Annette Zimpfer
Associate Professor of Pathology
Institute of Pathology
University Medical Center
Rostock, Germany

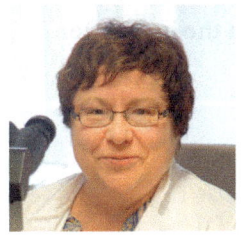

What does a pathologist do?

The pathologist is often referred to as the "doctor's doctor" or the "backbone of the hospital" due to the strong interaction with pretty much all clinical specialties. While not directly interacting with patients, the pathologist is still very actively involved in the course of the patient's care by diagnosing the nature of the patient's disease and, if necessary staging the malignancy identified on the patient's specimen. The findings will be correlated and communicated to treating clinicians and, if necessary presented at tumor boards to the radiologists, surgeons, oncologist and other members of the treatment team to find the best treatment for the individual patient.

Depending on the anatomic or clinical pathology track, clinical duties and responsibilities have a big variation from diagnostic work-up of surgical specimens (biopsies, surgical resections, intraoperative consultations for gross exams or frozen sections), autopsy services or managing laboratory services (hematology, chemistry, microbiology lab, transfusion medicine).

Training Requirements:
In order to become a general anatomic and/or clinical pathologist, candidates need to complete medical (US or international) or osteopathic medical school before entering a residency training program.
There are about 136 anatomic and clinical pathology programs in the United States offering training.

The residency program in the US offers multiple training pathways:
Anatomic Pathology (3 years of training)
Clinical Pathology (3 years of training)
Anatomic and Clinical Pathology (4 years of training)
Anatomic and Neuropathology (4 years of training)

Fellowship Programs:
ACGME-accredited programs:
Blood Banking/Transfusion Medicine
Chemical Pathology
Clinical Informatics
Cytopathology
Dermatopathology
Forensic Pathology
Hematopathology
Medical Microbiology
Molecular Genetic Pathology
Neuropathology Pediatric Pathology
Selective Pathology

*Note: Some clinical pathology specialties can also be entered through a different pathway certified by the American Board of Medical Specialties.

Non-ACGME Accredited Fellowship Programs (depending on the institution):
Breast Pathology
Gastrointestinal Pathology
Genitourinary Pathology
Renal Pathology
Surgical Pathology
Thoracic/Pulmonary Pathology
Perinatal Pathology

Contents

I Review of Histology

1. Inflammatory Pathology
- 1.1 Lobar Pneumonia 20
- 1.2 Acute Appendicitis 23
- 1.3 Acute and Chronic Cholecystitis 25
- 1.4 Chronic Gastric Ulcer 27
- 1.5 Meningitis 29
- 1.6 Gout (Foreign Body-induced Inflammation) 31

2. Infectious Diseases
- 2.1 Bacterial Myocarditis (Sepsis) 39
- 2.2 Esophageal Candidiasis 41
- 2.3 Fungal Pneumonia (Aspergillosis) 43
- 2.4 Pneumocystis Pneumonia 45
- 2.5 Cytomegalovirus (CMV) Pneumonia 48

3. Cellular Adaptation: Hypertrophy, Hyperplasia, Atrophy
- 3.1 Myocardial Hypertrophy 52
- 3.2 Benign Prostatic Hyperplasia 55
- 3.3 Thyroid Goiter (Hyperplasia) 57
- 3.4 Hydronephrosis (Atrophy) 59
- 3.5 Pulmonary Emphysema 62

4. Cell Death: Necrosis, Apoptosis
- 4.1 Coagulation Necrosis (Kidney Infarction) 68
- 4.2 Liquefactive Necrosis (Encephalomalacia) 71
- 4.3 Caseous Necrosis (Tuberculosis) 74
- 4.4 Fat Necrosis (Acute Pancreatitis) 77
- 4.5 Gangrenous Necrosis (Wet Gangrene, Peripheral Arterial Disease) 79

5. Circulatory Diseases and Disorders
- 5.1 Arterial Thromboembolism (White/Precipitation Thrombus) 83
- 5.2 Venous Thromboembolism (Red/Coagulation Thrombus) 85
- 5.3 Hyaline Microthrombi 87
- 5.4 Pulmonary Embolism 89

6. Vascular Pathology and Myocardial Infarction
- 6.1 Atherosclerosis (Aorta) 93
- 6.2 Atherosclerosis (Coronary Artery Disease) 96
- 6.3 Cystic Medial Degeneration/Necrosis 99
- 6.4 Myocardial Infarction 101

7. Immunopathology
- 7.1 Bronchial Asthma 107
- 7.2 Rheumatic Myocarditis 109
- 7.3 Lymphocytic Thyroiditis (Hashimoto's Thyroiditis) 111
- 7.4 Graves' Disease 113
- 7.5 Temporal/Giant Cell Arteritis 115
- 7.6 Vascular Rejection of Kidney Transplant 118

8. Pathologic Regeneration
- 8.1 Leukoplakia 122
- 8.2 Carcinoma in-situ and Squamous Cell Carcinoma of the Esophagus 123
- 8.3 Barrett's Esophagus 125
- 8.4 Barrett's Esophagus - Cancer (Adenocarcinoma) 127
- 8.5 Chronic Gastritis with Intestinal Metaplasia and Dysplasia 129
- 8.6 Cervical Intraepithelial Neoplasia, Grade 2-3 131

9. Epithelial Tumors
- 9.1 Papilloma (Oral) 140
- 9.2 Non-invasive Papillary Urothelial Carcinoma, low- and high-grade 142
- 9.3 Tubulovillous Adenoma of the Rectum with low-grade Dysplasia 143
- 9.4 Basal Cell Carcinoma (Nodular Type) 145
- 9.5 Prostate Cancer 147

10. Non-epithelial Tumors
- 10.1 Lipoma 152
- 10.2 Cavernous Hemangioma (Liver) 153
- 10.3 Leiomyoma (Uterine) 155
- 10.4 Leiomyosarcoma 157
- 10.5 Melanocytic Nevus (Compound Type) 159

11. Appendix
- List of Abbreviations 161
- References 164

1	Review of Histology
1	Inflammatory Pathology
2	Infectious Diseases
3	Cellular Adaptation: Hypertrophy, Hyperplasia, Atrophy
4	Cell Death: Necrosis, Apoptosis
5	Circulatory Diseases and Disorders
6	Vascular Pathology and Myocardial Infarction
7	Immunopathology
8	Pathologic Regeneration
9	Epithelial Tumors
10	Non-epithelial Tumors
11	Appendix

Review of Histology
Jessica Claus, L. Corey Hanley, Joyce Ou

I Review of Histology

Types of Epithelium	Function	Examples
Simple squamous epithelium	- Layer of flat and thin cells - Enables the passage of molecules via diffusion or filtration - Builds lining of blood vessels and body cavities	- Endothelium - Peritoneum - Glomeruli - Alveoli
Simple cuboidal epithelium	- Cube-shaped cells organized in a single (simple) layer - Often found in secreting/glandular cells - Lining (germinal) for ovaries, testes, seminiferous tubules	- Salivary, sweat glands - Pancreas, thyroid - Collecting ducts (kidney) - Mammary glands - Germinal lining
Simple columnar epithelium	- Layer of tall/slender cells with oval-shaped nuclei, ciliated or non-ciliated - **Non-ciliated:** Inner lining of GI-Tract - **Ciliated:** Promote transportation of fluids or other particles	**Non-ciliated:** - Esophagus, stomach **Ciliated:** - Respiratory epithelium - Fallopian tubes - Lining of cerebral ventricles
Stratified squamous epithelium	**Two components:** - Multiple layers of flat epithelial cells - One basal layer (contains stem cells) **Non-keratinizing:** - Forms the lining of mucosal tissue **Keratinizing:** - Skin	**Non-keratinizing:** - Mucosa of oral cavity or pharynx - Upper esophageal mucosa - Vaginal mucosa - Anal mucosa **Keratinizing:** - Epidermis - Metaplastic process
Stratified cuboidal epithelium	- Protective barrier - Occcurs in excretory ducts	- Sweat glands - Salivary ducts - Mammary glands - Pancreatic gland ducts
Stratified columnar epithelium	- Protects underlying tissue - Secretory function	- Conjunctival epithelium - Male Urethra
Pseudostratified columnar epithelium	- Epithelium, with one layer of cells - Cells organized in different levels, creating the appearance of stratified epithelium ('pseudo') - Can be ciliated-or non-ciliated	- Respiratory epithelium - Epididymidis - Vas deferens
Transitional epithelium	- Lines the urogenital tract - Expands and contracts	Urothelium of the: - Proximal urethra - Bladder - Ureter - Renal pelvis

I Review of Histology

Organ:	Skin
Stain:	Hematoxylin - Eosin

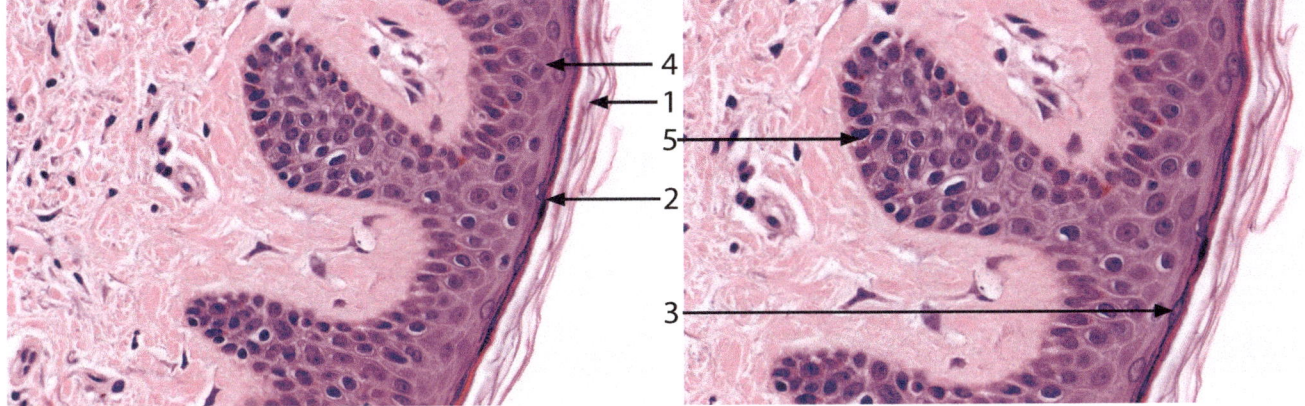

Microscopy: **Epidermis:**

- **Stratum corneum[1]:** Consists of keratinocytes, usually without nuclei
- **Stratum lucidum[2]:** Eosinophilic/pink cell layer with liquefied keratohyalin granules only on the ridged skin (palms, finger soles, toes)
- **Stratum granulosum[3]:** With keratohyalin granules and cell transformation into flattened corneocytes
- **Stratum spinosum[4]:** Polygonal cells and starting point of keratinization
- **Stratum basale[5]:** Iso- to high prismatic stem cells

Dermis:

- **Stratum papillare:** Loose connective tissue, Meissner's corpuscles, nerve endings, capillary loops and cells of the immune system
- **Stratum reticulare:** Tight connective tissue, hair follicles, Ruffini bodies, glands, blood and lymph vessels

Subcutis: Adipose and loose connective tissue, also contains nerves, blood vessels, Vater-Pacini corpuscles

Organ:	Adipose Tissue
Stain:	Hematoxylin - Eosin

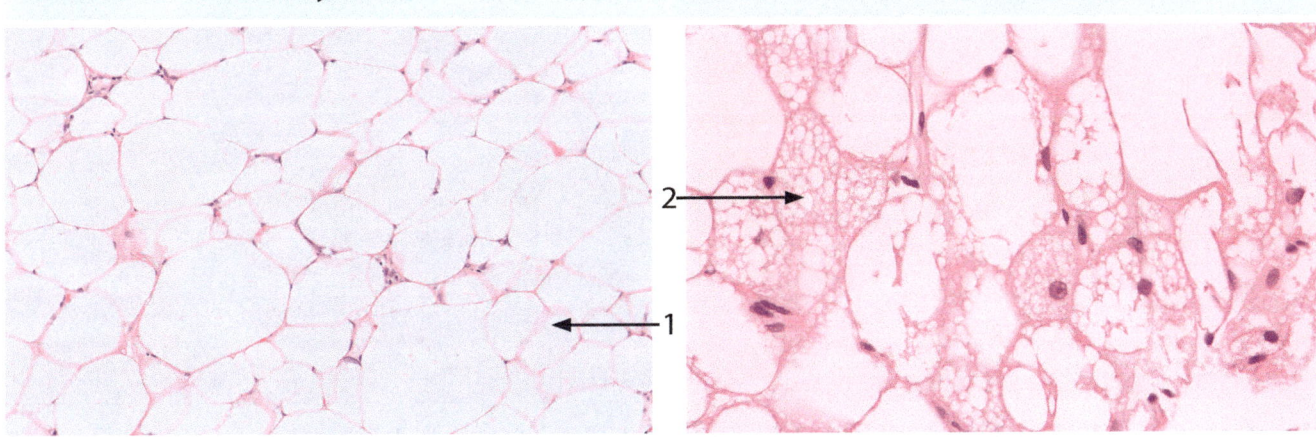

Microscopy:
- **White adipose tissue[1]:** One large fat vacuole in cell, cytoplasm appears clear, nucleus pushed to extreme edge of cell (unilocular), uniform appearing cells
- **Brown adipose tissue[2]:** Adipocytes are polygonal with abundant intracytoplasmic droplets (multilocular), polyogonal appearing cells

2

I Review of Histology

Organ: Skeletal muscle vs smooth muscle
Stain: Hematoxylin - Eosin

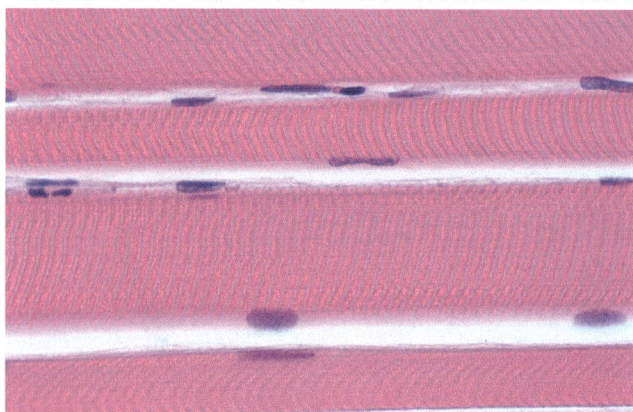 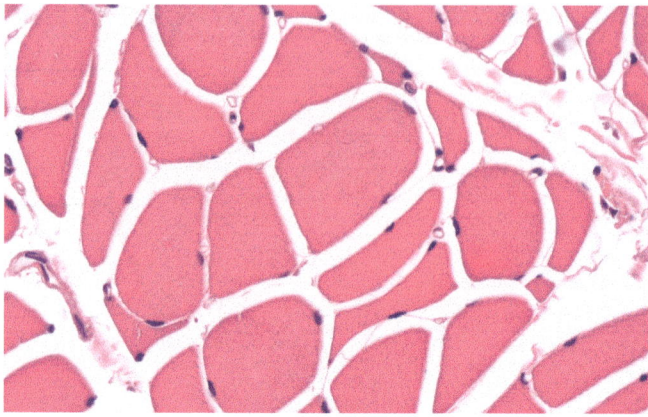

Microscopy: **Skeletal muscle:** Long cylindrical cells, striated, multinucleate, nuclei at cell edge

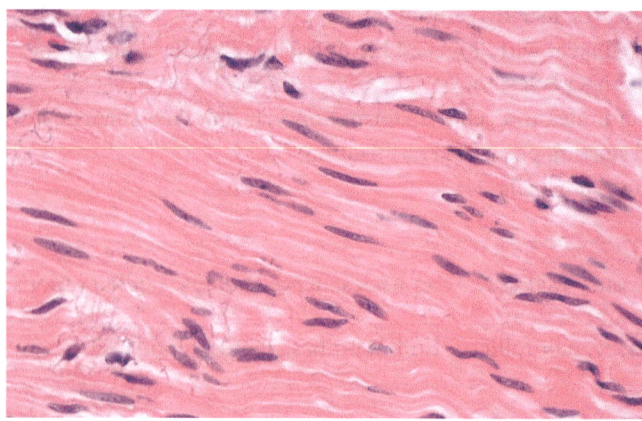 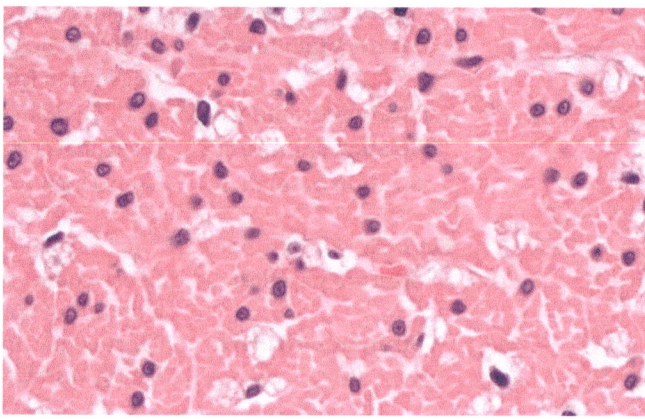

Microscopy: **Smooth muscle:** Shorter, spindle-shaped cells, no striations, nuclei are central

Organ: Heart muscle
Stain: Hematoxylin - Eosin

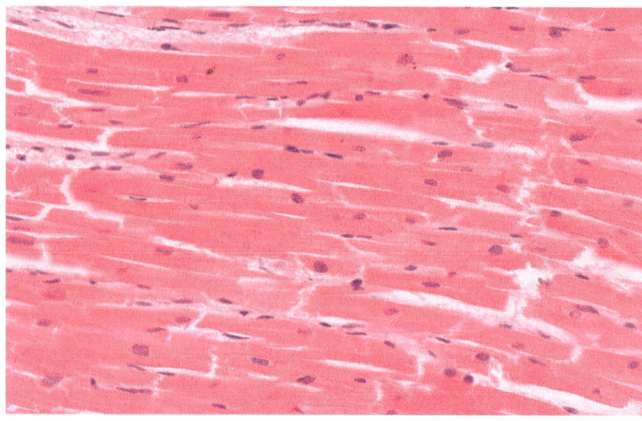 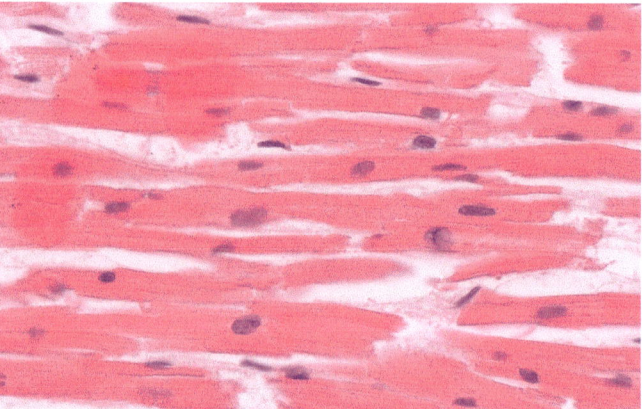

Microscopy: **Endocardium:** Inner layer of the heart (heart valves, atria, ventricles)
Lamina epithelialis (simple squamous epithelium)
Lamina propria (subendothelial loose connective tissue)
Myocardium: Short branched cells called "cardiomyocytes" with central nuclei, striated, longitudinal ends connected by intercalated discs (desmosomes, gap junctions)
Epicardium: Visceral layer of the pericardium with serosa (mesothelial cells)

I Review of Histology

Organ:	Aorta
Stain:	Hematoxylin - Eosin

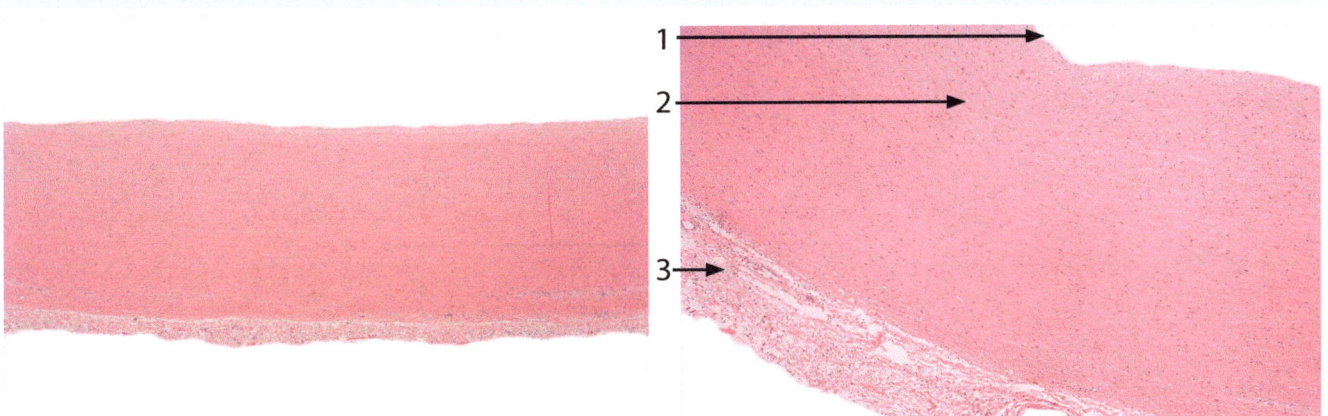

Microscopy:
- Intima[1]: Flat endothelium, basal layer, subendothelial layer, internal elastic lamina
- Media[2]: Circumferential smooth muscle with admixed elastic fibers, and external elastic lamina
- Externa[3]: Adventitia with connective tissue (fibroblasts, proteoglycans, elastic fibers6), collagen fibers, vasa vasorum(vessels of the vessel))

Organ:	Coronary arteries
Stain:	Hematoxylin - Eosin

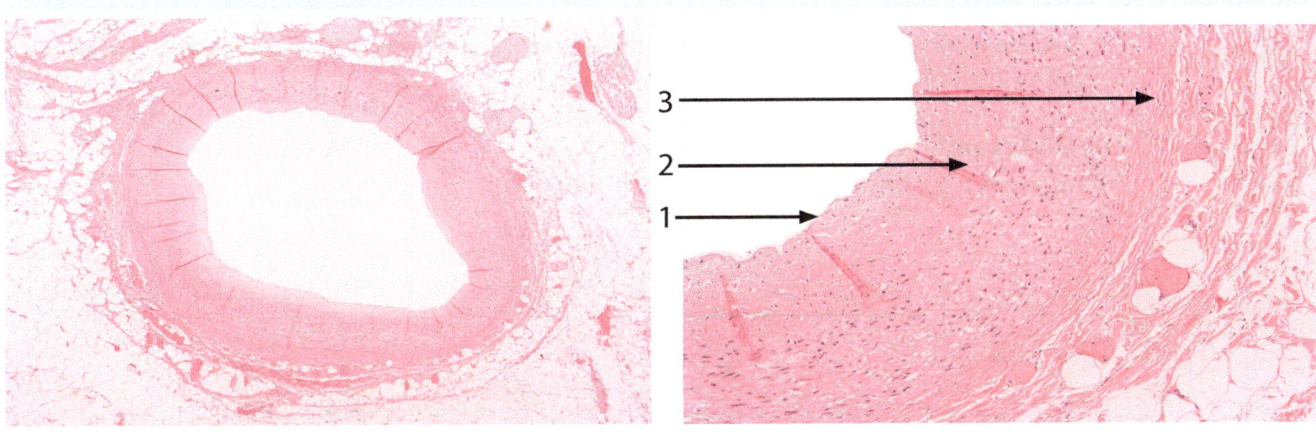

Microscopy: Similar to the aorta, coronary arteries have three layers:
- Intima[1], media[2] and externa[3]

I Review of Histology

Organ: Parathyroid Gland
Stain: Hematoxylin - Eosin

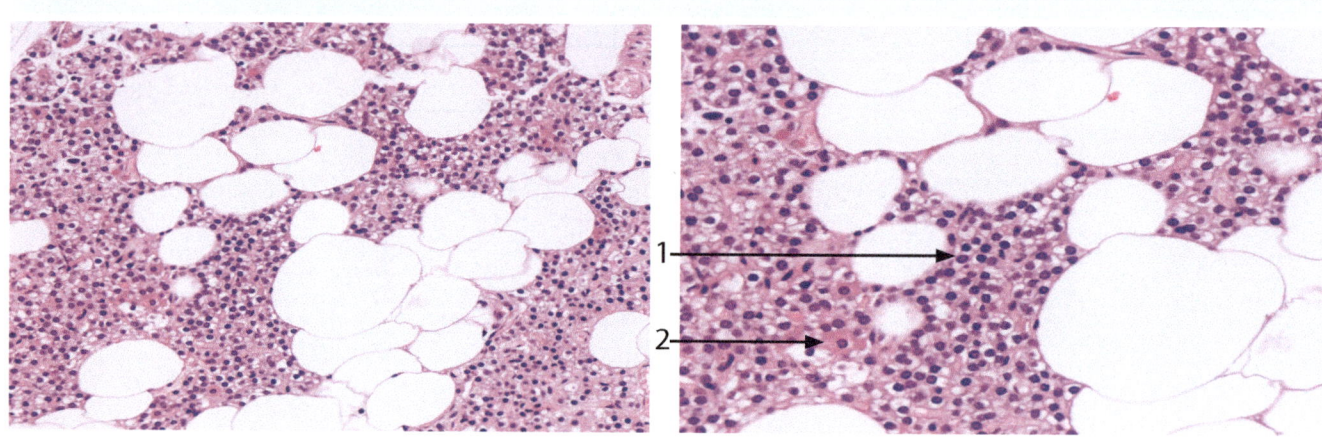

Macroscopy: Four small ovoid glands, approximately 5 mm in size, on posterior of thyroid

Microscopy: Parenchyma consists small cuboidal cells:

- **Chief cells[1]:** Main cell, hormone (parathyroid hormone, PTH) producer, cuboidal with round nucleus, cytoplasm pale (if high glycogen content) or basophilic

- **Oxyphil cells[2]:** Fewer in number, more eosinophilic cytoplasm, many mitochondria, produce low levels of PTH

Cells arranged in strands and clusters, with delicate fibrous connective tissue, capillaries, and admixed fat cells

Parathyroid hormone (PTH) important in calcium metabolism, acts in bone and kidney, increases calcium level and decreases phosphorus levels in serum

Organ: Thyroid gland
Stain: Hematoxylin - Eosin

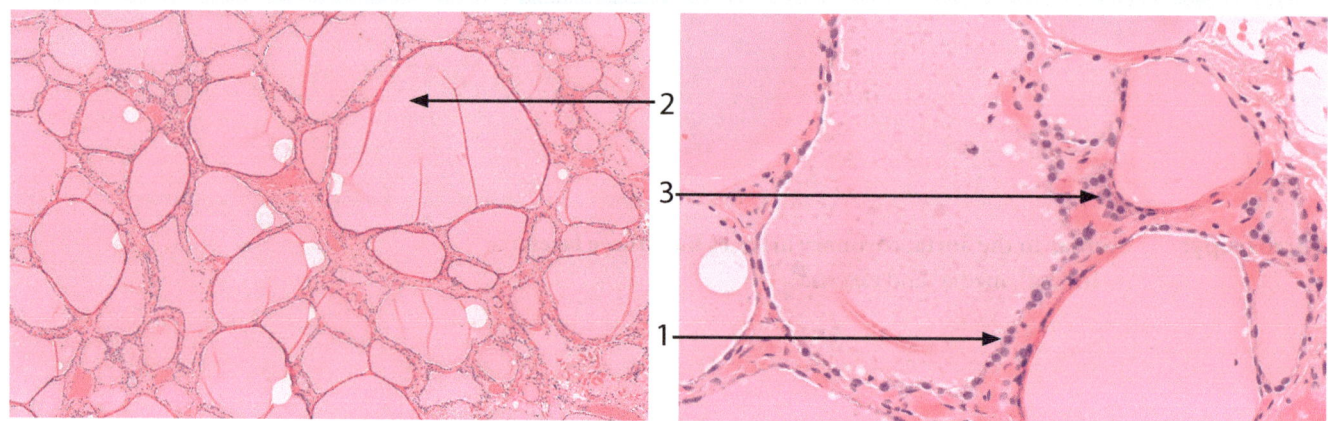

Microscopy: Normal adult weight: 20-25 g, consisting of two lobes connected by the isthmus
Follicles:

- Round cavities surrounded by a single layer of cuboidal epithelial cells[1] with colloid (acellular eosinophilic material) in the lumen
- **Colloid[2]:** Thyroglobulin, triiodothyronine/T3, thyroxine/T4 on protein bound
- **Follicular epithelium:** Iodinates and releases hormone, regulated by thyroid-stimulating hormone (TSH)
- Each follicle surrounded by basement membrane and many fenestrated capillaries with diaphragms

I Review of Histology

Microscopy: Gland composed of two endocrine cell types:
Thyroid epithelium = Follicular cells and C-cells

- **Follicular cells[1]:** Cuboidal cells, arranged in follicle structures around central colloid

- **C-cells[3]:** Also called parafollicular cells, indistinct polygonal cells found between follicles, stain positive for calcitonin (calcium metabolism, decreases blood concentration, inhibits osteoclasts), can appear single or grouped with follicle epithelium and basement membrane

Organ: Lung
Stain: Hematoxylin - Eosin

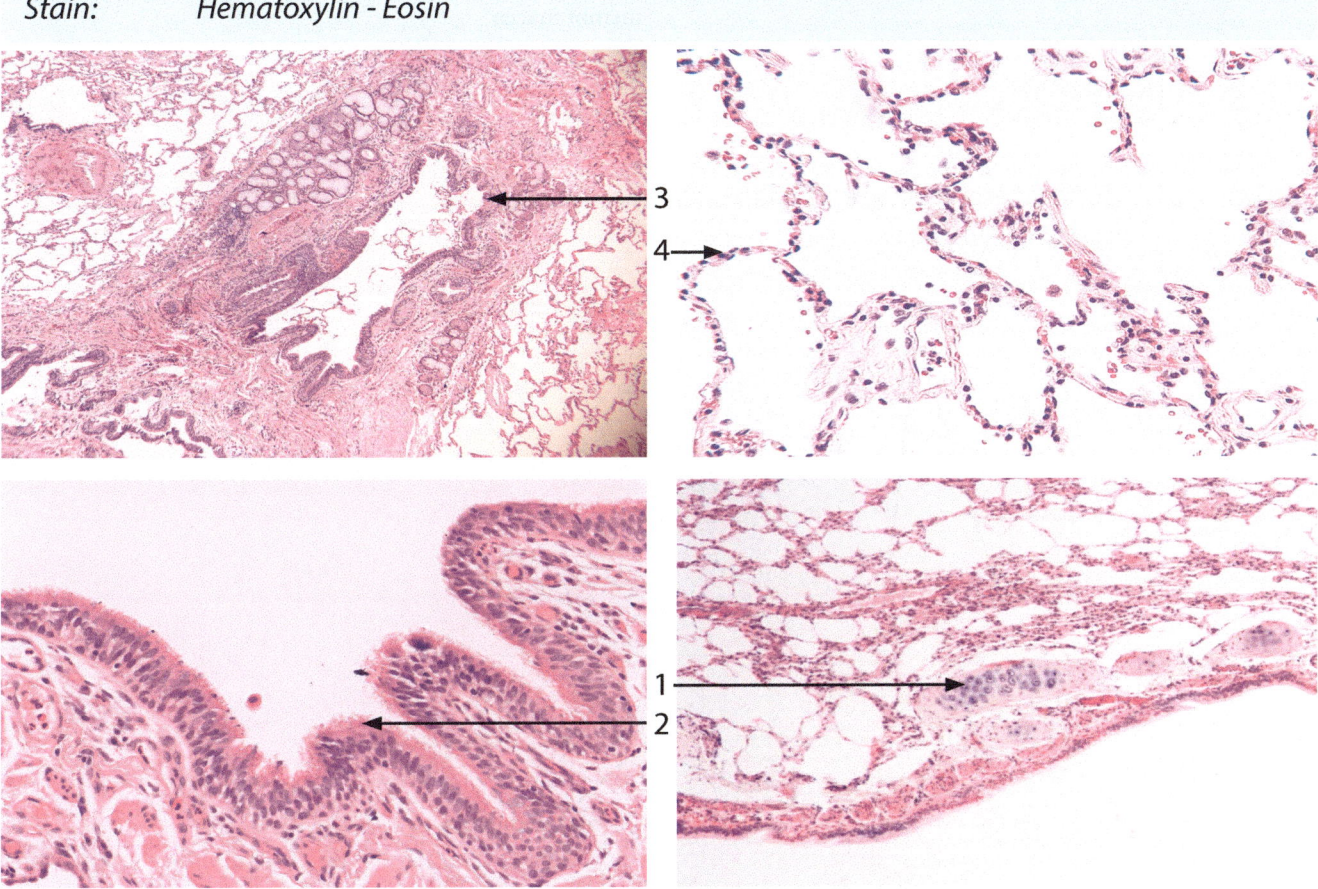

Microscopy:
- **Bronchus[1]:** Discontinuous plates of hyaline cartilage[1], with increasing amounts of smooth muscle as diameter narrows, ciliated pseudostratified columnar epithelium[2] and submucosal glands present

- **Bronchiole[3]:** Prominent smooth muscle with no cartilage and no submucosal glands, ciliated pseudostratified epithelium flattens from columnar to cuboidal to simple squamous at junction between respiratory bronchiole and alveolar structures

Alveolar pneumocytes:
- Type 1[3]: ~ 95% of alveolar lining, simple squamous, contributes to air-blood barrier for gas exchan
- Type 2: ~ 5% of alveolar lining, cuboidal, contain lamellar bodies with pulmonary surfactant

I Review of Histology

Organ: Trachea
Stain: Hematoxylin - Eosin

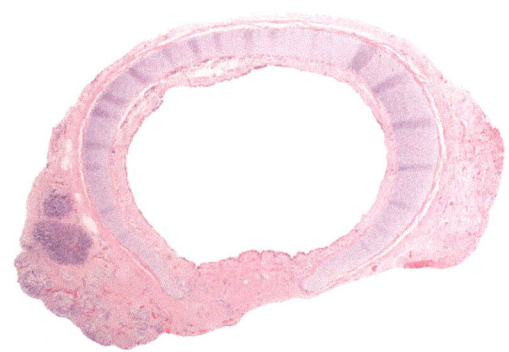

Microscopy:

Mucosa: Ciliated pseudostratified columnar epithelium
Submucosa: Contains glands and elastic tissue
Cartilaginous layer (tunica fibro-musculo-cartilaginea)
Adventitia

Posterior connecting tissue, connecting the cartilages = pars membranacea

Organ: General architecture of gastrointestinal tract:
Stain: Hematoxylin - Eosin

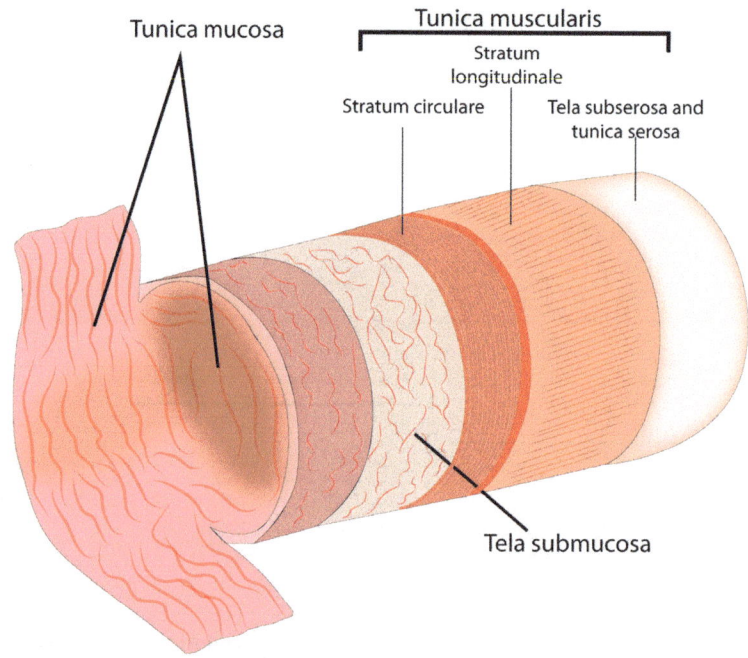

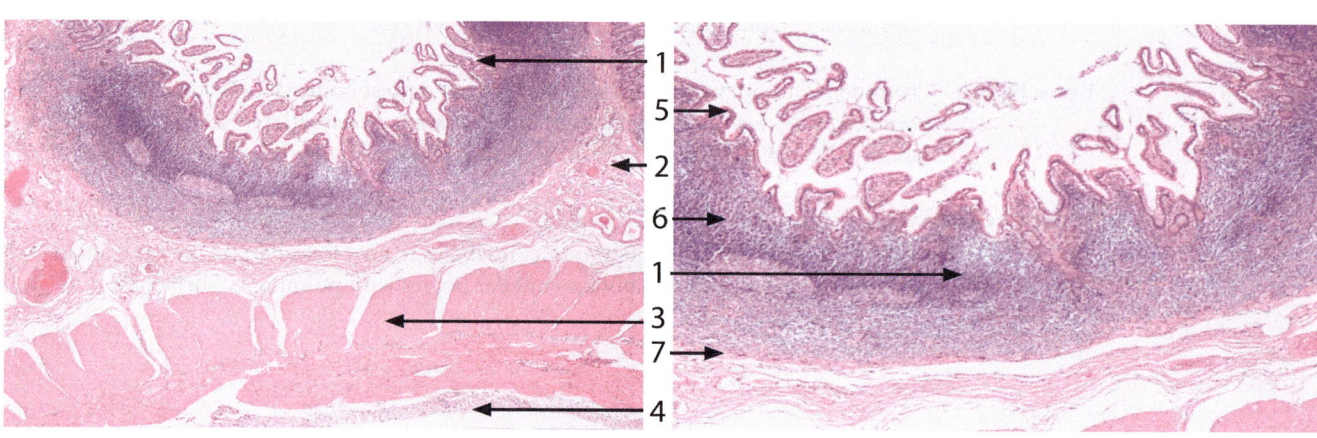

I Review of Histology

Microscopy: Layers of the gastrointestinal tract:

- **Mucosa[1]:** Epithelium[5], lamina propria[6] (loose connective tissue, inflammatory cells), muscularis mucosa[7]
  Regional variations: epithelial cell types, inflammatory cell population, architectural arrangement

- **Submucosa[2]:** Loose connective tissue, lymph and blood vessels, submucosal (Meissner's) plexus
  Regional variations: glands, lymphoid follicles, architectural arrangement

- **Muscularis propria[3]:** Smooth muscle, arranged into two layers, the circular and the longitudinal, myenteric (Auerbach's) plexus between layers
  Regional variations: Additional oblique layer in stomach

- **Serosa[4]:** Visceral peritoneum, consisting of thin, single-layered mesothelial cells, minimal loose connective tissue

*Lymph follicles:
- In the lamina propria mucosae and submucosa, lymphatic follicles protrude into the lumen, above that is follicle-associated epithelium (FAE) of the intestines,
- No crypts above the areas with lymphoid follicles
- Dome epithelium with M cells

Part of the gut-associated lymphoid tissue:
- GALT: gut-associated lymphatic tissue
- MALT: mucosa-associated lymphatic tissue

Organ: Esophagus
Stain: Hematoxylin - Eosin

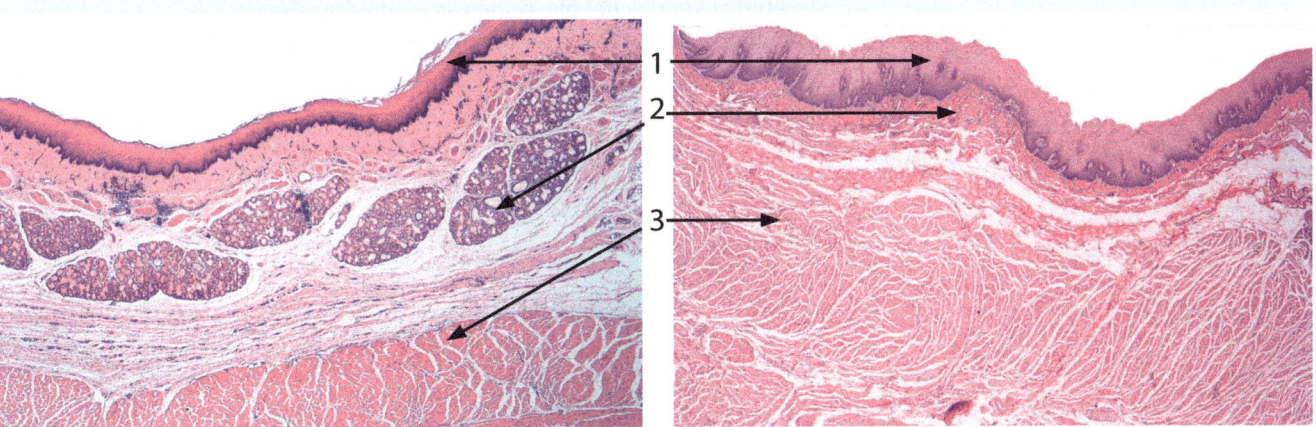

Microscopy:

- **Mucosa[1]:** Non-keratinizing stratified squamous epithelium, scant lamina propria (loose connective tissue), muscularis mucosa

- **Submucosa[2]:** Connective tissue, vessels, nerve plexus (Meissner's)

- **Muscularis propria[3]:** Two layers; inner circumferential layer, outer longitudinal.
  Upper third of esophagus has skeletal muscle
  Middle third converts from skeletal to smooth muscle
  Lower third is smooth muscle

- **Adventitia:** Connective tissue, blends with surrounding tissues

I Review of Histology

Organ: Stomach
Stain: Hematoxylin - Eosin

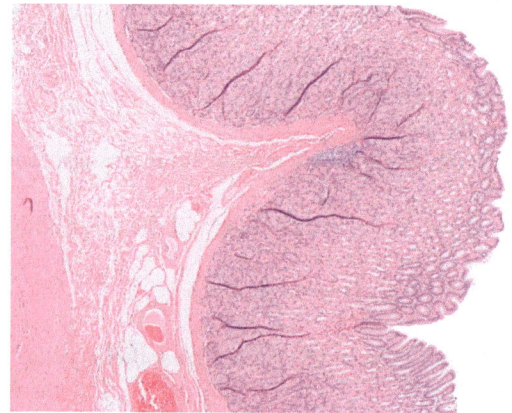 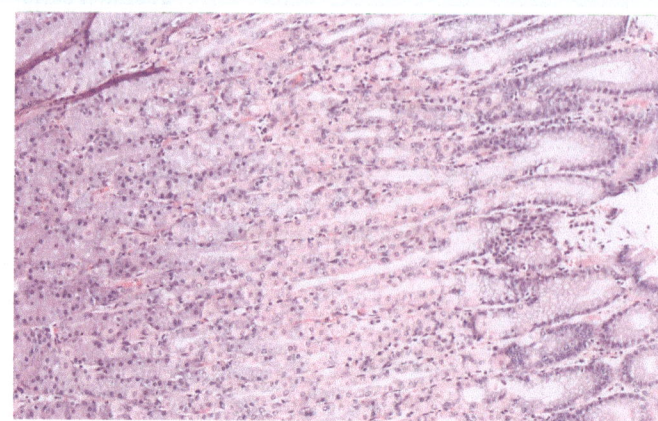

Microscopy:

Mucosa:	Simple columnar epithelium arranged in pits and glands, pits lined by foveolar cells (apical mucin caps), enteroendocrine cells scattered in glands. Cells of the glands vary by anatomic region:
Gastric cardia:	Epithelium with short pits, short mucus glands
Gastric fundus and body:	Epithelium with short pits and long glands, overall very pink ("oxyntic" mucosa); mid-gland with parietal cells (brightly eosinophilic, many mitochondria, secrete HCl and intrinsic factor in response to gastrin) Bottom of gland with chief cells (basophilic, secrete pepsinogen, lipase, and leptin in response to secretin)
Gastric antrum:	Epithelium with long pits, short glands with bland mucus cells
Submucosa:	Connective tissue, vessels, submucosal (Meissner's) nerve plexus
Muscularis propria:	Three layers of smooth muscle (oblique, circumferential, and longitudinal) Myenteric (Auerbach's) plexus between outer two layers
Serosa:	Scant connective tissue, layer of mesothelial cells (simple squamous)

Organ: Duodenum, Jejunum, Ileum
Stain: Hematoxylin - Eosin

Duodenum	Jejunum	Ileum
Long, small villi, with shorter of crypts	Long, slender villi (finger-shaped), deeper crypts	Shorter villi with increased distance to each other, deeper crypts
Brunner glands, especially in the duodenal bulb portion	Submucosa has no special adaptations, may have a few lymph follicles	Submucosa contains Peyer's patches (lymphoid aggregates - MALT)

I Review of Histology

Organ: Colon
Stain: Hematoxylin - Eosin

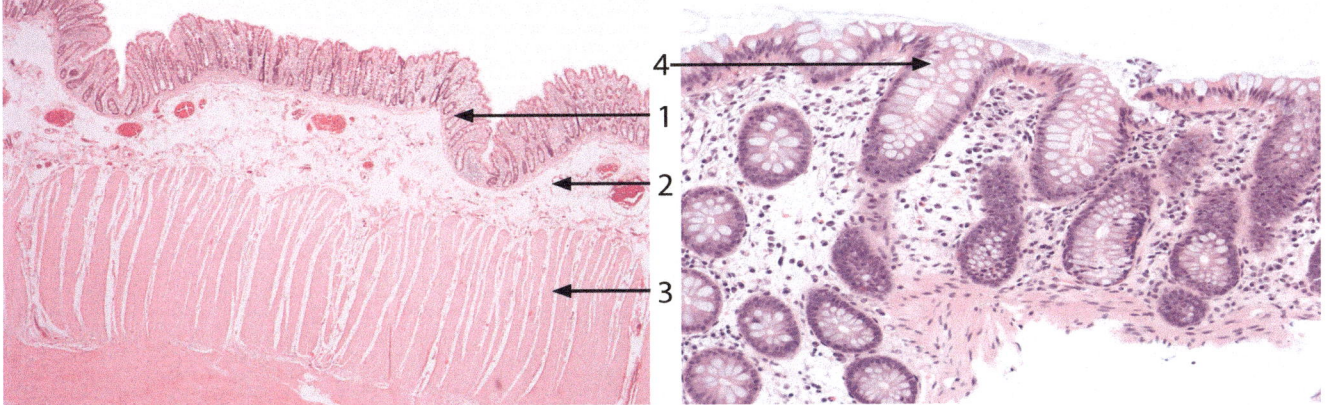

Microscopy:	Mucosa[1]:	Simple columnar epithelium arranged in crypts, enterocyte cells (have microvilli, visualized as "brush border") and goblet cells[4]; ratio of enterocyte to goblet cells decreases across the course of the colon Paneth cells found at base of crypts in cecum and ascending colon Scattered enteroendocrine cells
	Submucosa[2]:	Connective tissue, vessels, nerve plexus (Meissner's) Lymphoid aggregates (MALT)
	Muscularis propria[3]:	Two smooth muscle layers; inner circumferential, outer longitudinal Myenteric (Auerbach's) plexus between layers
	Adventitia/serosa:	Predominantly serosa (visceral peritoneum with mesothelial cells) Area attached to body wall (early ascending, rectum) has adventitia

Organ: Appendix
Stain: Hematoxylin - Eosin

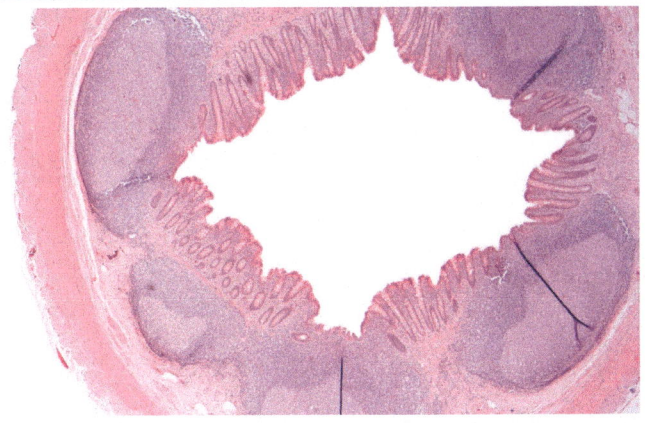 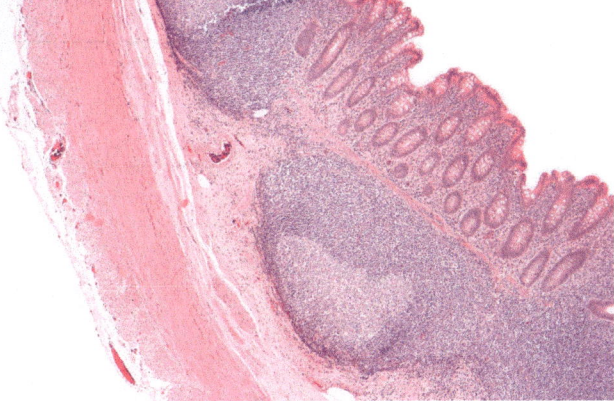

Microscopy:	Mucosa:	Simple columnar epithelium, enterocytes and goblet cells Scattered enteroendocrine cells, arranged in crypts
	Submucosa:	Connective tissue, vessels, nerve plexus, prominent lymphoid aggregates
	Muscularis propria:	Two layers of smooth muscle, inner circumferential and outer longitudinal
	Serosa:	Visceral peritoneum with mesothelial cells

I Review of Histology

Organ: Pancreas
Stain: Hematoxylin - Eosin

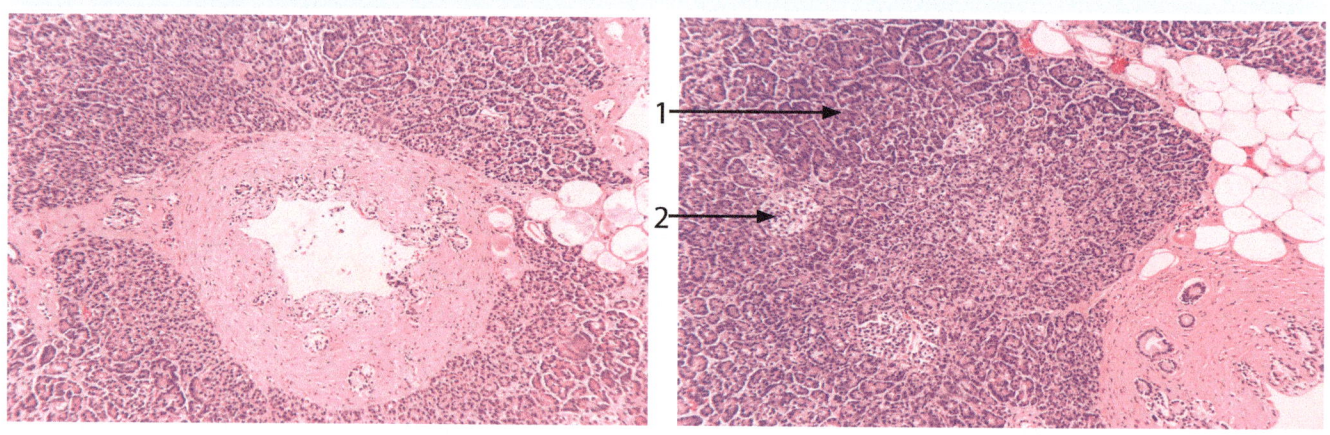

Microscopy:	Encapsulated and lobulated organ, both exocrine and endocrine functions, may contain fat cells

Exocrine:

Acinar cells[1]:	Cuboidal to columnar cells arranged in acini[1], contain zymogen granules (enzyme precursors) which are released in response to cholecystokinin
Intercalated ducts:	Bland cuboidal cells, secrete bicarbonate in response to secretin
Centroacinar cell:	A ductal cell that may appear centrally in acinar when tissue is sectioned, may help identify pancreas

Endocrine:

Islets of Langerhans[2]:	Pale cell clusters, scattered in parenchyma, more numerous in tail; contain variety of endocrine cells but all appear same on H&E:

Alpha cells make glucagon, beta cells make insulin, delta cells make somatostatin, PP cells make pancreatic polypeptide

Enriched in fenestrated capillaries with diaphragms, to enable circulation of endocrine products

Organ: Liver
Stain: Hematoxylin - Eosin

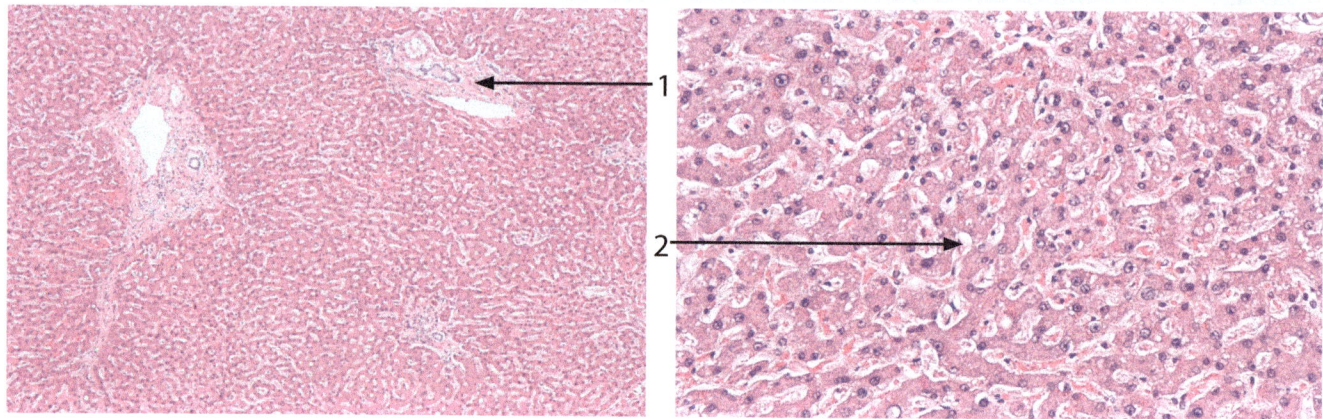

Microscopy:	Portal Triad[1]:	Contains artery (oxygen-rich blood from hepatic artery), vein (nutrient-rich blood from portal vein), and bile ductule (leads out to hepatic bile duct)
	Sinusoids[2]:	Discontinuous, slow-flow capillaries; blood flows through them from portal area to central vein
	Space of Disse:	Between wall of sinusoid and hepatocytes; hepatocytes project microvilli into this space
	Central vein:	Drains the sinusoids, leads to hepatic vein

I Review of Histology

Microscopy:
- **Hepatocytes:** Main cell of the liver; cuboidal epithelial cell with eosinophilic cytoplasm and central nucleus, arranged in cords along sinusoids; high metabolic activity, processes materials incoming from portal system and generates bile
- **Kupffer cells:** Macrophages of the liver, found along the space of Disse
- **Hepatic stellate cells:** Also called Ito cell, in space of Disse, inconspicuous; store fats and vitamin A

Organ: Breast
Stain: Hematoxylin - Eosin

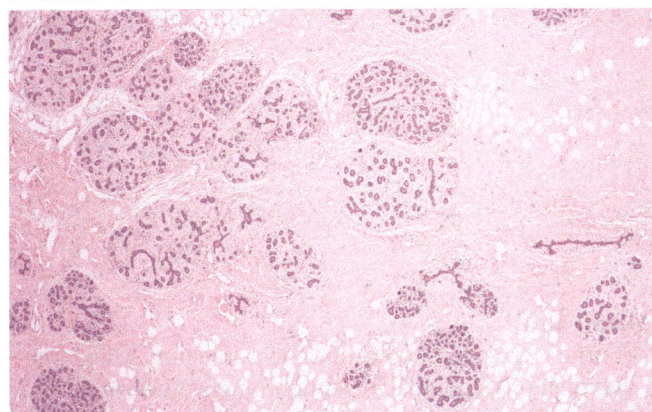 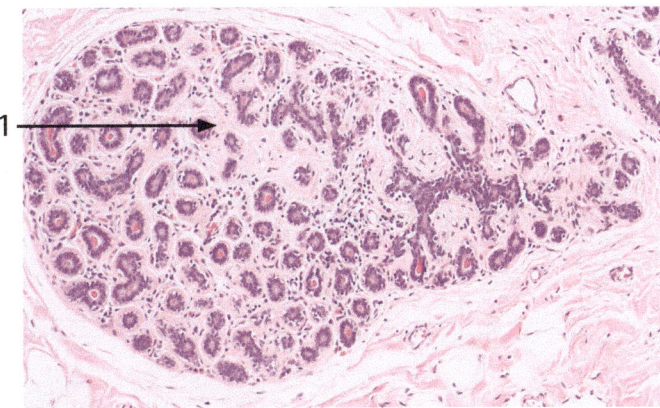

Microscopy:
- Mammary glands in a connective tissue stroma (fibrous connective tissue and fatty tissue)
- **Mammary gland:** from 10 to 20 individual gland structures, each opens to its excretory duct on the nipple, at the ends rudimentary end pieces (in non-lactating breast) arranged in groups called lobules
- **Terminal ductal-lobular unit[1]:** composed of the terminal duct and the lobule
- **Lobule and terminal ducts:** cuboidal epithelium inside and myoepithelial layer outside
- Epithelial cells arranged into small gland-like lobules that empty into ducts; background of fibrous tissue and fatty tissue

Organ: Fallopian Tube
Stain: Hematoxylin - Eosin

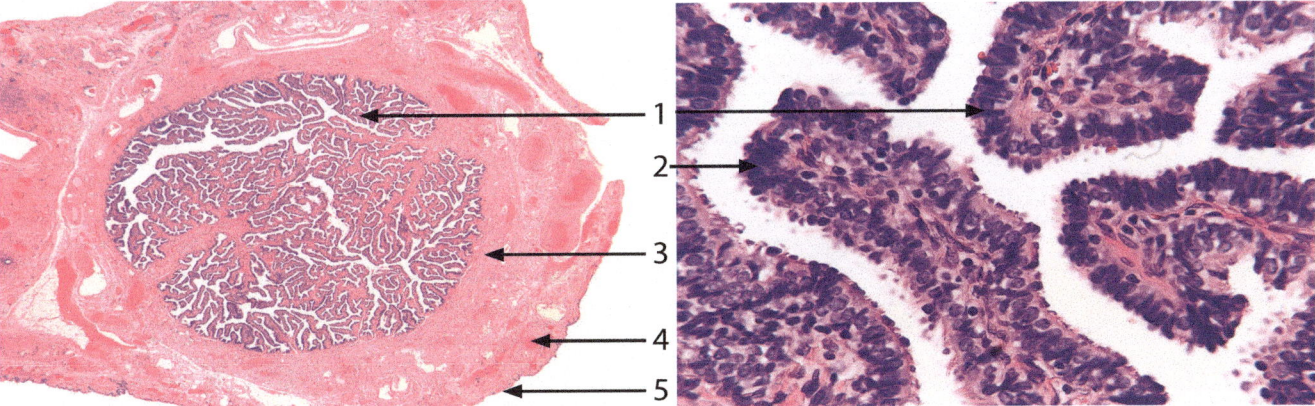

Microscopy:
- **Mucosa[1]:** Simple columnar epithelium[2] with cilia and scattered pale peg cells, arranged densely in folds (plicae[3]) supported by lamina propria (loose connective tissue)
  Plicae decrease toward the isthmus and intramural portion of the tube
  Plicae form the fimbriae at distal ends, here the lumen opens to peritoneal cavity
- **Muscularis[3]:** Smooth muscle, circumferentially to spirally arranged, increases in thickness towards the uterus
- **Subserosa[4]:** Contains vessels, nerves
- **Serosa[5]:** Thin layer of connective tissue, layer of mesothelial cells (simple squamous)

I Review of Histology

Organ: Ovary
Stain: Hematoxylin - Eosin

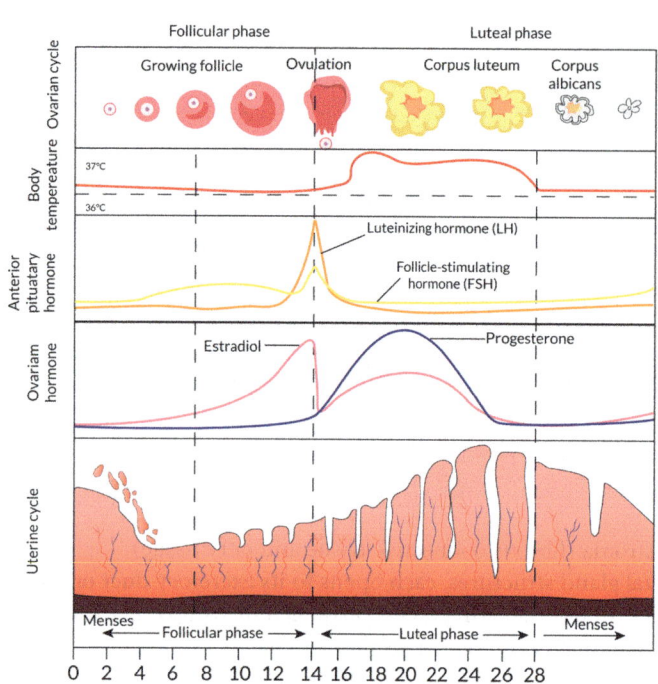

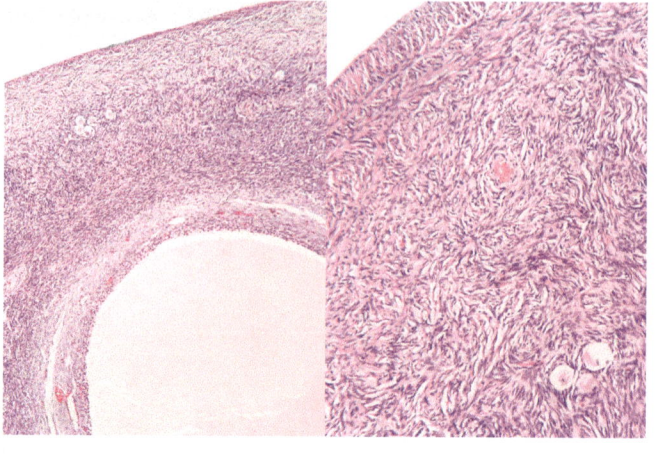

Microscopy:
- Surface epithelium (peritoneal mesothelium, Müllerian epithelium), cuboidal in young women, otherwise flat
- Narrow layer of connective tissue (tunica albuginea) beneath
- Cortical stroma with dense connective tissue in which the evolving follicles and related structures (corpus luteum, corpus rubrum, corpus albicans) are embedded
- Medulla and hilum with loose connective tissue and many blood vessels, groups of endocrine interstitial cells (hilar cells, correspond to Leydig cells of the testicle)

Organ: Uterus
Stain: Hematoxylin - Eosin

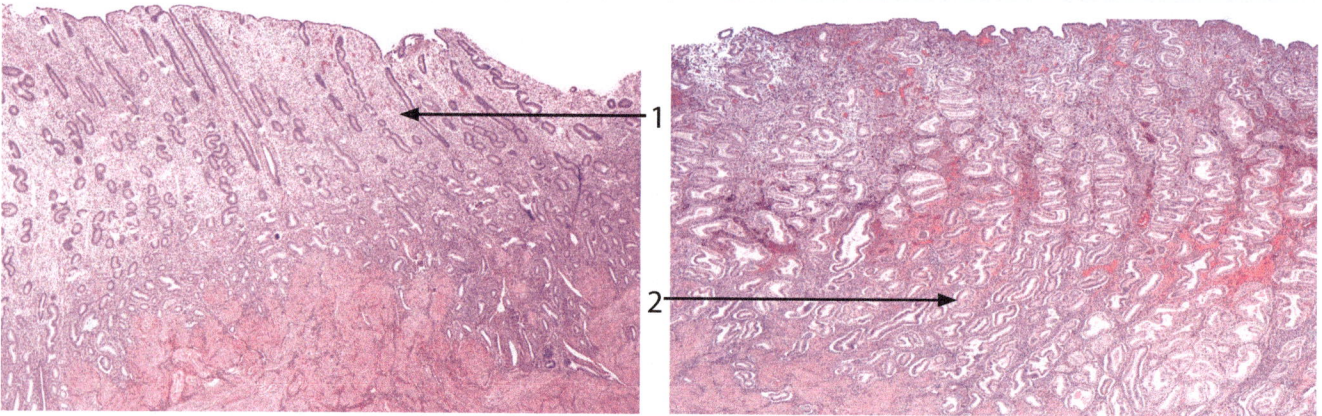

Microscopy: **Endometrium:** Contains endometrial glands, supported by endometrial stromal cells. Endometrium basalis layer is deepest, does not cycle, and is not shed. Remainder of the endometrium varies widely across the menstrual cycle, and is shed.

Proliferative phase[1] (pre-ovulatory):
Columnar cells with mitotic figures, initially in straight tubes, then beginning to corkscrew, stromal cells also mitotically active

Secretory phase[2] (post-ovulatory):
Corkscrew glands, columnar cells contain vacuoles that are secreted into gland lumens; stromal cells become plump and eosinophilic

I Review of Histology

Microscopy: Menstruation: disintegration and shedding of glands and stroma

    Myometrium: Thick wall of the uterus, composed of bundles of smooth muscle running in different directions
    Serosa: Scant connective tissue, layer of mesothelial cells (simple squamous)

Organ: Cervix
Stain: Hematoxylin - Eosin

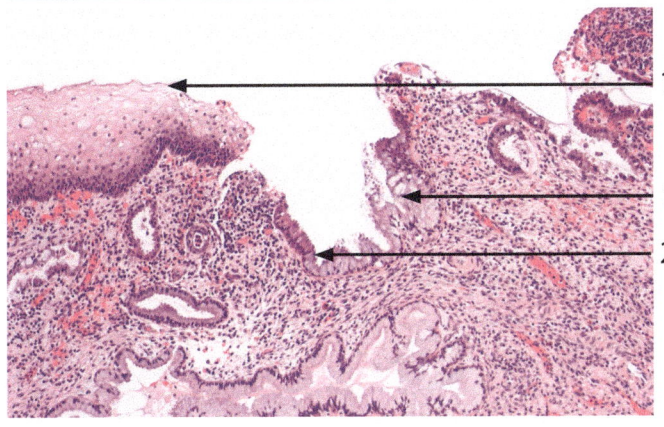
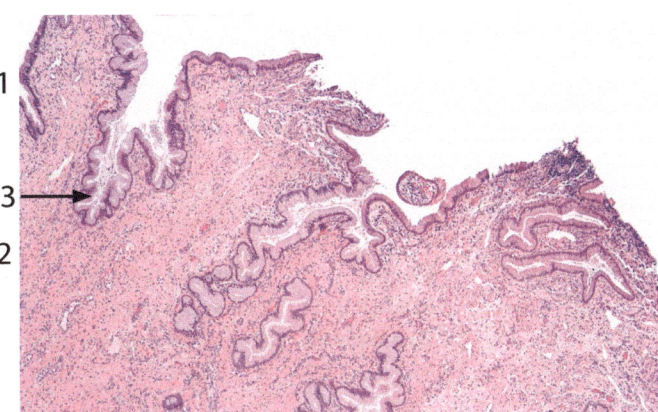

Microscopy:
- **Ectocervix[1]:** Non-keratinizing stratified squamous epithelium
- **Endocervix[3]:** Simple columnar cells, mucin-making, line the canal, and form deeper glands
- **Transformation zone[2]:** Site of conversion from squamous to columnar epithelium, typical location for HPV-related pathologic changes. Squamous metaplasia of the glandular epithelium progresses across reproductive age, transformation zone is thus deeper in the canal in older patients.
- **Stroma:** Connective tissue, occasional smooth muscle, vessels

Organ: Adrenal
Stain: Hematoxylin - Eosin

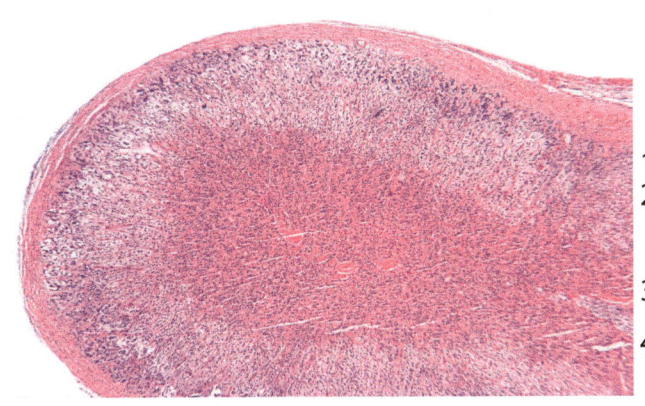
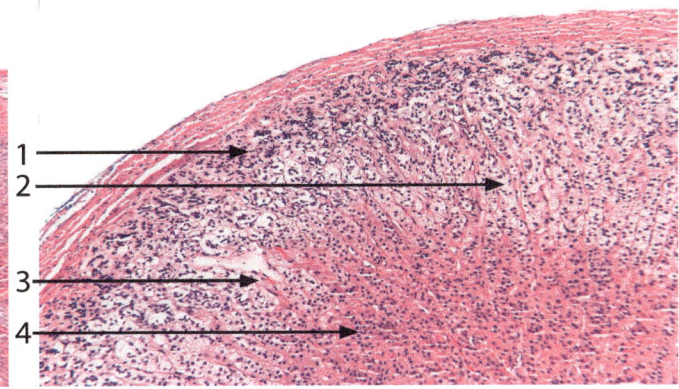

Microscopy: Subdivision into cortex (steroid hormone formation) and medulla (catecholamine formation)

Three cortex zones (from external to internal):
- 1. Zona glomerulosa[1] (mineralocorticoids)
- 2. Zona fasciculata[2] (glucocorticoids, majority of the cortex in adults)
- 3. Zona reticularis[3] (androgens)

Medulla[4]:
Medullary cells are part of the sympathetic nervous system (adrenaline, noradrenaline)
Heavily capillarized (fenestrated capillaries with diaphragms)

I Review of Histology

Organ: Kidney
Stain: Hematoxylin - Eosin

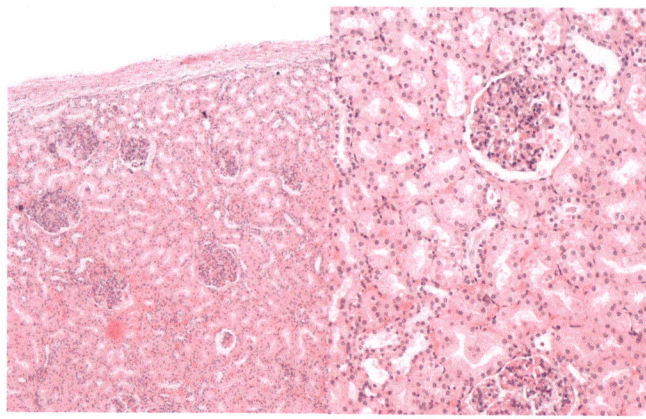
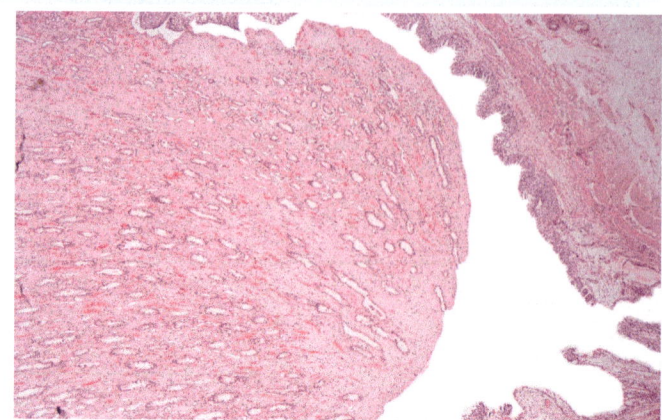

Microscopy:
- **Cortex:** Glomeruli, proximal convoluted tubules, distal convoluted tubules
- **Medulla:** Collecting ducts
- **Renal pelvis:** Transitional epithelium (urothelium)

Organ: Testes
Stain: Hematoxylin - Eosin

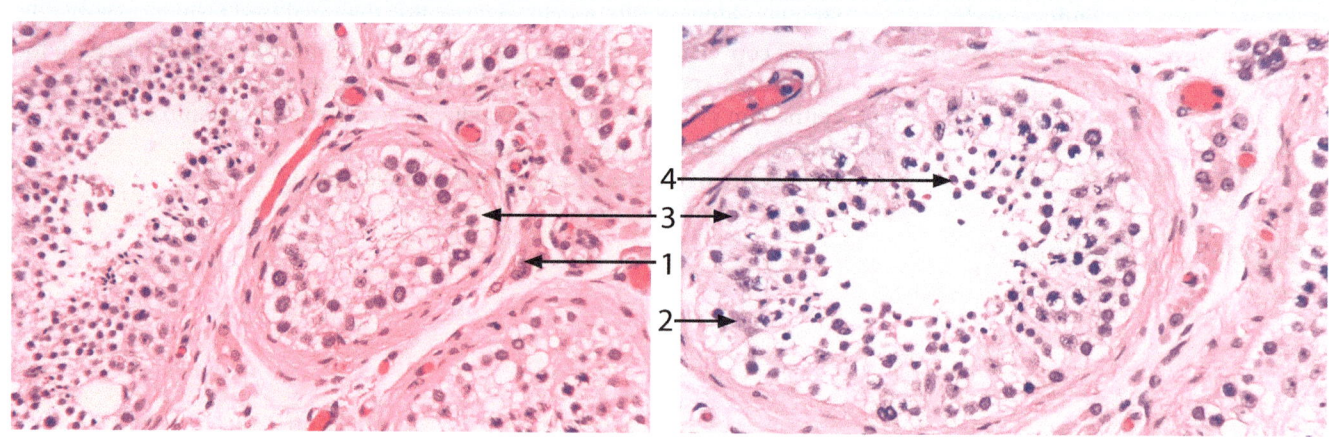

Microscopy:

- **Tunica albuginea:** Dense connective tissue capsule, encloses the testicle and focally the head of the epididymis, contains some smooth muscle cells, communicates with the mediastinum of the testicle

- **Testicular lobule:** Radial subdivision of the testicular parenchyma by delicate connective tissue septa (derives from tunica albuginea to the mediastinum), contains one or more seminiferous tubules
  Groups of Leydig cells[1] (generate testosterone) between seminiferous tubules

- **Seminiferous tubules:** Developing sperm and supporting Sertoli cells[2], which help create the blood-testis barrier.
  Primordial spermatogonia[3] are located basally, and the cells move towards lumen as they mature to spermatocytes[4]

- **Rete testis:** Straight duct-like structures, through which structurally mature sperm exit the testis

I Review of Histology

I Review of Histology

Organ: Ureter
Stain: Hematoxylin - Eosin

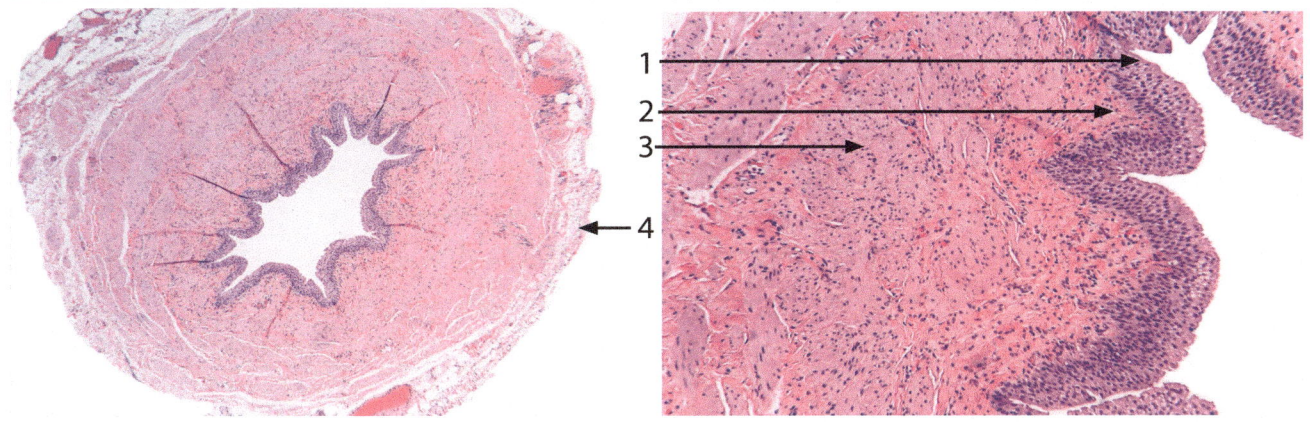

Microscopy:

- **Urothelium[1]:** Transitional epithelium, specialized epithelium with elastic properties

- **Lamina propria[2]:** Fibroelastic layer below the urothelium

- **Muscularis[3]:** Contains a longitudinal and circular muscle layer

- **Adventitia[4]:** Loose connective tissue with elastic properties, nerves and blood vessels

Organ: Lymph node
Stain: Hematoxylin - Eosin

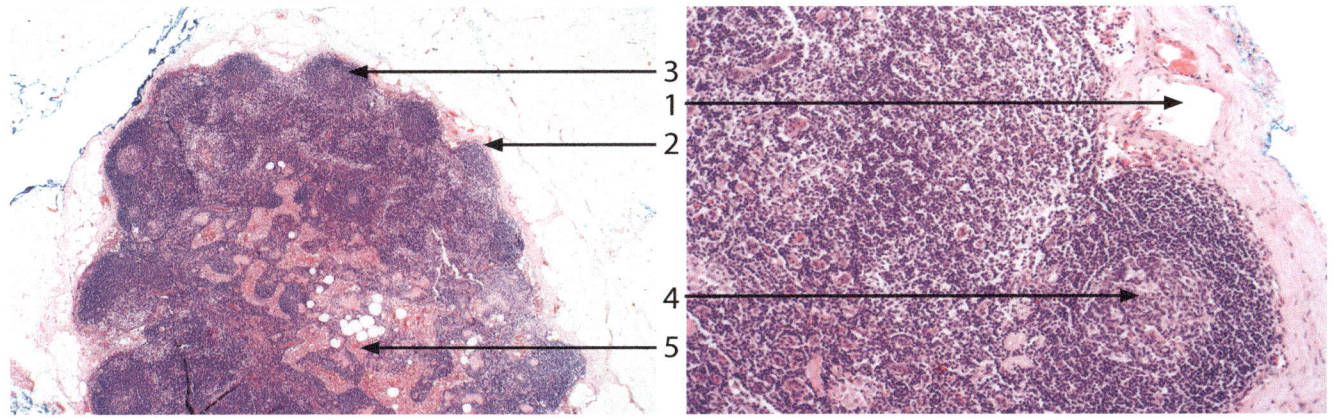

Microscopy: Encapsulated organ with cortex and medulla; feeder artery and draining vein enter/exit at the hilum.

- **Subcapsular sinus[1]:** Receives regional lymphatic drainage

- **Cortex[2]:** Follicles[3] (developing B-cells), with pale region of activated germinal center, and high endothelial venule for lymphocytes exiting blood, pale central cluster "germinal center[4];" interfollicular space (T-cell region)

- **Medulla[5]:** Sinusoidal capillaries; all cells collected to return to venous system

I Review of Histology

Organ: Spleen
Stain: Hematoxylin - Eosin

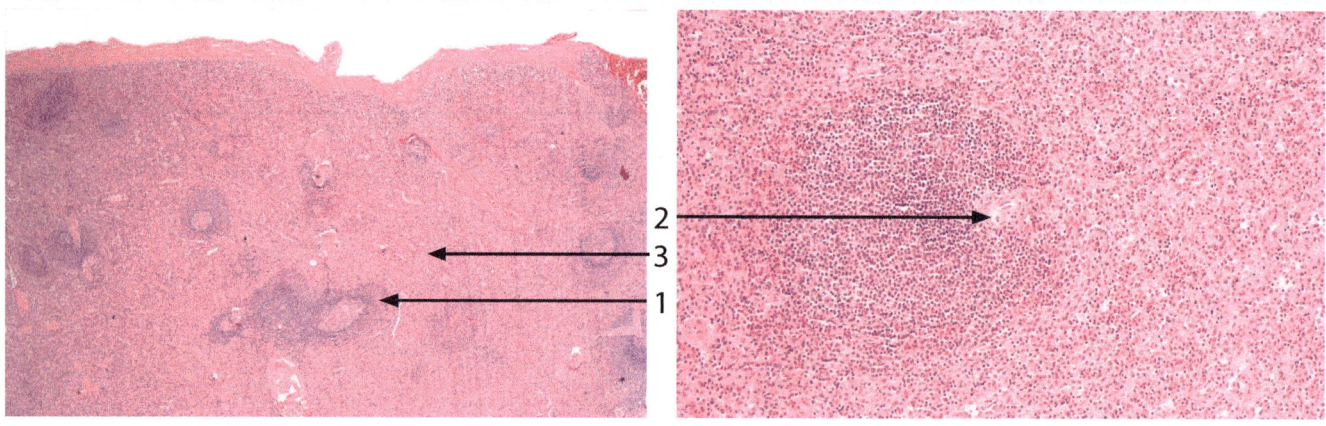

Microscopy: **White pulp[1]:**   Found around arterioles: the peri-arteriolar lymphoid sheath[2] (PALS) contain T-cells, follicles contain B cells; arterioles drain to sinusoidal capillaries (barrel-stave-shaped) and also directly into open space

                      Red pulp[3]:   Free blood, numerous macrophages; old RBCs are phagocytized and recycled here

Organ: Thymus
Stain: Hematoxylin - Eosin

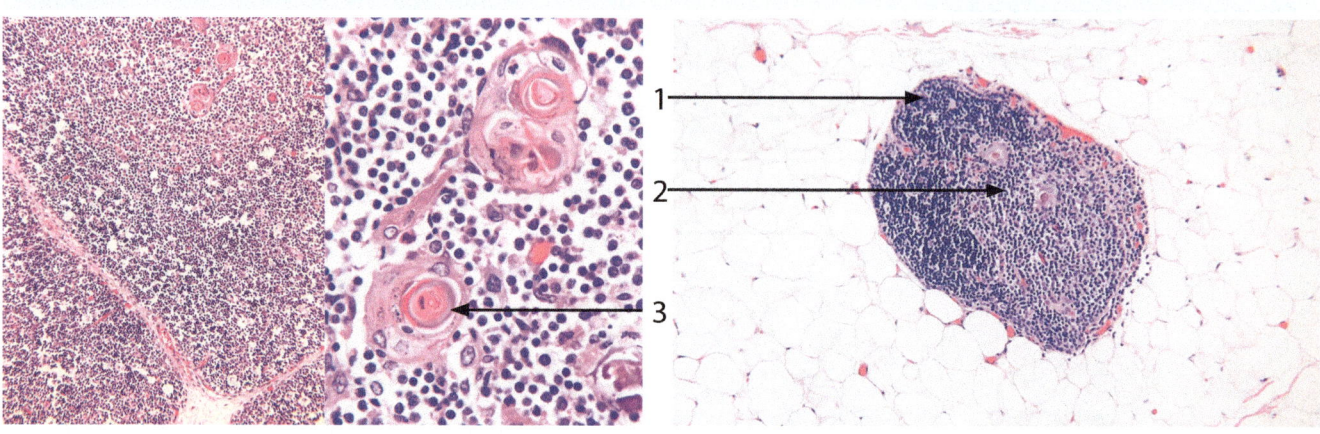

Microscopy: Primary lymphatic organ, located in the upper mediastinum and promotes proliferation and maturation of T-lymphocytes, lobulated and encapsulated

         Cortex[1]:   Location of immature T-lymphocytes and thymic nurse cells (epithelial component, regulates access to antigens, positive and negative selection of T-lymphocytes)
More basophilic appearance

         Medulla[2]:   Location of mature T-lymphocytes, macrophages, histiocytes and epithelial cells, has Hassall's corpuscles[3] (epithelial cells with onion-skin or concentric arrangement and central keratin debris)

         Positive selection: Transfer of T-lymphocytes from cortex to medulla after phenotype selection CD4 positive ($CD4^+CD8^-$) or CD8 positive ($CD4^-CD8^+$)

         Thymic involution: Regression and fatty replacement of the thymus as part of age-related changes

Inflammatory Pathology

Shivali Marketkar, Abigail Alexander, Ann Ding, Jao Ou

1.1　Lobar Pneumonia

1.2　Acute Appendicitis

1.3　Acute and Chronic Cholecystitis

1.4　Chronic Gastric Ulcer

1.5　Meningitis

1.6　Gout (Foreign Body-induced Inflammation)

1 Inflammatory Pathology

Inflammation is often seen in response to bacteria, viruses, fungi, protozoa, parasites, physical stress or damage, or chemical damage. Inappropriate or dysregulated inflammation can itself be a disease state.

Depending on the type of inflammation, pathophysiological and cellular changes may differ significantly. This chapter will present common, representative diseases that involve an inflammatory response.

Cardinal Signs of Acute Inflammation

Rubor - redness
Calor - heat
Tumor - swelling
Dolor - pain

Described by Celsus and Galen

Functio laesa - impaired function

Fifth symptom, added by Rudolf Virchow

Infections can be spread through:

Direct extension - from one tissue to another by direct spread
Lymphatic system
Blood system

Inflammatory Processes

Types of Inflammation	Time Frame	Involved Processes	Involved Cells	Examples
Acute - exudative (fibrinous, hemorrhagic, purulent) - lymphocytic - necrotic	Immediate	**Vascular processes** Release of vasoactive mediators (e.g. cytokines, leukotrienes, histamine), promotes increased blood flow, vasodilatation. Vascular permeability may greatly increase if endothelium damaged **Neutrophil response:** Margination Rolling Chemotaxis/migration **Monocyte/macrophage response:** Phagocytosis	**Leukocytes** - Neutrophils - Eosinophils - Monocytes/ macrophages **Lymphocytes** - B-lymphocytes - T-lymphocytes	- Acute Appendicitis - Acute Cholecystitis - Acute Pancreatitis - Bacterial Meningitis - Some Pneumonias
Chronic	Slower	**Lymphocytic reaction** **Infection can cause granulation tissue:** - Fibrosis - Capillarization **Granulomatous changes:** - Macrophages become epithelioid cells or form multinucleated giant cells - Multinucleated giant cells may also consist of lymphocytes, fibroblasts etc **Can be related to:** - Infections - Immunologic processes - Reactions to foreign material (crystals, calcifications, silica dust)	Lymphocytes Macrophages Fibroblasts	Chronic lymphocytic thyroiditis: - Hashimoto - Grave's disease) - Chronic gastric ulcer - Chronic pancreatitis - Tuberculosis - Sarcoidosis - Giant cell arteritis - Gout - Crohn's disease

Inflammatory Pathology

Entity:	1.1 Lobar Pneumonia
Stain:	Hematoxylin - Eosin

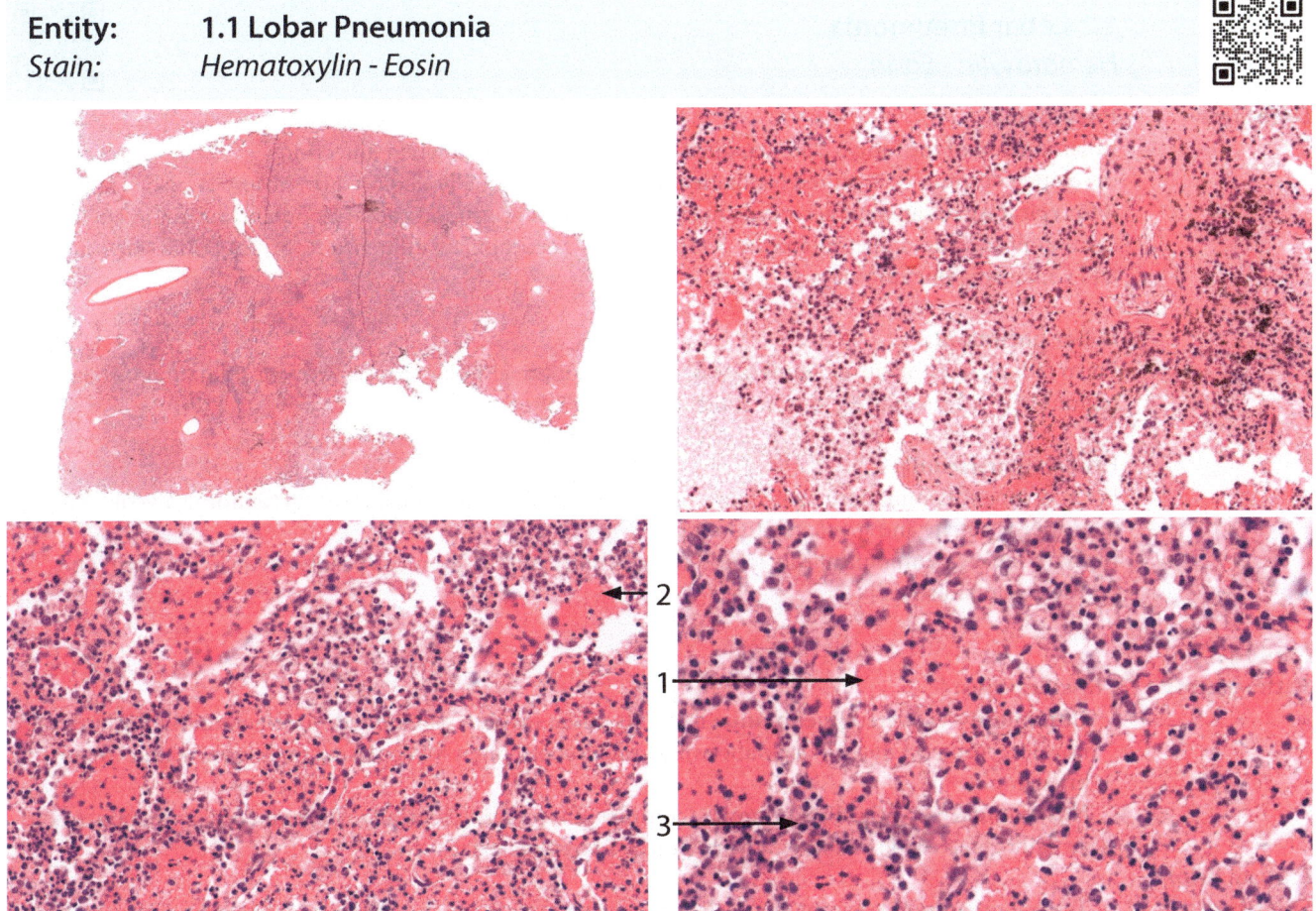

Macroscopy: Depending on the stage of the lobar pneumonia, lobes may be firm

Microscopy: Tissue/organ: Lungs with increased volume (liver-like firm consistency = hepatization)
Lungs with relatively dry, brittle reddish, gray or gray-yellow cut surface

Histological Stages of Pneumonia	Time Frame	Pathophysiological Features
Coupling Stage 1	1st day	Lung capillaries bulging with erythrocytes, alveolar spaces with only scant inflammatory cells
Red hepatization Stage 2	2nd - 3rd day	Copious erythrocytes spilling into alveolar spaces
Gray hepatization Stage 3	4th - 6th day	Intra-alveolar exudate of fibrin, dense fibrin network in the alveolar spaces
Yellow hepatization Stage 4	7th - 8th day	Intra-alveolar fibrin with numerous neutrophils, which break down into pus
Lysis Stage 5	From day 8	If the disease resolves, dissolution of inflammatory exudate, is absorbed and/or expectorated - restitutio ad integrum

The attached photo shows stage 3, gray hepatization:
- Alveoli[1] with intra-alveolar fibrin[2] (homogeneous, somewhat fibrillary eosinophilic material) and neutrophils[3]
- Dilated, congested capillaries containing responding granulocytes (leukostasis)
- Alveolar macrophages or "dust cells" containing black pigment is part of anthracosis (repeated exposure to soot/smoking); this finding is not necessarily part of lobar pneumonia

1 Inflammatory Pathology

Entity:	1.1 Lobar Pneumonia
Stain:	Hematoxylin - Eosin

Definition

Pneumonia:
Inflammation of the lung tissue, classified by location of patient when infection develops: community-acquired (outpatient) versus nosocomially-acquired (in hospital); also classified into typical versus atypical according to clinical features. Common causative organisms in the US for community acquired pneumonia are Streptococcus pneumoniae, influenza A, Mycoplasma pneumoniae and Chlamydia pneumoniae.

Lobar pneumonia:
Form of lung inflammation; numerous neutrophils in the alveolar spaces, with consolidation into large regions of involvement (e.g. one or more entire lung lobes)

Bronchopneumonia:
Form of lung inflammation; neutrophils involving bronchi and immediately surrounding alveolar tissue, may appear patchy and involve both lungs
In short, lobar pneumonia affects lobes, whereas bronchopneumonia is patchy involving bronchi and peribronchiolar areas.

Etiology/Pathogenesis:

Classifications:
- **Community-acquired pneumonia:** in adults, often involves pneumococci, (Haemophilus influenzae now less common due to vaccinations); in adolescents, often Mycoplasma pneumoniae and Chlamydia pneumoniae
- **Nosocomially-acquired pneumonia** (contracted inpatient): typically Staphylococci and gram-negative pathogens (e.g. Pseudomonas aeruginosa, Enterobacteriaceae)

Clinical Info/Symptoms:
- **Typical pneumonia:** Symptoms such as fever, productive cough with purulent sputum, abnormal lung sounds (crackles, egophony, dullness to percussion)
- **Atypical pneumonia:** more subtle symptoms and clinical features

Diagnostics: Auscultation, consolidation on CXR, elevated CRP and ESR (non-specific), procalcitonin (high specificity for bacterial infection), blood gas, blood culture, sputum gram stain and culture

CURB-65 score: Estimation of mortality from community-acquired pneumonia, score helps determine whether inpatient vs outpatient treatment	
Parameter	CURB-65 Scoring
C = confusion	Clinical confusion
U = uremia	BUN > 19 mg/dL
R = respiratory rate	Respiratory rate ≥ 30/min
B = blood pressure	Diastolic blood pressure ≤ 60 mmHg or Systolic blood pressure <90 mmHg
65 = 65 years	Age ≥ 65 years

Mortality Score:
0 to 1 points = 1% (outpatient treatment recommended)
2 points = 9% (inpatient vs outpatient)
3+ points = 22% mortality (inpatient treatment; consideration of ICU admission for 4-5)

Diagnosis indicated by: 1) consolidation noted on chest imaging and
2) clinical diagnosis (cough, fever, shortness of breath, sputum)

Supporting labs: leukocytosis, bandemia, procalcitonin, sputum culture

Inflammatory Pathology

Entity:	1.1 Lobar Pneumonia
Stain:	Hematoxylin - Eosin

Therapy:

Treatment of Pneumonia			
	Mild Pneumonia	**Moderate Pneumonia**	**Severe Pneumonia**
Level of Care	Outpatient	Inpatient	Inpatient
Respiratory therapy	+	+	+
Mode of administration	PO	IV	IV
Beta lactam	Firstline	Firstline	-
Beta lactam with lactamase inhibitor + macrolide	Firstline with comorbidities	Firstline	-
Respiratory fluoroquinolones	With penicillin allergy	With penicillin allergy	Alternative
Piperacillin- tazobactam	-	-	Add if concerned for pseudomonas
3rd generation cephalosporins	-	-	With penicillin allergy
Vancomycin	-	-	Add if concerned for MRSA

Radiology:

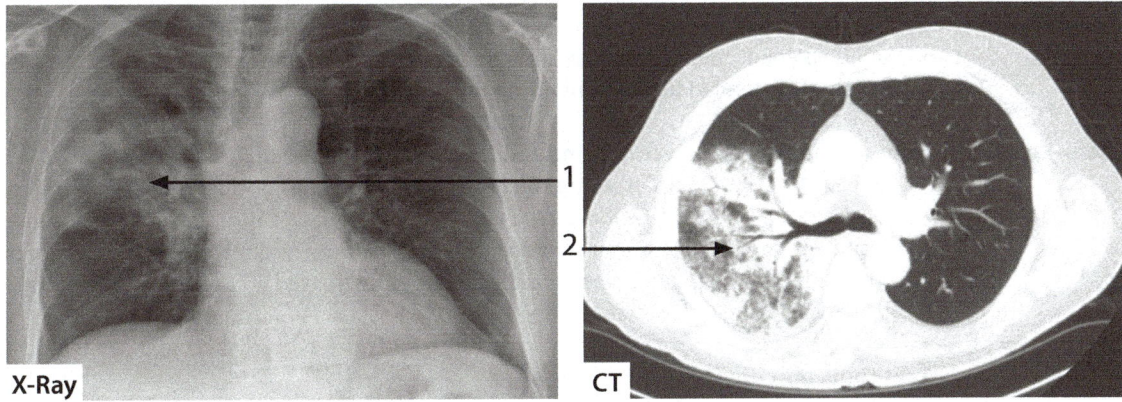

Radiographs[1]:
- Consolidation without collapse/volume loss: homogeneous opacification of the right upper lobe; represents the fibrinosuppurative filling of the parenchyma

CT (corresponding cross-sectional images in the same patient)[2]:
- Abnormal densities, notably sparing the underlying airways, characteristic of an "air bronchogram"

1 Inflammatory Pathology

Entity: 1.2 Acute Appendicitis
Stain: Hematoxylin - Eosin

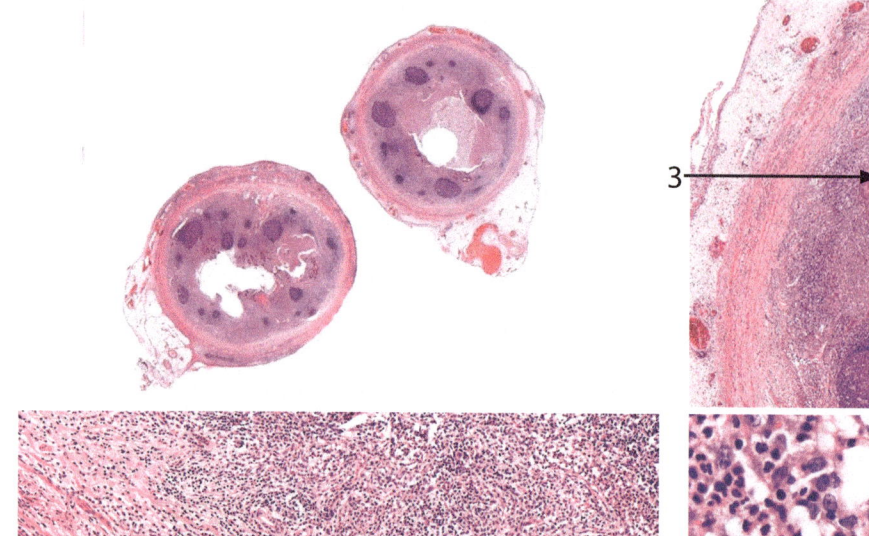

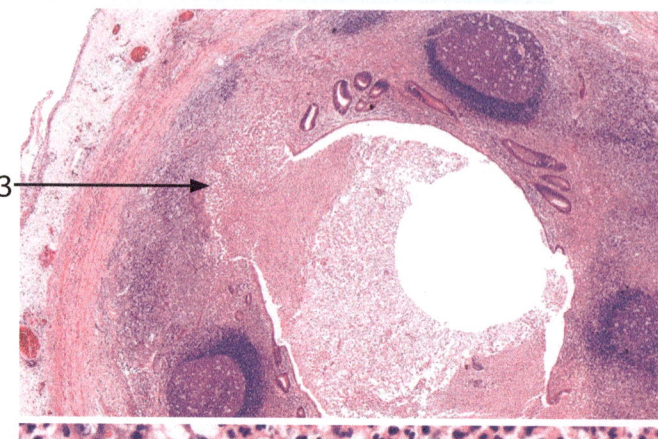

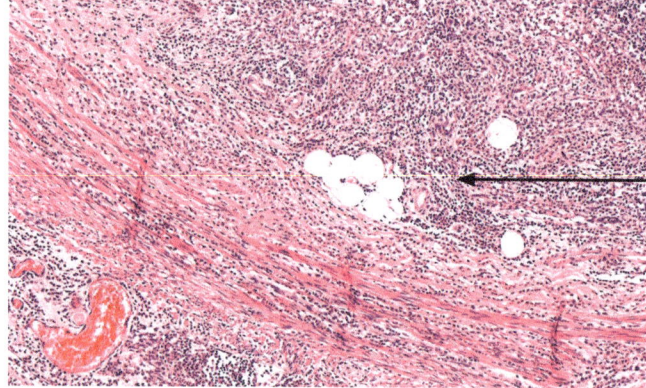

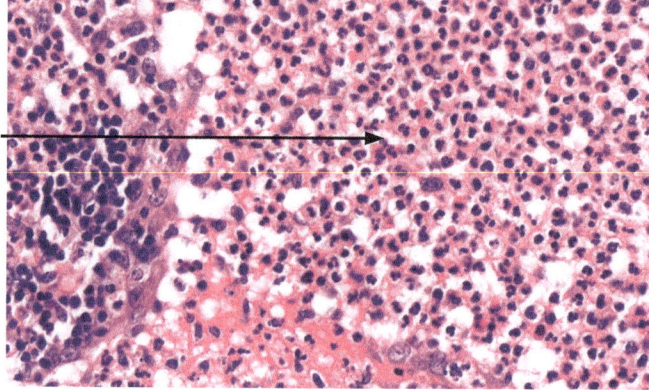

Macroscopy:
- Dull serosa; if serosa directly involved may show white-yellow deposits (pus)
- Wall thickened, edematous, may show yellow deposits (pus)
- May show distended lumen containing fibrinopurulent exudate and debris

Microscopy: Tissue/organ: Appendix vermiformis (GIT and lymphatic tissue)
- Attached to cecum, lumen contiguous with cecal lumen at the appendiceal orifice
- Layers similar to colon - colonic-type mucosa, submucosa, muscularis propria, subserosa and serosa.
- Prominent lymphoid aggregates in deep mucosa/submucosa, may show germinal centers
- Mucosal lymphocytes and plasma cell population increased compared to colonic mucosa
- Presence of acute inflammation is pathologic

Acute appendicitis:
- Clusters and/or sheets of many neutrophils[1] and some eosinophils
- Inflammation seen in all layers[2]; rarely only in mucosa (+/- crypt abscesses[3]).
- Neutrophils may extend into periappendiceal fat, called "periappendicitis."

Interval or subacute appendicitis:
If antibiotic treatment precedes surgery, may see few neutrophils, and eosinophils, focused in the muscularis propria. Sometimes chronic lymphohistiocytic aggregates may be noted in interval appendicitis.

Chronic appendicitis:
Rare, difficult to determine based only on histology.

Definition: **Appendicitis:** Inflammation of the appendix vermiformis

Inflammatory Pathology

Entity:	1.2 Acute Appendicitis
Stain:	Hematoxylin - Eosin

Etiology/Pathogenesis: Commonly present in childhood, can lead to perforation with peritonitis; older patients may have atypical course with few symptoms; classification is according to stages of inflammation. May be further classified into acute, interval/subacute, and very rarely chronic.

Clinical Info/Symptoms:
- Classic presentation is periumbilical pain that migrates over time to the right lower quadrant
- Nausea/vomiting
- Fever generally occurs later in course of illness

Diagnostics:
- CT, ultrasound, or MRI
- Elevated WBC count, elevated C-reactive protein (CRP, non-specific)

Appendicitis Sign	Description
McBurney's point tenderness	Pain at one third of the distance from anterior superior iliac spine to umbilicus
Obturator sign	Right lower quadrant pain with flexion of right hip/knee and internal rotation of right leg; indicates pelvic appendicitis
Rovsing sign	Palpation in the left lower quadrant elicits pain in the right lower quadrant; indicates right-sided peritoneal irritation
Psoas sign	Right lower quadrant pain elicited by right hip extension; indicates a retrocecal appendicitis

Therapy: Appendectomy, but also can consider conservative monitoring with antibiotics and IV hydration

Radiology:

General:
- CT is most useful for diagnosis and assessment of complications
- Ultrasound and MRI may be used for pediatric and pregnant patients to avoid ionizing radiation

CT:
- Dilated (>6 mm diameter), blind-ending tubular structure at the base of the cecum, filled with fluid, with poorly defined walls, and edema of surrounding fat
- The underlying etiology of inflammation is obstruction by a tiny appendicolith

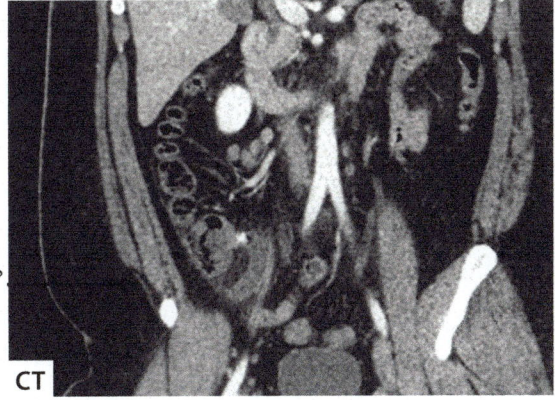

CT

1 Inflammatory Pathology

Entity: 1.3 Acute and Chronic Cholecystitis
Stain: Hematoxylin - Eosin

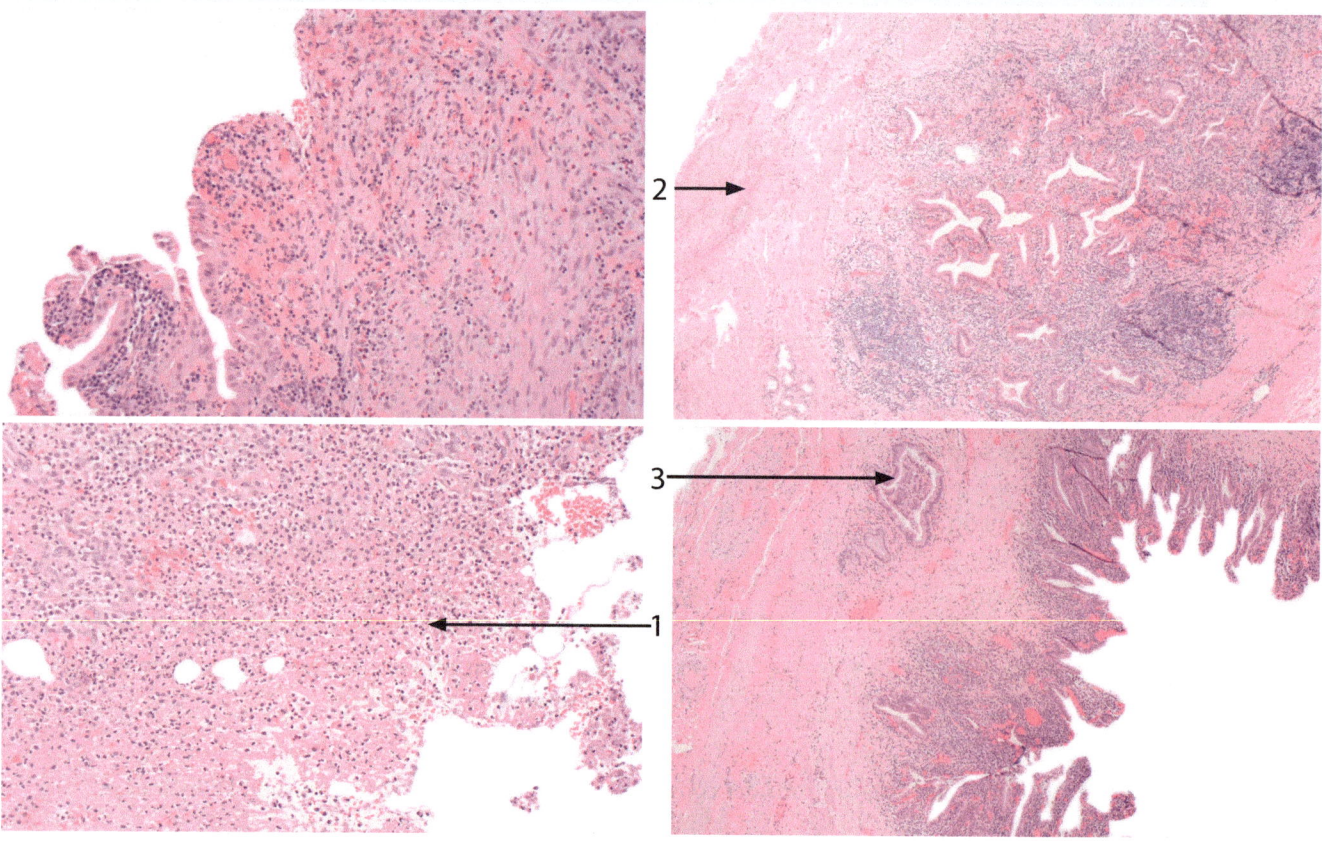

Macroscopy: Variable gross appearance: normal size, or distended due to bile or stones, or shrunken due to fibrosis; possible gallstones or biliary sludge in the lumen; dull, shaggy mucosa; normal or thickened wall
  If acute, possible gross purulence in wall or on serosa
  If gangrenous, wall often grossly thinned, blackened

Microscopy: Tissue/organ: Gallbladder

Acute Cholecystitis	Chronic Cholecystitis:
- Acute inflammation[1] (neutrophils, possibly eosinophils) - Involves entire wall (mucosa through muscularis propria, possibly to serosa) - May show fibrinopurulent exudate and vascular proliferation - May also show changes of background chronic cholecystitis - Acute gangrenous cholecystitis will also show necrosis of the wall[2]	- Plasma cells and lymphocytes (may be in follicles) - Involves entire wall (mucosa through muscularis propria) - Rokitansky-Aschoff sinuses[3], can be deep and confused with an invasive process such as carcinoma (desmoplastic reaction can help indicate a carcinoma) - Pyloric metaplasia can be seen - If mostly plasma cells, consider IgG4-related chronic cholecystitis

Definition/Etiology/Pathogenesis:

Acute cholecystitis:
  Often due to mechanical obstruction of outlet due to stones, more rarely due to altered bacterial flora causing changes in pH

Chronic cholecystitis:
  May be due to recurrent acute cholecystitis, or motility issues that result in improper emptying of bile

Inflammatory Pathology

Entity:	1.3 Acute and Chronic Cholecystitis
Stain:	Hematoxylin - Eosin

Clinical Info/Symptoms: Sharp pain referred to right shoulder/upper back, often following fatty meal
Fever, nausea, vomiting
Murphy's sign: deep palpation to the right upper quadrant with deep inspiration causes patient to catch their breath and causes worsening pain

Diagnostics: Labs: Leukocytosis, may have elevated liver function tests

Imaging:
RUQ Ultrasound: gallbladder wall thickening, pericholecystic fluid, edema, "sonographic Murphy's sign"
HIDA Scan: obtain if unequivocal US; nonvisualization of gallbladder is diagnostic of acute cholecystitis

Therapy: Conservative therapy: IV fluids, pain control, IV antibiotics
Surgical: Cholecystectomy

Radiology:

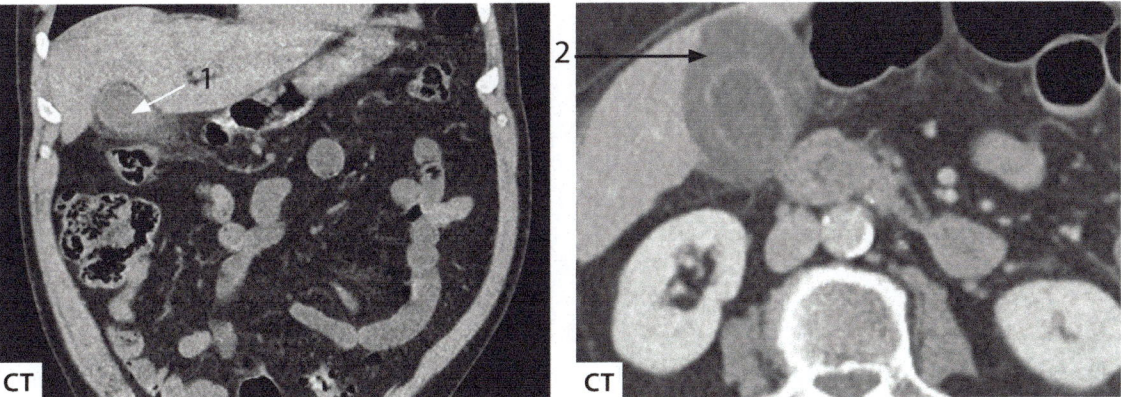

General: Multiple modalities depict various elements of the gallbladder and biliary system in complementary fashion.

CT:
- Has advantage of showing regional inflammatory changes and complications
- Acute inflammation: Gallbladder distention, wall thickening, and surrounding edema[1]
- Chronic inflammation: Marked wall thickening[2]

Ultrasound (US):
- Best detects gallstones and biliary duct dilation
- A gallstone lodged in the neck of the gallbladder, which is distended and shows intramural edema[3] indicating acute inflammation
- The historically purported value of the "sonographic Murphy's sign" is markedly overstated.

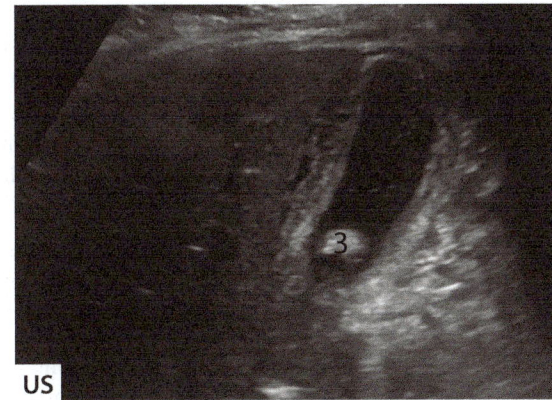

Inflammatory Pathology

Entity: 1.4 Chronic Gastric Ulcer
Stain: Hematoxylin - Eosin

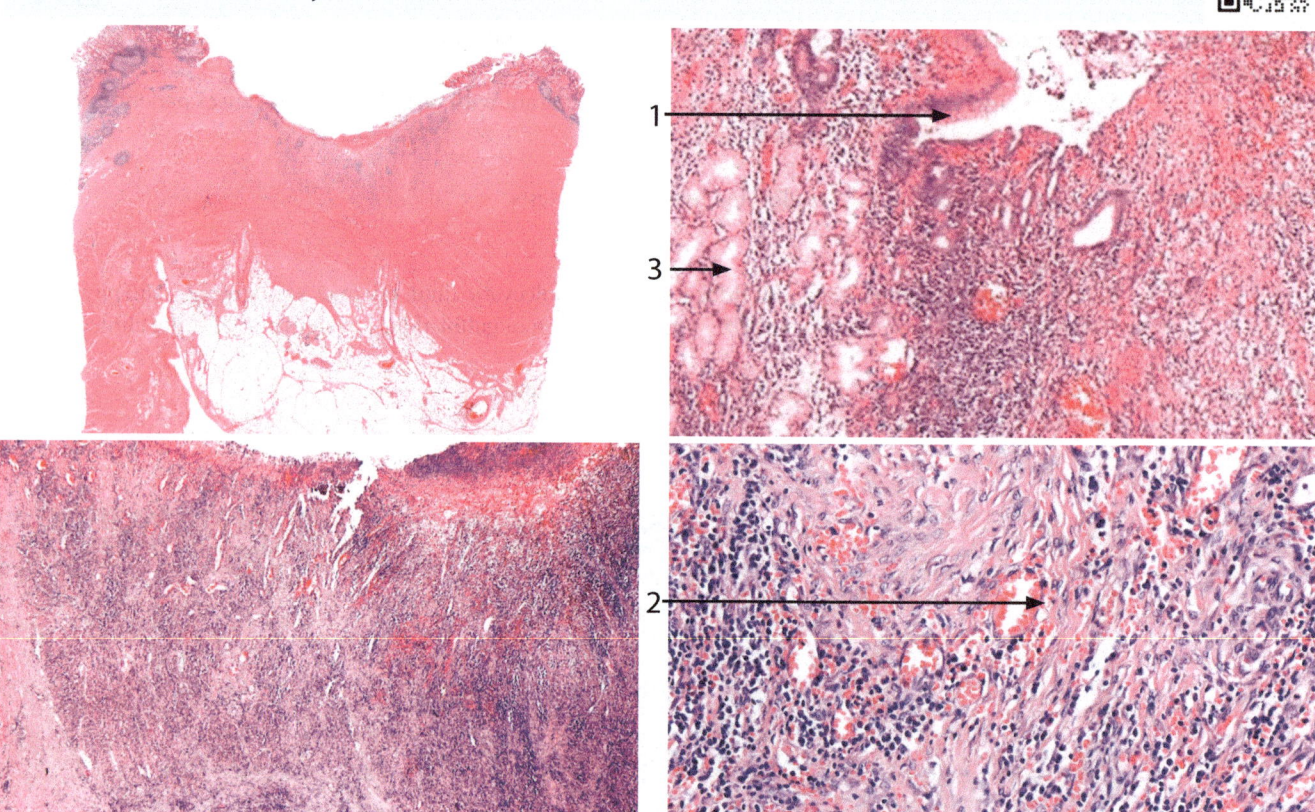

Macroscopy:	**Acute gastric ulcer:** Punched out round/ovoid defect with sharply demarcated edges, bleeds on contact
	Chronic gastric ulcer: Rounded, crater-shaped mucosal defect, rough edge and base, possible hypertrophic folds of mucosa around the edge

Microscopy: Tissue/organ: Stomach
- Gastric mucosa with hyperplastic foveolar epithelium[1] and lamina propria fibrosis[2]
- Regenerative changes of the mucosa
- Possible intestinal metaplasia[3]
- Acute phase: Neutrophils with fibrinopurulent deposits
- Helicobacter pylori may be visualized on H&E or by immunohistochemistry

Definition: **Erosion:** Defect in the mucosa (muscularis mucosa is intact)
Ulcer: Defect through the muscularis mucosa, exposing the submucosa

Etiology/Pathogenesis:

Ulcer development:
- Initially acute inflammation with mucosal defect (erosion); if persistent there is deeper mucosal sloughing extending deeper and exposing the submucosa (ulceration)
- Superficial fibrin with necrotic debris, with admixed neutrophils
- After an acute phase, lymphocytes arrive and may form lymphoid follicles
- May see formation of granulation tissue, rich in fibroblasts and blood vessels
- Eventual scar tissue, with collagen fibers deposited at the base of the ulcer
- May show prominent small arteries deeper to the base

Peptic ulcer: Deep defect in the wall of stomach or duodenum
- Often due to increased hydrochloric acid production
- Acid repeatedly damages tissue, ulcer deepens/progresses
- Common causes: Helicobacter pylori, NSAIDs, stress

ABC Classification of Gastritis

Type A	Autoimmune (autoantibodies)
Type B	Bacterial (H. pylori)
Type C	Chemical (Ethanol, NSAIDS)

Inflammatory Pathology

Entity:	1.4 Chronic Gastric Ulcer
Stain:	Hematoxylin - Eosin

Clinical Info/Symptoms: Epigastric pain, postprandial pain (if gastric ulcers present), bleeding, vomiting blood (hematemesis), tarry stool (melena). Of note, duodenal ulcers may have improved pain after a meal, though pain often will recur several hours later.

Complications: Bleeding (Dieulafoy's lesion is a rare cause of severe bleeding from superficial angiodysplasia), perforation to peritoneal cavity

Diagnostics:
- Esophagogastroduodenoscopy with biopsy (gold standard)
- Assessment for Helicobacter pylori: rapid urease test, 13-C breathing test, or most commonly stool H. pylori antigen detection
- Of note, patients need to be off of proton pump inhibitor (PPI) therapy for 1-2 weeks prior to testing for H. pylori

Forrest Classification of Upper GI Bleeding, 1974:
(stratifies severity of upper GI bleed according to endoscopic findings)

Forrest I = active bleeding	A = active arterial bleeding, spurting B = active venous bleeding, oozing
Forrest II = inactive bleeding	A = non-bleeding visible vessel B = adherent clot C = flat pigmented spot
Forrest III = lesion with no signs of bleeding	Clean ulcer base

Therapy: All patients with evidence of active infection with H pylori should be offered treatment.

Eradication therapy for Helicobater pylori

Bismuth quadruple therapy	Proton pump inhibitor + Bismuth + Tetracycline + Metronidazole
Clarithromycin triple therapy	Proton pump inhibitor + Clarithromycin + (Amoxicillin or Metronidazole)
Levofloxacin triple therapy	Proton pump inhibitor + levofloxacin + (Amoxicillin or Metronidazole)

Radiology:

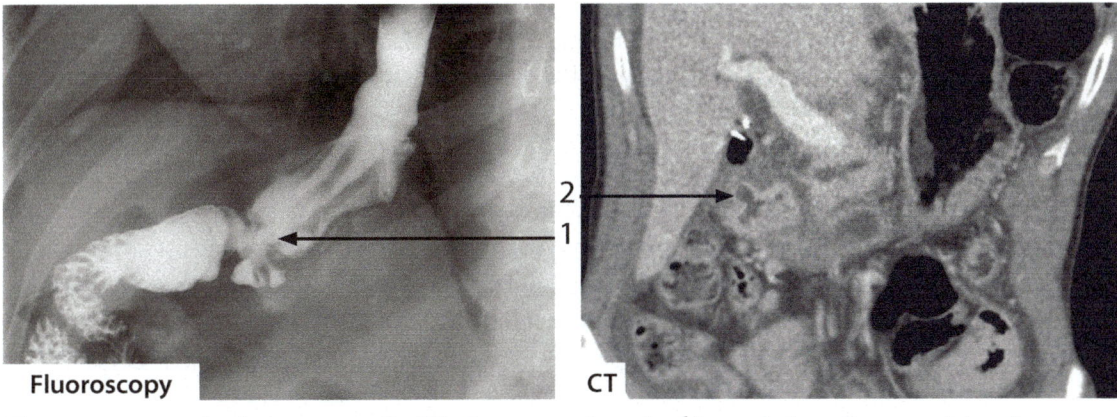

Fluoroscopy CT

Fluoroscopy: Oral contrast media fills the crater of an ulcer[1] located along the gastrojejunal anastomosis of a bariatric surgery (marginal ulcer)

CT: A deep outpouching occuring along the antropyloric stomach[2], with an adjacent extraluminal gas locule indicating a developing perforation

1 Inflammatory Pathology

Entity: 1.5 Meningitis
Stain: Hematoxylin - Eosin

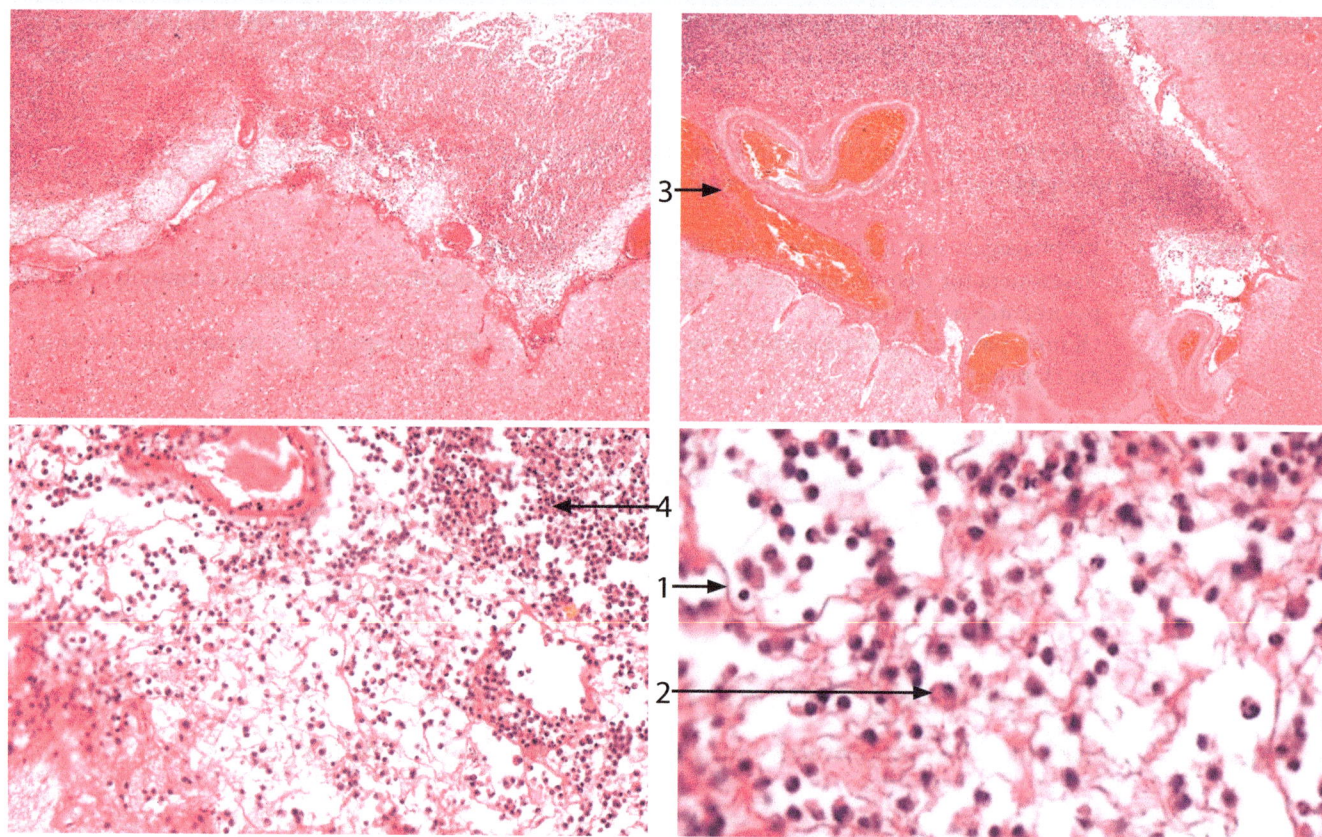

Macroscopy: Acute meningitis: Meninges are thickened, whitish-yellowish, may be frank pus, vasculature appears prominent, possible hemorrhage

Microscopy: Tissue / Organ: Meninges
 The pia mater has fine collagen fibers[1] and elastic/reticulin fibers, and epithelioid meningeal cells[2]
 Bacteria typically invade from the bloodstream[3], and often have pili or fimbriae which promotes bacterial colonization
 Massive buildup of fibrin and neutrophils[4] in the subarachnoid space

Definition: **Meningitis:** Inflammation of the meninges (Greek meninx = "skin"), often viral, but may be bacterial (with purulence) or tuberculous. The disease may transition to meningoencephalitis when cortical tissue also becomes involved

Etiology/ Pathogenesis:

Dominant Pathogens:	
Neonate to 6 months:	Group B streptococcus (now decreased due to maternal testing/prophylaxis), E. coli, Listeria
Young children:	S. pneumoniae, N. meningitidis (meningococci), H. influenzae type B (decreased due to vaccination), Group B Streptococcus, Enteroviruses
Older children to adult:	S. pneumoniae, N. meningitidis, Enteroviruses, HSV
Older adults (>60 years):	S. pneumoniae, N. meningitidis, H. influenzae type B, Group B Streptococcus, Listeria

Inflammatory Pathology

Entity:	1.5 Meningitis
Stain:	Hematoxylin - Eosin

Clinical Info/ Symptoms:
- Obtain CBC, electrolytes, coagulation studies (to assess for concomitant DIC), and blood cultures
- Obtain CSF before starting antibiotics, unless patient is clinically decompensating
- If concerned for a mass lesion in brain or increased ICP, obtain CT brain before lumbar puncture due to concern for cerebral herniation after removal of large amounts of CSF ("First CT, then CSF!")
- Send CSF for opening pressure, cell count and differential, glucose, protein, gram stain culture, and other specific tests depending on clinical suspicion (e.g. HSV PCR, Enterovirus PCR, fungal cultures

Diagnostics:

	Bacterial	Viral	Fungal
Opening Pressure	High	High or normal	High
Appearance	Turbid	Clear	Variable
Protein	High	Normal/low/high	Normal
Glucose	Low	Normal	Normal
Gram Stain	+	-	-
WBC	Very high	High	High
Predominant Cell Differential	Neutrophils	Lymphocytes	Lymphocytes

Therapy:
- If concerned for bacterial meningitis in adults and children: 3rd general cephalosporin (Ceftriaxone or Cefotaxime) + Vancomycin at meningitic dosing to cover Strep pneumo, Neisseria meningitidis, Haemophilus influenzae, MRSA + IV steroids (dexamethasone) to help prevent neurologic complications of bacterial meningitis
- Acyclovir if there is clinical suspicion for HSV
- Ampicillin if adult >50 years old and also in neonates to cover Listeria monocytogenes
- In neonates: Ampicillin + Aminoglycoside (usually gentamicin) + 3rd/4th generation cephalosporin to cover E. coli, Group B Strep, Listeria +/- Vancomycin if concerned for MRSA
- In immunocompromised patients: consider treatment for fungal meningitis
- Excepting HSV (where you would give acyclovir), if concerned for other viral meningitis: typically supportive care

Radiology:

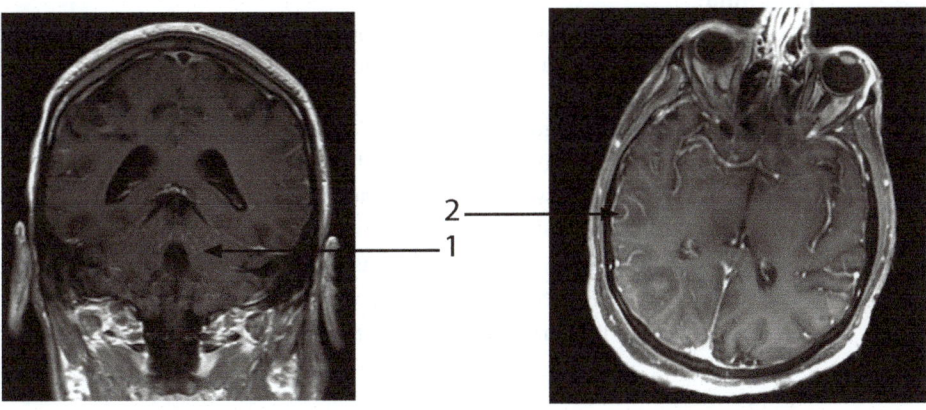

General:
- Radiologic imaging: Not sensitive or specific in obtaining a direct diagnosis of meningitis, may be useful in assessing for contraindications to lumbar puncture (intracranial bleeding or masses), or to identify complications in clinically confirmed cases
- Contrast enhancement of the meninges may be seen on CT or MRI, such as along the cerebellar folia in a case of cryptococcal meningitis[1]
- Severe cases of pyogenic infection can have contiguous spread to the brain proper, resulting in cerebritis and abscess formation[2]

Inflammatory Pathology

Entity: 1.6 Gout (Foreign Body-induced Inflammation)
Stain: Hematoxylin - Eosin

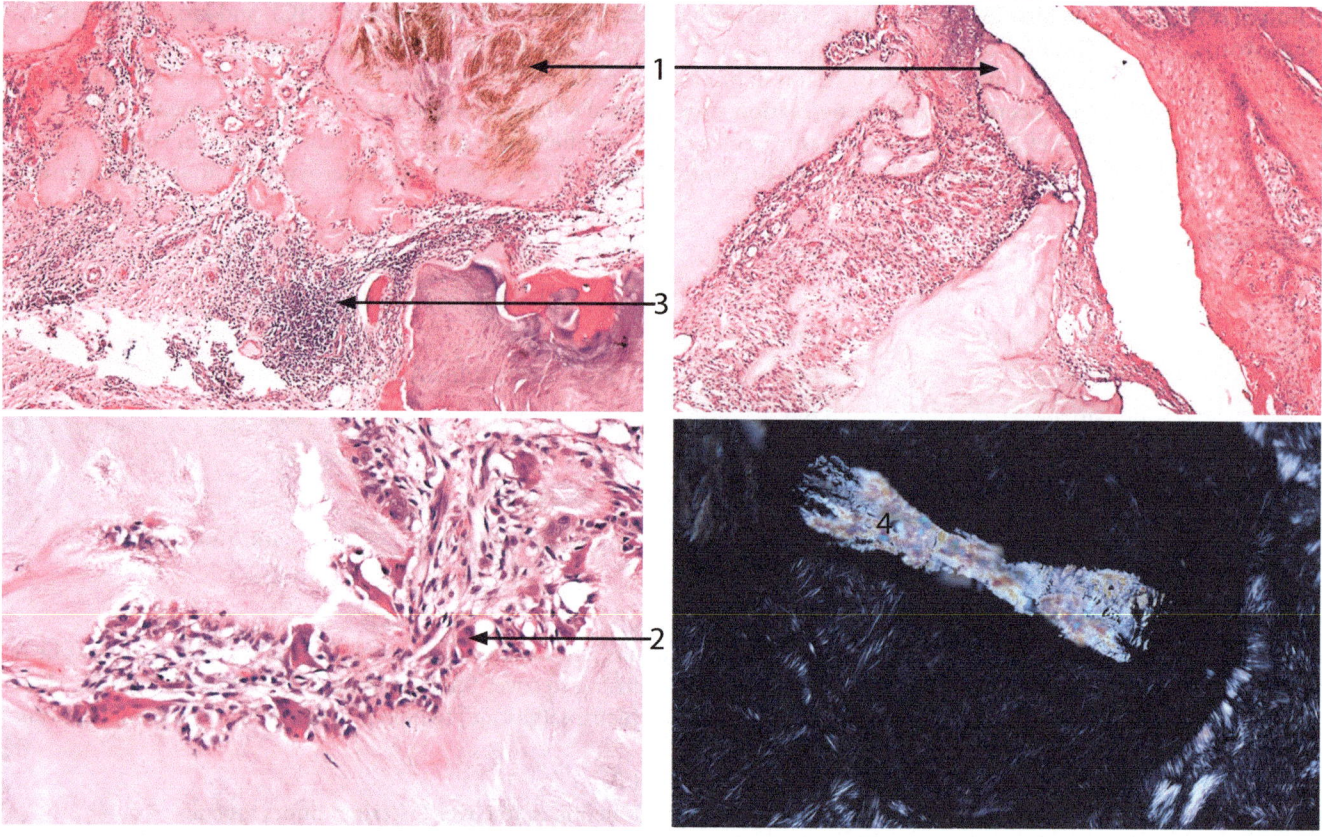

Macroscopy: Swollen and reddened skin and soft tissues around a joint, may be overlying skin ulceration; aspirated joint fluid may be cloudy, or gritty with gout tophi (whitish grains)

Microscopy:

Tissue/organ: Soft tissue/bone

Joint fluid:
- Grossly cloudy synovial fluid, microscopically shows crystals (true gout has needle-shaped urate crystals, pseudogout has polygonal calcium pyrophosphate crystals). These can be seen best under polarized light.

Skin and subcutis (true gout):
- Subcutaneous deposition of urate crystals[1] → bundles of needle-shaped crystals, or artifactual spaces[1] where crystals have dissolved during tissue preparation
- Often prominent fibrosis
- May show foreign body-type granulomas: multinucleated foreign body giant cells[2] surround urate crystals (Giant cells predominantly with disordered nuclei), rimmed by lymphocytes[3]
- Under polarized light, monosodium urate (MSU) crystals are birefringent[4], may be seen in bundle

Remember!	
Urate Crystals (True Gout)	**Calcium Pyrophosphate Crystals (Pseudogout)**
Negatively birefringent needle-shaped crystals	Positively birefringent rhomboid shaped crystals

Inflammatory Pathology

Entity:	1.6 Gout (Foreign Body-induced Inflammation)
Stain:	Hematoxylin - Eosin

Definition: **Gout:** A form of inflammatory arthritis caused by an elevated level of uric acid in the blood and accumulation of monosodium urate (MSU) crystals in the joints or soft tissue.

Etiology/Pathogenesis:

Increased uric acid due to:
- Overproduction of uric acid (e.g. in malignancy)
- Decreased uric acid breakdown (enzyme defects such as Lesch-Nyhan Syndrome - deficiency of hypoxanthine-guanine phosphoribosyltransferase (HGPRT)
- Decreased uric acid excretion (renal)

Pathogenesis:
- High concentration of urate → crystal deposition in synovium or soft tissue → overwhelms phagocytosis → release of mediators → foreign body giant cell reaction → further inflammation → cartilage or other soft tissue destruction and reparative fibrosis
- 90% primarily due to genetic predisposition, 10% secondary to hyperuricemia
- Hyperuricemia may be due to reduced excretion or increased formation of uric acid

Clinical Info/Symptoms:
- Typically monoarticular but can be polyarticular
- Joint pain and swelling; overlying skin hot and reddened.
- Most common joints: base of great toe (first metatarsophalangeal joint, known as podagra), knee, ankle, wrist, finger; uncommon for axial joints to be involved
- Gouty tophi (grossly visible, granular collections of crystals)
- Factors provoking gout flare: anything causing increased uric acid levels, such as trauma, surgery, starvation, fatty foods, dehydration, alcohol consumption

Diagnostics:
- Joint fluid aspiration for microscopic examination: send for cell count, gram stain and culture, and crystal analysis
- Uric acid crystals (true gout): negatively birefringent needle-shaped crystals
- Calcium pyrophosphate crystals (pseudogout): positively birefringent rhomboid shaped crystals
- Can also obtain serum uric acid testing but this level may be normal in an acute gout flare
- Can also consider X-Ray, CT, ultrasound

Therapy:

Acute gout flare:
- Oral glucocorticoids
- Oral NSAIDs
- Oral colchicine
- Intra-articular glucocorticoid injection

Preventive gout treatment:
- Indicated in patients with 2+ flares per year, clinical/radiographic signs of severe gout (e.g. structural joint damage or tophaceous deposits), or high risk of severe gout
- Allopurinol is firstline, other options include febuxostat, pegloticase, probenecid
- Patients of Chinese, Thai, or Korean ethnicities should be tested for HLA-B*5801 prior to starting allopurinol, due to risk of severe cutaneous adverse reactions in this group
- Target serum uric level <6 mg/dL
- During initiation of urate-lowering therapy, patient should also receive low doses of colchicine or NSAID to decrease/prevent recurrence of gout flare

Inflammatory Pathology

Entity: 1.6 Gout (Foreign Body-induced Inflammation)
Stain: Hematoxylin - Eosin

Radiology:

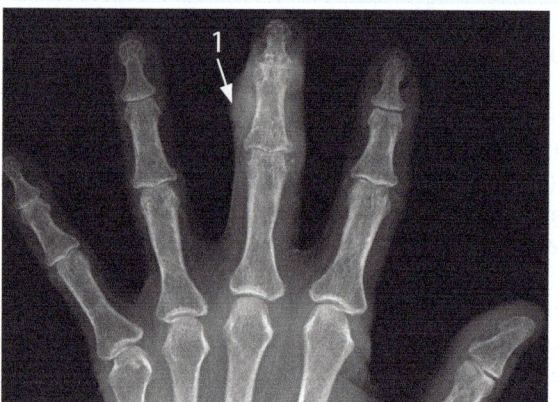
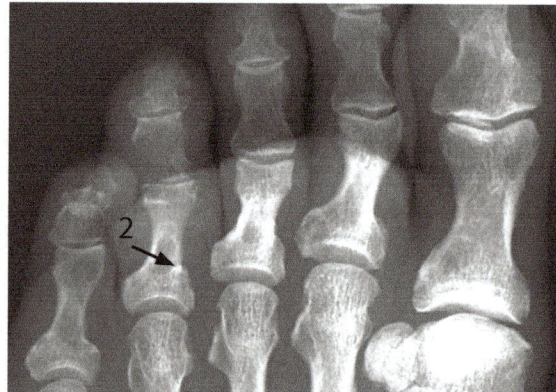

Conventional radiographs are used for diagnosis and monitoring
Classic features: Cloud-like soft tissue densities surrounding the joint representing tophi (middle finger[1]) and periarticular erosions with a sharp "overhanging edge" (medial aspect of the proximal interphalangeal joint of the 4th toe[2])

CT[3]:
Modern dual-energy techniques allow for crystal composition analysis
3D volume rendering of the foot shows an area of monosodium urate deposition (color-coded as green) adjacent to the great toe metatarsal head

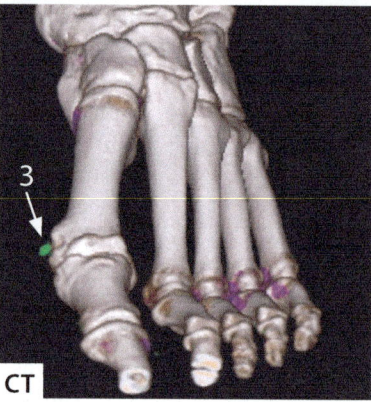
CT

Infectious Diseases

Tao Hong, Diana Treaba, Miguel Carabaño, Ann Ding, Carsten Fechner

2.1   Bacterial Myocarditis (Sepsis)

2.2   Esophageal Candidiasis

2.3   Fungal Pneumonia (Aspergillosis)

2.4   Pneumocystis Pneumonia

2.5   Cytomegalovirus (CMV) Pneumonia

2 Infectious Diseases

In this chapter we present selected infectious diseases that are commonly encountered in clinical practice and are either caused by bacteria, fungi or viruses. The human body is susceptible to infection by microorganisms, and a variety of organ systems may be involved. The following selected pathologies represent a review of some typical examples of viral, bacterial, and fungal infections, including histopathologic findings and the typical immune response seen within the affected tissues.

Sepsis:
- Pyogenic bacteria (e.g. Staphylococcus, Streptococcus, Pseudomonas)
- Mostly hematogenously spread of pathogens in the context of a septic pyemia
- Rarely via direct extension starting for example from bacterial endocarditis or pericarditis
- Pneumonia is the most common source for bacteremia/sepsis for adults; other sources are abdominal, urinary tract and skin/soft tissue infections

According to consensus criteria, sepsis (Greek σήψη ("sipsi") = putrefaction) is a life-threatening condition due to organ dysfunction, defined as a misdirected immune response to an infection.
- Risk stratification using the SOFA score
- Decrease in blood/pathogen culture before giving antibiotics
- Inflammation parameters (CRP, procalcitonin, IL-6)
- Lactate for assessing organ dysfunction due to disrupted microcirculation
- Organ and circulatory parameters

Simplified sepsis criteria = qSOFA	
Tachypnea:	> 22 breaths / minute
Hypotension:	Systolic BP <100mmHg
Neurology:	Vigilance reduction, confusion

Bacterial Infections:
- Staphylococcus aureus
- Streptococcus pneumoniae
- Enterococcus species
- Escherichia coli
- Klebsiella species
- Pseudomonas species
- Acinetobacter species
- Neisseria meningitidis
- Salmonella,
- Anaplasma
- Ehrlichia species
- Proteus...

Fungal Infections:
- Candida albicans
- Aspergillus fumigatus
- Cryptococcus
- Blastomycosis
- Histoplasma capsulatum
- Sporothrix schenckii
- Mucor
- Malassezia furfur...

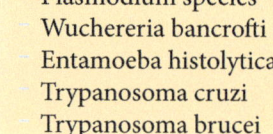

Parasitic Infections:
- Babesia species
- Plasmodium species
- Wuchereria bancrofti
- Entamoeba histolytica
- Trypanosoma cruzi
- Trypanosoma brucei
- Ascaris lumbricoides
- Echinococcus species
- Ancylostoma species (hookworm)....

Viral Infections:
- Hepadnaviridae (HBV)
- Hepeviridae (Hepatitis E)
- Coronaviridae
- Flaviviridae (HCV, dengue, yellow fever)
- Orthomyxoviridae (Influenza)
- Picornaviridae (Hepatitis A)
- Poxviridae
- Retroviridae (HIV-1 and 2, HTLV-1 and 2)....

Infectious Diseases

Overview of Gram-positive and negative Bacteria
Both Gram-positive and Gram-negative bacteria can cause sepsis. Gram-positive bacteria feature a thick layer of peptidoglycan which retains the purple-colored dye used in Gram stain procedure. In contrast, Gram-negative organisms have a thin layer of peptidoglycan, does not retain the purple dye (thus "Gram-negative"), and will be stained only by the pink counterstain.

The most common organisms causing sepsis:

Gram positive organisms:	Staphylococcus aureus, Staphylococcus epidermidis, Streptococcus pneumoniae, Enterococcus species
Gram negative organisms:	Escherichia coli, Klebsiella species, Pseudomonas species, Acinetobacter species

Some Gram-positive organisms can be further identified by appearance and enzyme activity:

Differences in Gram stain morphology:

Gram-positive cocci appearing in groups like bunches of grapes: Staphylococci

Gram-positive cocci appearing in linear strands: Streptococci

Differences in catalase reaction:

Catalase positive:	Staphylococci
Catalase negative:	Streptococci

Further differentiating Staphylococci:

Coagulase positive:	Staphylococcus aureus
Coagulase negative:	Staphylococcus epidermidis (novobiocin sensitive)
	Staphylococcus saprophyticus (novobiocin resistant)

Further differentiating Streptococci:
Depends on degree of hemolysis on blood agar

Alpha hemolysis (partial):	Streptococcus pneumoniae (encapsulate)
	Streptococci, viridans group (no capsule, Str. mutans, Str. mitis)
Beta hemolysis (complete):	Group A strep (Streptococcus pyogenes)
	Group B strep (Streptococcus agalactiae)
Gamma hemolysis (no hemolysis):	Enterococcus (E. faecium, E. facalis, grow in 6.5%Nacl, and PYR positive)
	Non enterococcus: Streptococcus bovis

Differentiating Gram-positive rods:

Aerobic:	Listeria, Bacillus, Corynebacterial
Anaerobic:	Clostridium, Cutibacterium

Differentiating Gram-positive branching/filamentous:

Aerobic:	Nocardia
Anaerobic:	Actinomyces

Infectious Diseases

Gram-negative organisms may be differentiated based on their Gram stain morphology:

Gram-negative diplococci:

Maltose fermentation negative:	Neisseria gonorrhea, Moraxella
Maltose fermentation positive	Neisseria meningitidis
Gram-negative coccobacillus:	Hemophilus influenza, Pasteurella, Brucella, Acinetobacter baumannii, Fransicella tularensis

Gram-negative bacilli differentiation by enzyme activity:

Lactose fermentation positive:	E. coli, Klebsiella pneumoniae, Enterobacter, Citrobacter, Serratia
Lactose fermentation negative, oxidase negative:	Salmonella, Shigella, Proteus, Yersinia
Lactose fermentation negative, oxidase positive:	Pseudomonas, Burkholderia

Curved Gram negative rod, oxidase positive:

Grow at 42°C	Campylobacter
Grow in alkaline media	Vibrio
Strong urease producer	Helicobacter

Of note, bacteria frequently colonize the human body (e.g. skin, colon, vagina) without causing any diseases. However, when the normal barrier of host defense (intact skin, mucous membrane, immune system) fail, an infection may occur. This table lists some common organisms and the infection/diseases they may cause.

Pathogen	Diseases
Staphylococcus aureus	Leading cause of nosocomial (hospital or nursing home-acquired) infections, soft tissue infections, bacteremia, endocarditis, osteoarticular infections, septic arthritis, often colonized in nasal mucous membrane. Methicillin-resistant Staphylococcus aureus (MRSA) is the most commonly identified multidrug-resistant organism. Uncommonly causes meningitis and pneumonia.
E. coli	Normal flora of large intestine, most common cause of urinary tract infection, also causes neonatal meningitis, bacteremia/sepsis. Pathogenic strains may cause diarrhea.
Streptococcus pneumoniae	Most common cause of community-acquired pneumonia, also bacteremia, meningitis (usually children <5 or adult > 65 year old). Asymptomatic colonization by this organism is common.
Group A Streptococcus	Streptococcus pharyngitis, skin and soft tissue infections, scarlet fever, necrotizing fasciitis, bacteremia, pneumonia, toxic shock syndrome. Postinfectious sequelae may include rheumatic fever and rheumatic heart disease, and glomerulonephritis.
Group B Streptococcus	Colonizes the GI and genital tract in 25-35% of individuals; may cause infections in neonates (meningitis, bacteremia, pneumonia). Adult infections include the female genital tract, pneumonia, bacteremia, arthritis, osteomyelitis, skin and soft tissue infections, meningitis, urinary tract infection.
Viridans Streptococci	Normal microbiota of oropharynx, skin, and GI tract. Major cause of bacterial endocarditis, abscesses, bacteremia, meningitis, septic arthritis.
Klebsiella pneumonniae	Mostly a nosocomial infection, seen as urinary tract infections, pneumonia, and bacteremia. Can also cause infection in healthy, immunocompetent individuals.
Neisseria meningitidis	Meningitis, bacteremia, pneumoniae, septic arthritis

Infectious Diseases

Pathogen	Diseases
Neisseria gonorrhea	Sexually transmitted infection causing male and female urogenital tract infection, also rectal infection, pharyngeal infection, pelvic inflammatory disease, disseminated gonococcal infection, neonatal and pediatric infections
Pseudomonas aeruginosa	Most common pathogen for nosocomial infections, such as ventilator-associated pneumonia and catheter-associated urinary tract infection, wound infections and burn infections.
Haemophilus influenzae	Meningitis, pneumonia, bacteremia, cellulitis, septic arthritis
Pasteurella	Most common cause of skin and soft tissue infection after an animal bite or scratch
Acinetobacter baumannii	Major cause of nosocomial infection, including ventilator-associated pneumonia, intravascular catheter associated bacteremia, surgical site infection, urinary tract infection, meningitis after surgery, soft tissue infection after burns
Staphylococcus saprophyticus	Urinary tract infection
Salmonella	Bacteremia, gastroenteritis
Shigella	Dysentery: bloody diarrhea with straining and painful defecation
Campylobacter	Diarrhea, bacteremia
Listeria monocytogenes	Fetuses are particularly at risk; maternal food-borne exposure may lead to transplacental spread of Listeria, causing severe complications including fetal loss, preterm labor, or neonatal infections such as meningitis and bacteremia. In adults, may cause acute gastroenteritis.
Brucella species	Brucellosis, a bacteremia commonly associated with animal contact and consuming unpasteurized cheese.
Mycobacterium tuberculosis	Pulmonary tuberculosis
Nocardia species	Pulmonary infection, skin infection
Actinomyces species	Oral-cervicofacial infection, pulmonary infection, pelvic infection
Clostridium difficile	Clostridium difficile infection (CDI) is an acute diarrheal disease due to colitis; the illness is often preceded by antimicrobial use, disturbing the normal colonic flora and allowing C. difficile to overgrow. The bacteria forms a toxin that damages human tissues. Common complication: Pseudomembranous colitis, can result in megacolon.
Corynebacterium diphtheriae	Pharyngeal diphtheria and cutaneous diphtheria. The incidence of diphtheria is very low due to widespread use of toxoid vaccine.

2 Infectious Diseases

Entity: 2.1 Bacterial Myocarditis (Sepsis)
Stain: Hematoxylin - Eosin

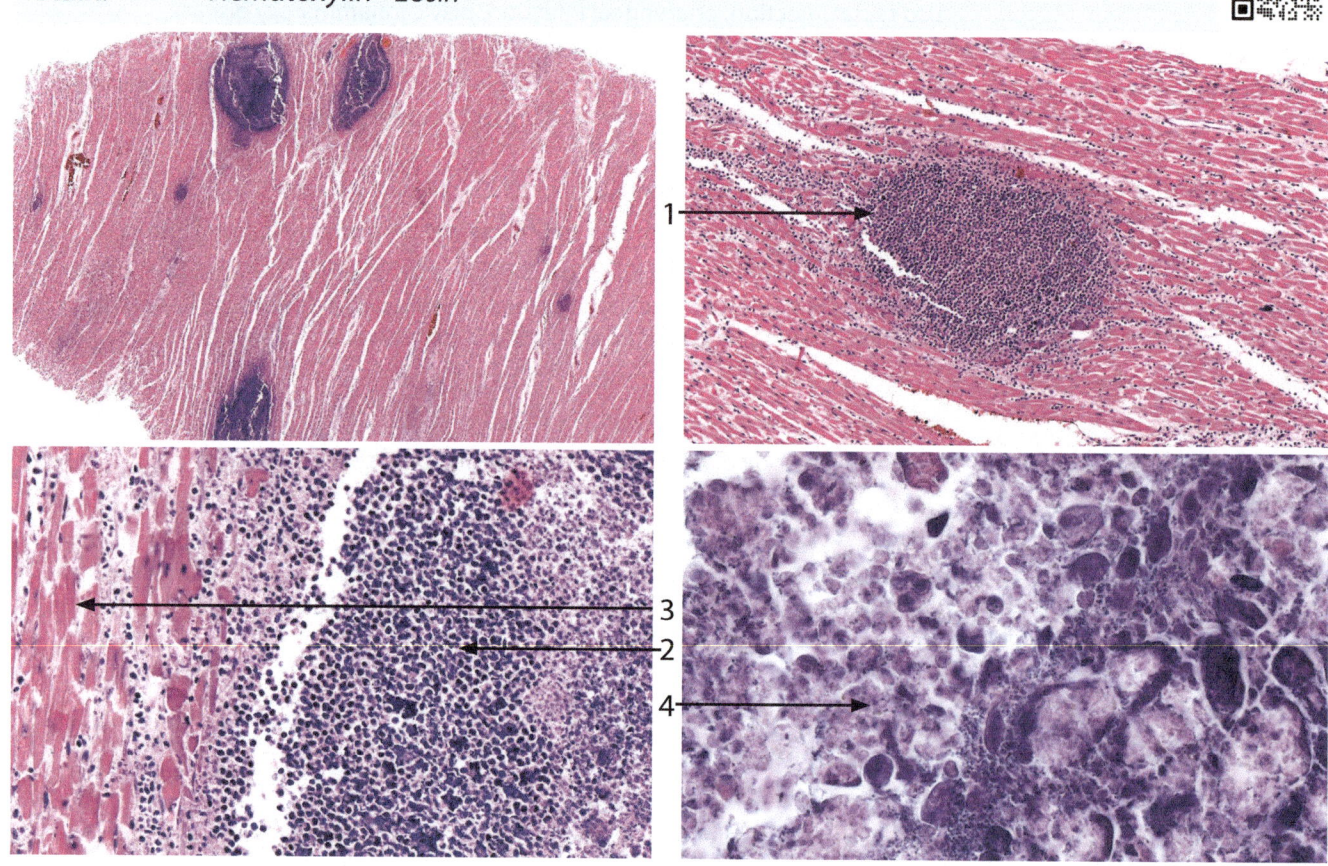

Macroscopy: Acute myocarditis: yellow-brown to yellow-gray foci, foci of discolored myocardium

Microscopy: Organ/tissue: Heart/myocardium
- Aggregates[1] (focused collections) of neutrophils[2] in the myocardium
- Remnants of necrotic cardiomyocytes[3] recognizable at the border of the inflammatory cell collections
- Dark blue/basophilic bacterial colonies[4]

Definition: **Myocarditis:** Inflammation of the heart musculature
Can be divided in three stages: acute, subacute with activation of lymphocytes or chronic with possible fibrosis, cardiomyopathy, chronic heart failure

Etiology/Pathogenesis:
- Most common etiology for myocarditis is viral (diffuse, lymphocytic response)
- Less often, bacteria can colonize myocardium (focal, neutrophilic response)
- Usually by hematogenous spread from elsewhere
- Pathogens: Staphyococci spp, Streptococci spp, Neisseria menigitidis, Salmonella spp, Campylobacter species, Brucella spp, etc
- Bacterial endocarditis can also invade the local myocardium as a complication
- Parasitic: Chagas disease - Trypanosoma cruzi (protozoa)
- Other causes of myocarditis: toxic substances (e.g. cocaine), immune-mediated, allergic/hypersensitivity (e.g. clozapine), immune checkpoint inhibitors, sarcoidosis

Infectious Diseases

Entity:	**2.1 Bacterial Myocarditis (Sepsis)**
Stain:	*Hematoxylin - Eosin*

Clinical Info/ Symptoms:
- If viral: general symptoms of malaise, fever; may show mild EKG changes or mild troponin elevation
- If bacterial: usually nidus of infection elsewhere, or sepsis; may be mild troponin elevation
- Acute: Sympoms less than 30 days, can be fulminant at presentation, increased inflammatory infiltrate
- Chronic: Symptoms more than 30days, often heart failure at presentation

Diagnostics:
- ECG: May show ST-segment elevation, tachycardia or bradycardia, arrhythmias.
- Cardiac biomarkers: Troponins, creatinine kinase-MB
- Other imaging studies: See below under Radiology

Therapy:
- Supportive management, oxygen
- Temporary pacemakers or AICD (automated implantable defibrillator) for arrhythmia
- Chronic heart failure management

Radiology:

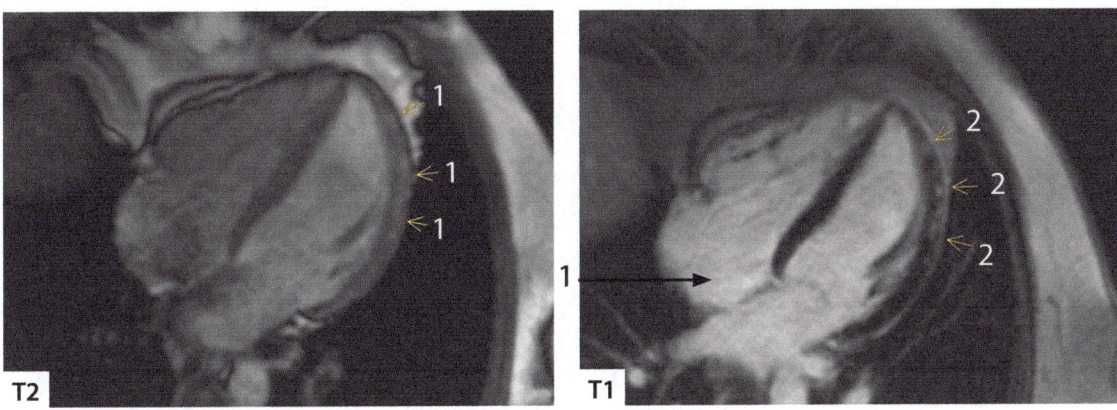

General:
- Myocarditis results in diffuse edema and hyperemic enhancement of the myocardium; later is fibrosis with late enhancement. Wall motion abnormalities can sometimes be seen.

Ultrasound:
- Often only functional abnormalities seen, such as left ventricular systolic dysfunction or diastolic dysfunction, regional wall motion abnormalities, pericardial effusion.

MRI:
- T2 hyperintense myocardial edema[1], myocardial hyperemia with early gadolinium enhancement or irreversible myocardial fibrosis with gadolinium late enhancement[2].

Lake Louise consensus criteria 2018: One T1 and T2 criterion has to be fulfilled.
T2-weighted:
- Regional high signal[1]
- Signal intensity ratio (myocardium/skeletal muscle) ≥2 increased
- T2 relaxation times in T2 mapping

T1-weighted:
- Subepicardial or mid myocardial late enhancement[2]
- Increased T1 relaxation times or extracellular volume in native T1 mapping

Supportive criteria: pericardial effusion, late enhancement, wall motion abnormalities

2 Infectious Diseases

Entity: **2.2 Esophageal Candidiasis**
Stain: *GMS (silver stain)*

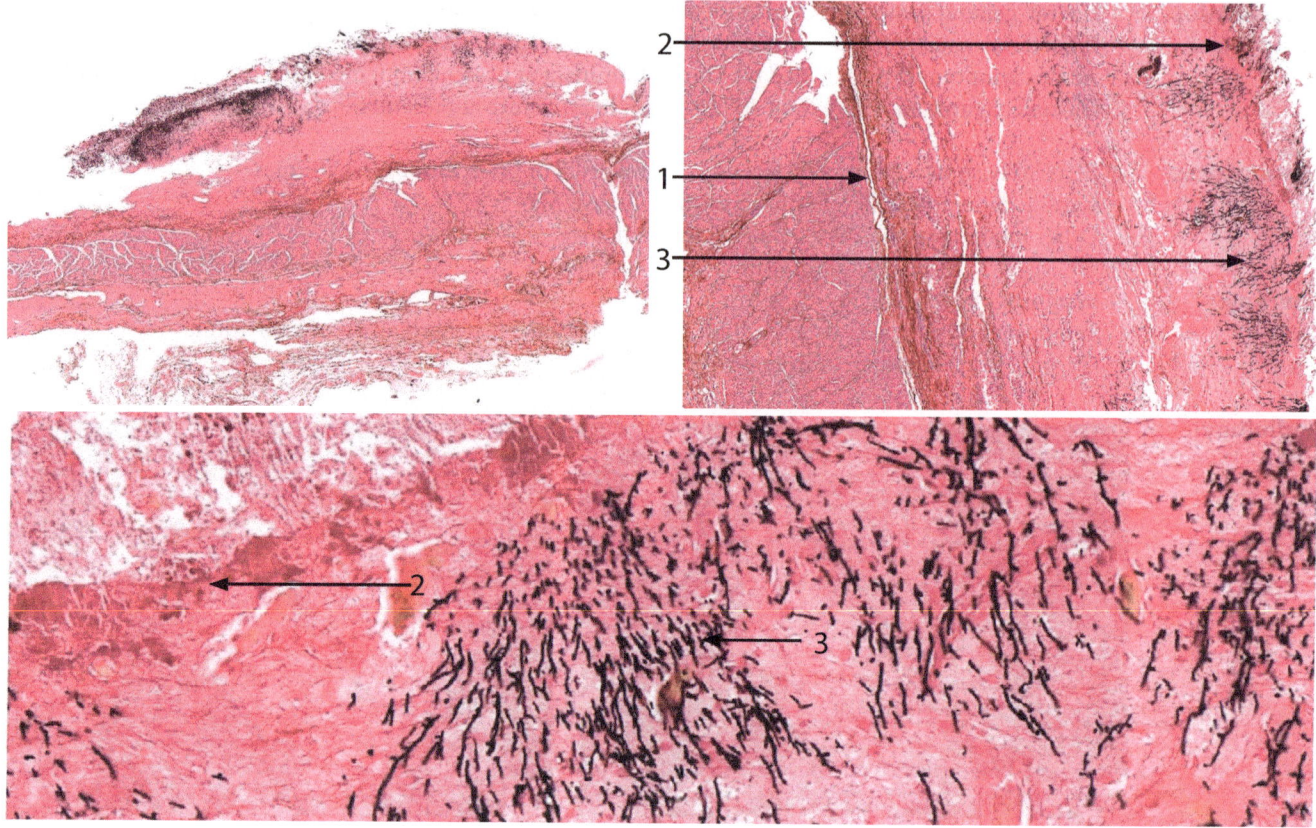

Macroscopy:	Esophageal mucosa with white to yellow-white deposits, hyperemia, associated erosions/ulcers
Microscopy:	Tissue/organ: Esophagus – Nonkeratinizing squamous epithelium, muscularis propria[1] (circumferential and longitudinal muscle (proximal is skeletal muscle, distal is smooth muscle) – Demarcated mucosal necrosis[2] – Fungal spores and pseudohyphae (black on silver stain) may penetrate deeply[3]
Definition:	**Candidiasis:** Fungal infection caused by Candida ssp. (yeast), e.g. Candida albicans
Etiology/ Pathogenesis:	– Often in immunosuppressed patients (AIDS), or patients with inhalative corticosteroid therapy, or following antibiotic therapy that disrupts normal oral flora – Often seen in patients with neutropenia/agranulocytosis due to medications/chemotherapy: E.g. thyreostatika (methimazole, carbomazole), cytostatics
Clinical Info/ Symptoms:	– Classification according to location: skin mycoses, intertriginous candidiasis, nail candidiasis, thrush stomatitis, thrush esophagitis, thrush vaginitis, thrush balanitis, diaper thrush, etc. – Thrush esophagitis is one of the more than 20 AIDS-defining diseases (HIV stage C); list of diseases defining AIDS can be found on the Centers for Disease Control and Prevention webpage
Diagnostics:	– Visual diagnosis: on mucosa, grossly uninflamed with yellowish-gray coatings; on skin shows erythematous macules, may be satellite foci – Pathogen identification via microscopy or culture or detection of antigen from body fluids
Therapy:	– Treatment of immunosuppressive disease and antifungal drugs – Systemic antifungal (e.g. fluconazole, caspofungin, liposomal amphotericin B) – Topical antifungal (e.g. ointments with ciclopirox, clotrimazole, nystatin)

Infectious Diseases

Entity:	2.2 Fungal Pneumonia (Aspergillosis)
Stain:	*Hematoxylin and Eosin*

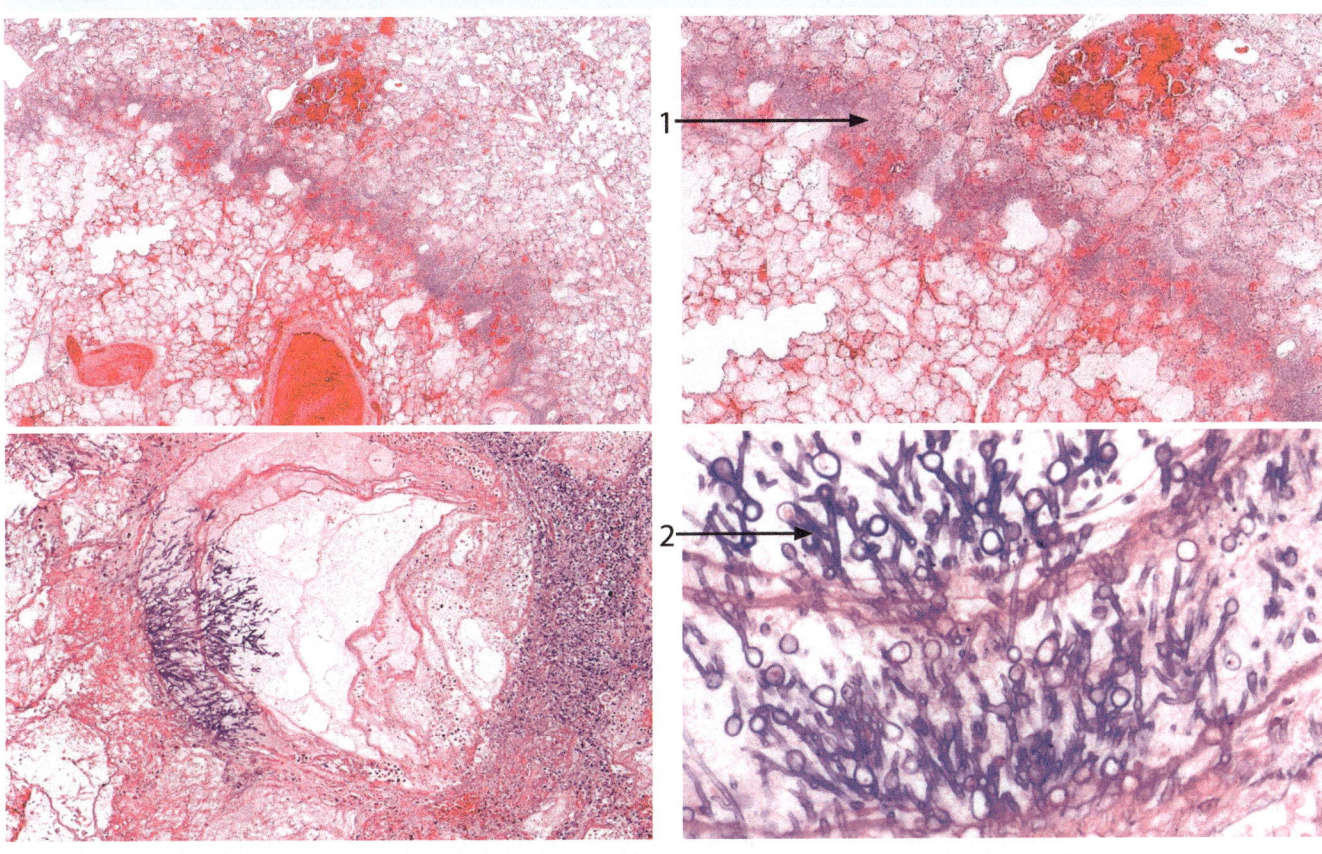

Macroscopy:	Presence of a circumscribed nodule (called mycetoma or aspergilloma, see below), grossly gray-white/light-brown with a soft to moderately firm consistency
Microscopy:	– ABPA (see below): dilation of the large bronchi, mucous plugs in the lumen – Aspergillus pneumonia: sharply or indistinctly demarcated, rounded gray or dark red foci of necrosis, often with hemorrhagic margins – Hemorrhagic infarcts indicate vascular invasion (e.g., invasive aspergillosis)
Microscopy:	Tissue/organ: Lungs – Necrosis with rim of granulocytes[1] – Mycelia[2] of septate hyphae with dichotomous (typical branching angle 45°) – Spore-bearing fruiting body (specialized hyphae) are rarely seen
Definition:	**Aspergillosis:** Fungal infection caused by Aspergillus spp. that mostly affects patients with weakened immune reponse
Etiology/ Pathogenesis:	– Aspergillus ssp. (e.g. Aspergillus fumigatus (mold)) – Fruiting body (specialized hypha) rarely seen, occurs in aerobic environment – Has high allergenic potential, e.g. allergic bronchopulmonary aspergillosis (ABPA) – Aspergillosis: Collective name for fungal diseases caused by Aspergillus spp. – Aspergilloma: Collection of Aspergillus surrounded by inflammatory cells (e.g. in preformed cavities, lung parenchyma or paranasal sinuses)
Clinical Info/ Symptoms:	More common in immunosuppressed, a descending spread occurs via inhalation or aspiration from the mouth into the body, less often due to haematogenous spread in sepsis Dry cough, hemoptysis, respiratory failure, with immunosuppression pneumonia, sepsis

2 Infectious Diseases

Entity: 2.3 Fungal Pneumonia (Aspergillosis)
Stain: Hematoxylin - Eosin

Diagnostics:

Rosenberg-Patterson Criteria (most acknowledged criteria):	
Major Criteria	Minor Criteria
- Asthma history - Pulmonary infiltrates - Aspergillus skin test (immediate hypersensitivity to Aspergillus fumigatus) - Elevated IgE levels - Aspergillus antibodies - Eosinophilia - Ectasia of the proximal or central bronchi (bronchiectasis)	- Positive Sputum Culture - Brownish sputum plugs/flecks - Delayed skin reactivity (Arthus-type)

Therapy: Antifungal drugs (voriconazole, amphotericin B, flucytosine); surgical excision of large aspergillomas

Radiology:

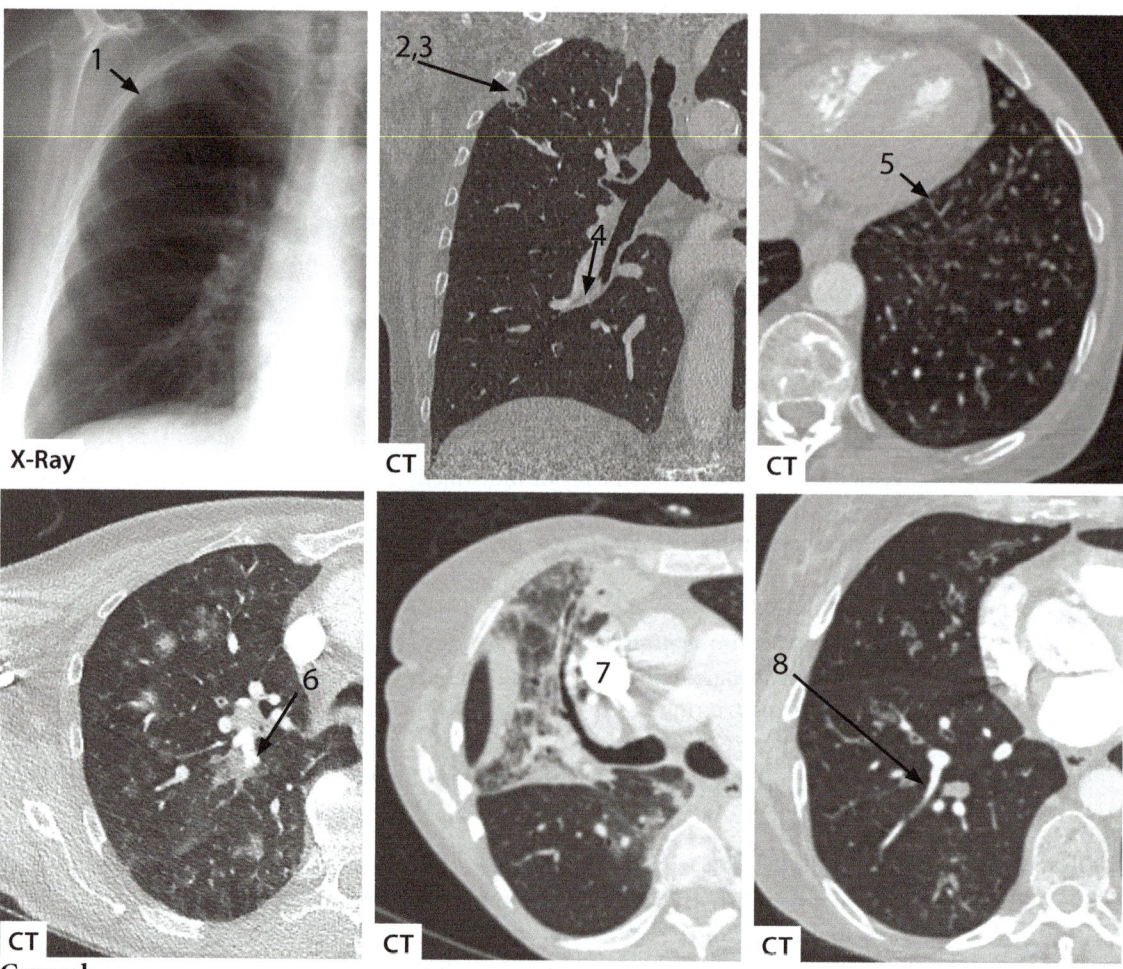

General:
Varies, dependent on immune status of patient; pulmonary aspergillosis manifests regionally in the immunocompetent, and often as diffuse invasive in the immunocompromised, with upper lobe predominance.

Immunocompetent:
Aspergilloma, dense round fungal ball[1] inside of pre-existing cavity[2] with air crescent sign (Monod sign[3]) on X-Ray and CT
Aspergillus nodules may appear smaller and without the air crescent sign on CT

Infectious Diseases

Entity:	2.3 Fungal Pneumonia (Aspergillosis)
Stain:	Hematoxylin - Eosin

Immunocompromised with invasive aspergillosis (Has three different entities):
- Airway-invasive aspergillosis: Bronchial wall thickening[4] and centrilobular nodules/tree in bud sign[5], transitions into peribronchial consolidations[6] on CT.
- Angioinvasive aspergillosis: Pulmonary nodules/masses[6] with a ground glass halo[7] of hemorrhage on CT. Peripheral wedge-shaped consolidations represent hemorrhagic pulmonary infarcts.
- Subacute invasive pulmonary aspergillosis: Pulmonary opacities developing central necrosis and forming cavities with or without a central mycetoma / aspergilloma1 on CT.

Allergic bronchopulmonary aspergillosis (ABPA) (immunocompetent):
- Bronchiectasis with mucus plugging[8] and vague centrilobular opacities, predominantly in the upper lobes in the CT.

Chronic pulmonary aspergillosis (CPA) (immunocompromised):
- Cavity forming changes, aspergillosis, or lung fibrosis in the upper lobes on CT.

Aspergillosis involving the heart:

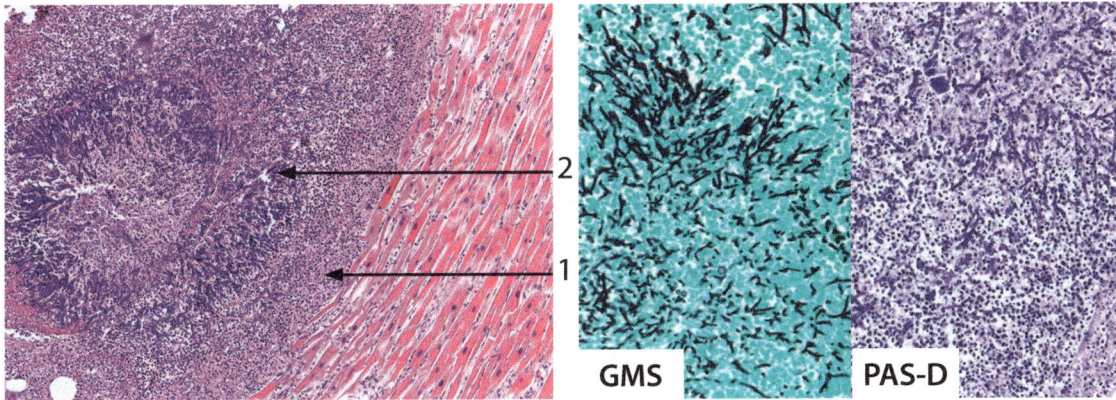

Tissue/organ: myocardium
- Necrosis with granulocytic demarcation[1], Mycelia[2] of septate hyphae with dichotomous parts development and typical branching angle of 45° or rarely with a spore-bearing fruit head (specialized hyphae), necrotic cardiomyocytes
- Fungal structures stain black on the GMS stain, and less distinctly as purple on the PAS stain

PAS stain: Periodic Acid-Schiff stain, stains fungal cells and mature spores

GMS stain: Grocott methenamine silver stain, used for staining of fungal forms

2 Infectious Diseases

Entity: 2.4 Pneumocystis Pneumonia
Stain: Periodic acid-silver methenamine (PASM) counterstained with H&E

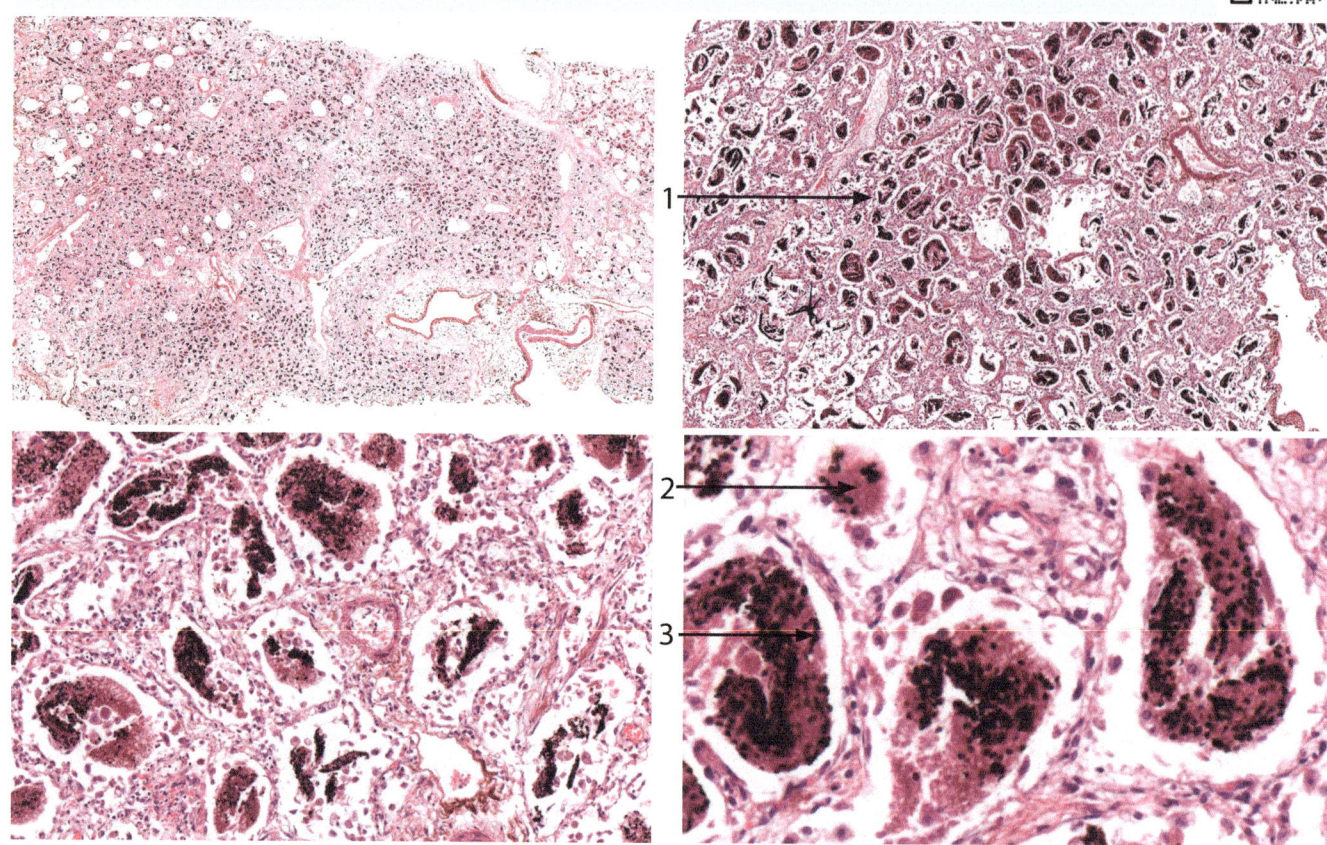

Macroscopy: Mostly heavy, solidified lungs

Microscopy: Tissue/organ: Lungs
- Diffuse interstitial pneumonia: widening of the interstitial lung framework[1] by edema and inflammatory cells (lymphocytes and plasma cells)
- Increased amount of pathogen in immunocompromised patients, possibly less of an inflammatory response
- Alveoli show foamy masses of pathogen, this is weakly eosinophilic or rust-colored, this exudate[2] contains round-oval to coffee bean-shaped organisms[3] (cyst with several intracystic bodies)
- Organisms can be highlighted on silver stain (e.g. Grocott-methenamine silver)

Definition: **Pneumocystis jiroveci (described by Otto Jirovec, 1907-1972):**
A causative agent of interstitial pneumonia

Etiology/Pathogenesis:
Most often seen in immunosuppressed, Pneumocystis Pneumonia (PcP) one of the more than 20 AIDS defining diseases (HIV stage 3), also seen on infant wards
Cysts are inhaled → burst → intracystic bodies are released → trophic form (trophozoite) most predominant (1-8 μm oval to elongated shapes) around → yeast anchors on pneumocytes → two haploid merge to form a zygote → formation of a cyst with intracystic bodies (= spores) → cycle starts again

Infectious Diseases

Entity:	2.4 Pneumocystis Pneumonia
Stain:	Hematoxylin - Eosin

Clinical Info/Symptoms: Subfebrile temperature, chronic progressive dyspnea, dry cough

Diagnostics: Typical increase in LDH (non-specific), radiologic imaging, visualizing organisms in a bronchoalveolar lavage specimen

Therapy: High-dose treatment with cotrimoxazole (trimethoprim + sulfamethoxazole, TMP/SMX), possibly glucocorticoids in addition for resp. Insufficiency, clarification / treatment of any underlying immuno-suppressive disease

Radiology:

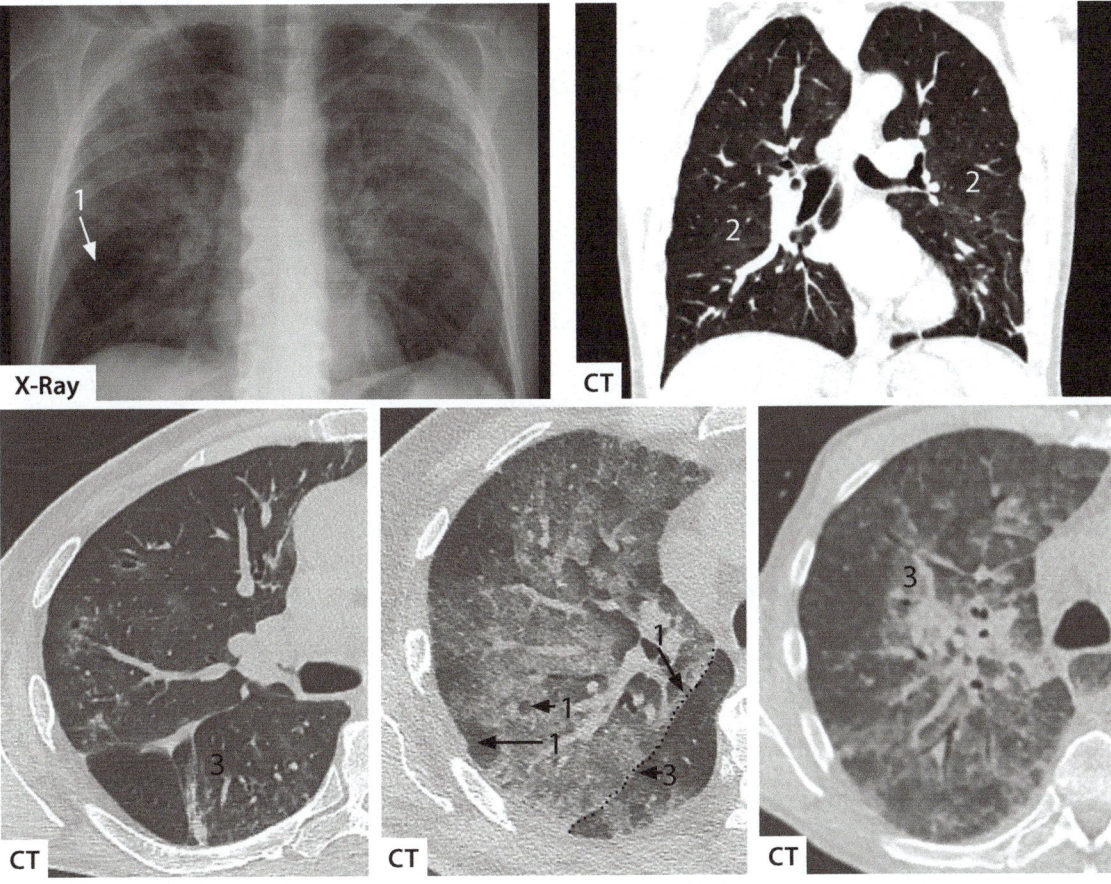

General:
- Diffuse alveolar damage generated by pneumocystis in immunocompromised (often HIV) patients

X-Ray:
- Small pneumatoceles[1] (thin air-filled cyst/s), subpleural blebs and fine reticular interstitial changes in a predominantly perihilar distribution

CT:
- Diffuse areas of ground glass[2] with or without septal thickening (crazy paving[3]) in the perihilar and mid zones
- Small pneumatoceles[1] may be seen
- Atypical features may include consolidation in patients with a recovering immune system

Infectious Diseases

Other Common Fungal Infections

Fungus	Geographic Distribution/Origin	Morphologic Characteristics	Associated Diseases	Treatment
Blastomyces	Environmental: Moist soil, decomposed plant matter; Worldwide: Mostly Canada, India, and Africa; US: Ohio and Mississippi River valleys.	Dimorphic fungi growing as: 1. Molds that produce asexual spores (conidia) or large chlamydospores, 2. Yeast	Blastomycosis: - Pulmonary - Cutaneous - Osseous - Genitourinary - CNS - Disseminated	Mild-moderate: Itraconazole Severe: Amphotericin B
Cryptococcus	Environmental: Moist soil, decaying wood, in tree hollows, in bird droppings Worldwide	Cryptococcus neoformans: Polysaccharide capsule, forms melanin, and has urease activity. Forms hyphae and basidiospores carried by club-shaped basidium with hyphae with a complex septate	Cryptococcosis: - Pulmonary - CNS (Immuno suppressed) - Disseminated (immunosuppressed)	Mild-moderate: Fluconazole Severe/CNS: Amphotericin B + flucytosine
Coccidioides	Environmental: Dust and soil in in Mexico, and South America. US: Arizona, California, Nevada, New Mexico, Texas, and Utah.	Thick-walled spherules: 20 to 80 micrometers in diameter.	Valley Fever (Coccidioidomycosis): - Pulmonary - Night sweats - Cutaneus - Musculoskeletal - CNS	Mild-moderate: Fluconazole Severe/Immunocompromised: Amphotericin B
Dematiaceous fungi	Environmental: Soil, wood, and dead decaying plant debris Geographic: Tropical and subtropical climates	Heterogenous: Cell walls contain melanin	- Chromoblastomycosis - Eumycotic mycetoma - Phaeohyphomycosis - Cutaneous infections	Surgery/thermotherapy/laser therapy/photodynamic therapy, itraconazole or voriconazole
Histoplasma capsulatum	Environmental: Soil Geographic: Africa, Asia, Australia, Central and south America US: Central and eastern states, most commonly in Ohio and Mississippi River Valleys	Dimorphic fungi: 1. Mold: Ship's wheel morphology (globose/tuberculate macroconidia and ovoid microconidia 2. Yeast: Small oval to round, budding yeasts	Histoplasmosis: - Pulmonary - CNS - Disseminated	Itraconazole or Amphotericin B
Mucor	Organic Substrates (fruits and vegetables), soil, dung	Class of Zygomycetes Filamentous fungi	Mucormycosis: - Cutaneous - Gastrointestinal - Pulmonal - Rhinocerebral (black lesions on nose and in oral cavity) - Disseminated	Amphotericin B, isavuconazole, posaconazole

Infectious Diseases

Entity:	2.5 Cytomegalovirus (CMV) Pneumonia
Stain:	Hematoxylin - Eosin

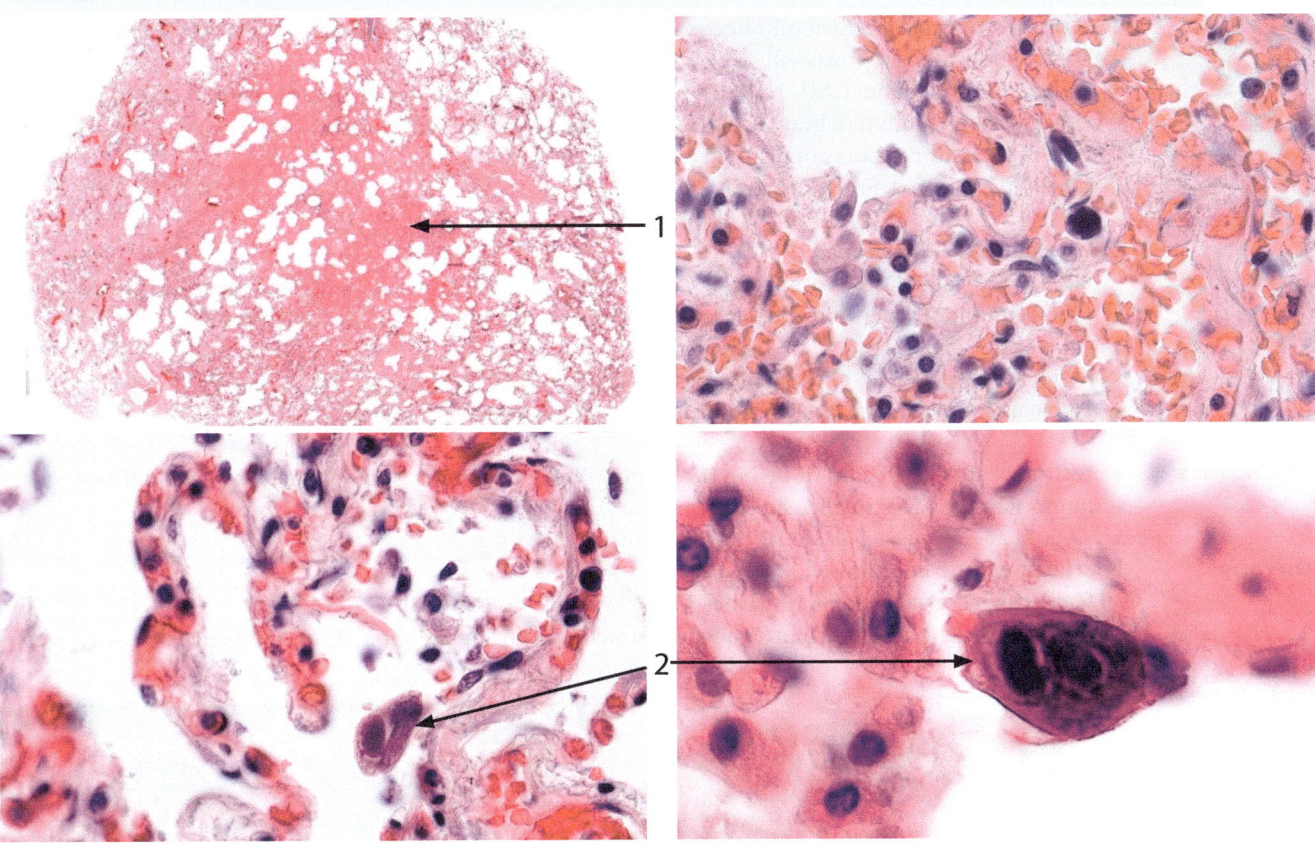

Macroscopy:	Focal or diffuse solidified lung parenchyma (interstitial pneumonia) – Macroscopic picture similar to that of Pneumocystis pneumonia (if diffuse alveolar disease (DAD) is present) – Rarely seen as numerous small hemorrhagic nodules – Very rarely seen as circumscribed solidified nodule (interstitial pneumonia)
Microscopy:	Tissue/organ: Lungs – Overall over-inflated appearance on tissue sections – Broadening of the septa, with edema[1] and scant inflammatory response – Pathognomonic cells: "owl-eye" cells[2] which are enlarged (up to 30 μm) pneumocytes with up to 10 μm nuclear inclusion bodies
Definition: Etiology/ Pathogenesis:	Viral infection, caused by the cytomegalovirus (human herpes virus 5) – Immunocompetent patients: high infection rate in the population, approx. 90%, usually asymptomatic – Immunosuppressed patients: atypical interstitial pneumonia with 50% lethality, CMV esophagitis, colitis, retinitis with risk of blindness – Infection through body fluids (blood, saliva, urine, semen, breast milk) or trans-placental
Clinical Info/ Symptoms:	90% asymptomatic (immunocompetent), dyspnoea and respiratory insufficiency (immunocompromised) Initial infection: – Immunocompetent children / adults: asymptomatic, but virus persistence! – Immunocompromised mothers: fetal death, generalized infection in newborns!

Infectious Diseases

Entity:	**2.5 Cytomegalovirus (CMV) Pneumonia**
Stain:	Hematoxylin - Eosin

Reactivation may occur when immune system compromised (immunodeficiency, AIDS, organ transplantation with immunosuppression):
- Generalized infection, CMV retinitis (blindness possible!), Especially liver (hepatitis) and Lungs (interstitial pneumonia), brain (encephalitis), gastrointestinal ulceration
- One of the leading causes of death in patients with
- One of the AIDS-defining diseases

Congenital CMV infection:
- CNS (hydrocephalus, periventricular calcifications, bleeding into the ventricles, microcephalus), eye (chorioretinitis), gastrointestinal tract (hepatosplenomegaly, jaundice, acholic stools)

Long-term consequences of congenital CMV infection:
- Hypacusis, eye damage, psychomotor deficits with intellectual disability

Diagnostics: Detection of anti-CMV IgM or IgG in the serum, PCR, p65 antigen, owl-eye cells in affected tissue, immunostain for CMV in affected tissue

Therapy: For the immunocompromised:
- Ganciclovir, valganciclovir, foscarnet, CMV hyperimmunoglobulin
- Prophylaxis with letermovir after allogeneic stem cell transplantation, if CMV positive

Radiology:

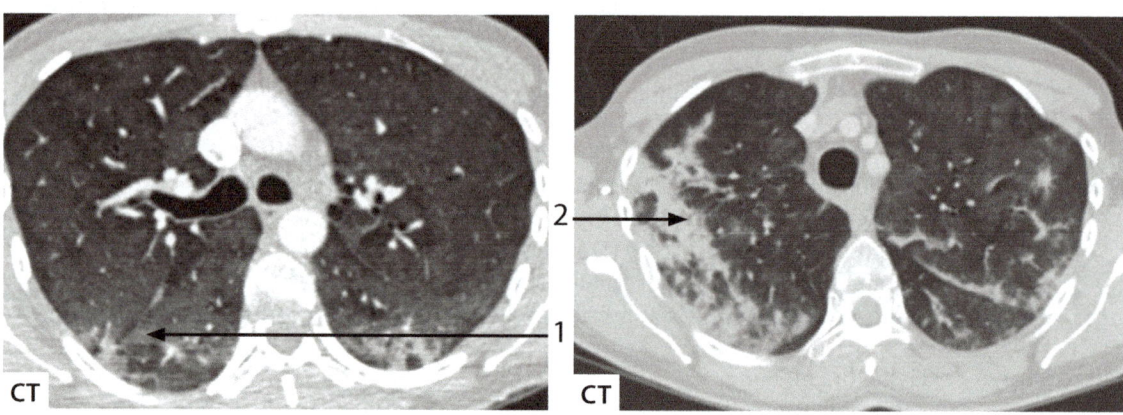

General: Diffuse alveolar damage in immunocompromised (stem cell transplant and HIV) patient.

CT: Areas of ground glass[1] with consolidations transitioning to confluent consolidations[2], predominantly involving the lower lobes.

Cellular Adaptation: Hypertrophy, Hyperplasia, Atrophy

Mariana Canepa, Ann Ding, Carsten Fechner

3.1 **Myocardial Hypertrophy**

3.2 **Benign Prostatic Hyperplasia**

3.3 **Thyroid Goiter (Hyperplasia)**

3.4 **Hydronephrosis (Atrophy)**

3.5 **Pulmonary Emphysema**

3 Cellular Adaptation: Hypertrophy, Hyperplasia, Atrophy

Cells and tissues are able to adapt in response to changes in their local environment and to meet the changing needs of the organism. Cells may respond by modifying biochemical pathways, altering gene expression, replicating, or dissembling unneeded internal structures. The terms used to describe these changes are below, and the chapter presents some classic examples of these adaptations.

In hypertrophy, the cells increase in size to accommodate more organelles to do more work; this is typically seen in tissues where the cells cannot divide, such as the myocardium. Increased work demand on the heart results in cardiomyocyte hypertrophy (larger cells). This overall increase in cell size is appreciated grossly as myocardial hypertrophy (larger heart). In hyperplasia, the need to do more work leads to cell replication, increasing the number of cells present to do the increased work. This change is often seen in hormone-responsive tissues, where increased hormones signal more work is needed, and the cells increase in number; thyroid goiter and benign prostatic hyperplasia are examples.

Atrophy occurs when work demand decreases, hormones are withdrawn, or there are external pressures that render the cells unable to do work. Organelles may be broken down if unneeded, and cell size and/or cell number decreases. This "shrinking" of tissue with smaller cells can be seen in kidney parenchyma that is under pressure from hydronephrosis. The cells are unable to do work properly, and will break down and repurpose extraneous organelles; decreasing cell size in the process. The lung tissue in emphysema may also be described as functionally atrophic (decreased functional volume), although the tissue arrives there via necrosis/apoptosis due to chemical insult (smoking).

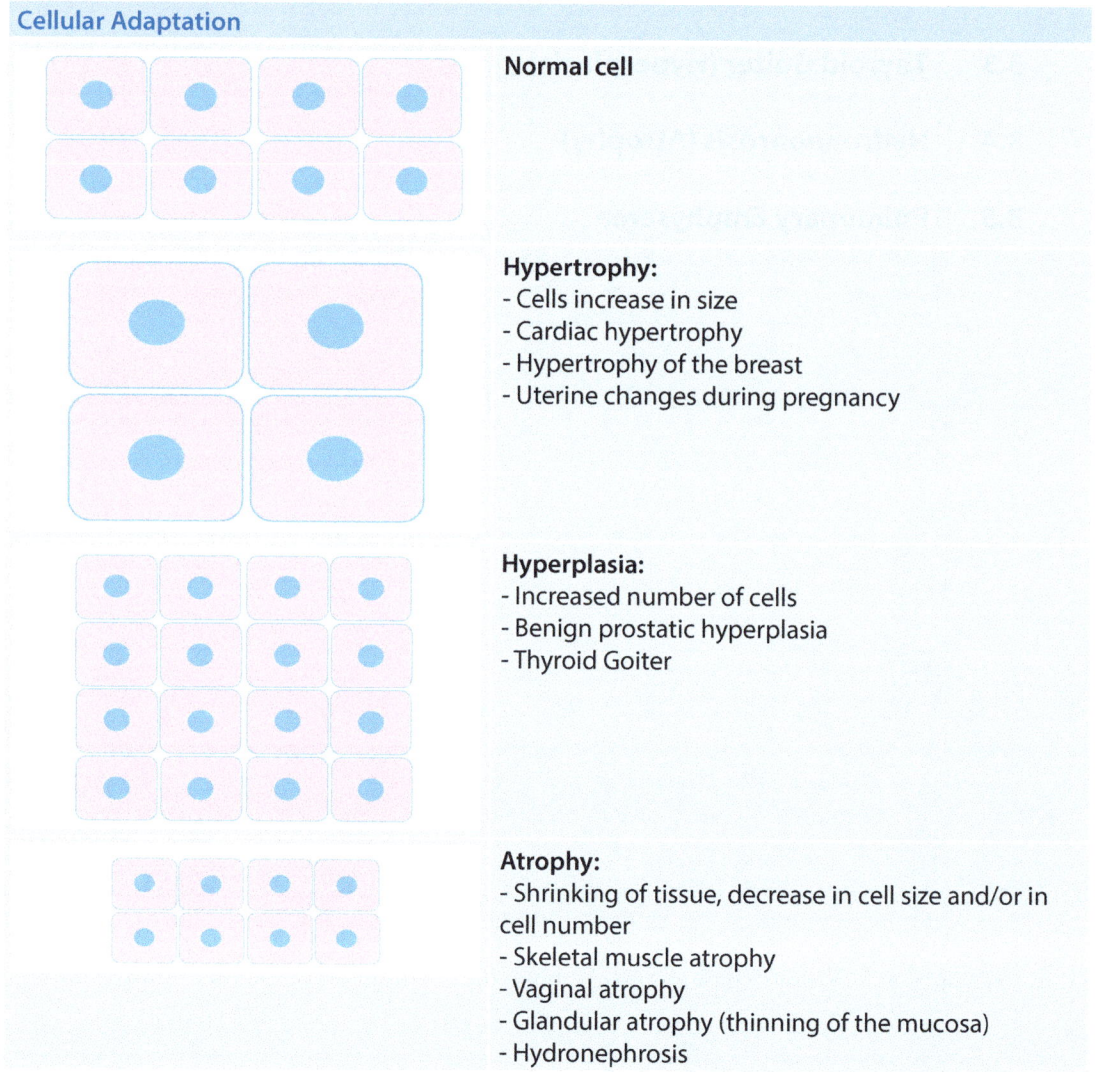

Cellular Adaptation

Normal cell

Hypertrophy:
- Cells increase in size
- Cardiac hypertrophy
- Hypertrophy of the breast
- Uterine changes during pregnancy

Hyperplasia:
- Increased number of cells
- Benign prostatic hyperplasia
- Thyroid Goiter

Atrophy:
- Shrinking of tissue, decrease in cell size and/or in cell number
- Skeletal muscle atrophy
- Vaginal atrophy
- Glandular atrophy (thinning of the mucosa)
- Hydronephrosis

Cellular Adaptation: Hypertrophy, Hyperplasia, Atrophy

Entity: 3.1 Myocardial Hypertrophy
Stain: Hematoxylin - Eosin

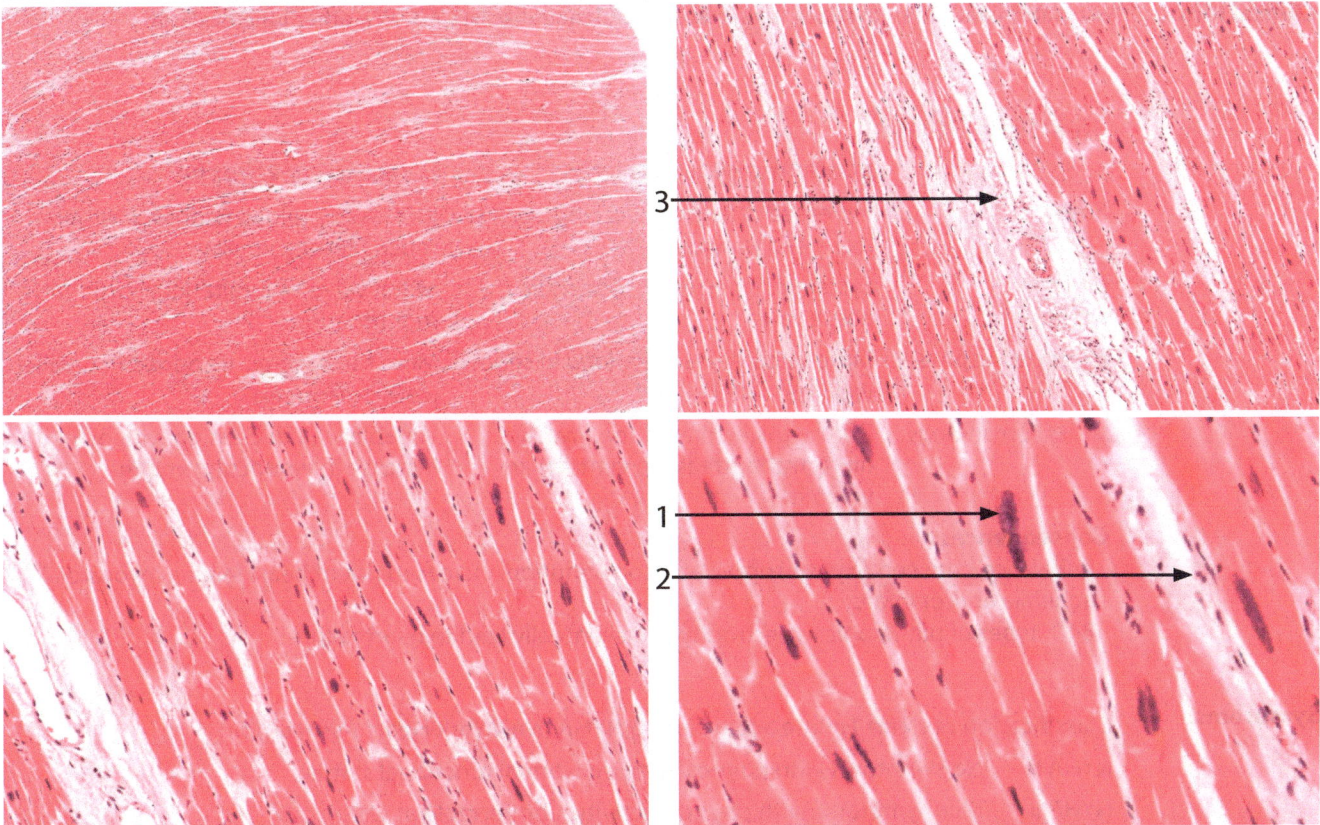

Macroscopy:
- Weight of normal heart: female 250-330 g, male 300-350 g; left ventricle wall thickness 1.4 ± 0.1 cm, right ventricle wall thickness 0.4 ± 0.1 cm; Rule of thumb: 4 g heart weight per kg body weight
- Hypertrophic heart: enlarged heart called "cardiomegaly", if > 500 g may be called "cor bovinum,"; left ventricular wall thickness> 1.4 cm, right chamber wall thickness> 0.4 cm
- Concentric hypertrophy: Uniform wall thickening, narrowed ventricular chamber space, apex may appear more pointed; usually due to pressure overload; heart is overall larger and more "chunky"
- Eccentric hypertrophy: Irregular wall thickening, with associated dilation of the chamber, apex may appear more rounded; usually due to volume overload; heart is overall larger and more "flabby"
- Cor pulmonale: Hypertrophy and dilation of the right heart only, due to increased pulmonary resistance from a primary lung disease. Sudden cardiac death due to an arrhythmia is possible!

Microscopy: Tissue/organ: Myocardium
- Cells are imperceptibly larger; but "boxcar nuclei"[1] can be recognized
- Possible decrease in overall myocyte count, with increased proportion of fibroblasts[2] which histologically may appear as small angular scars[3] between myocytes (interstitial fibrosis)

Definition: Hypertrophy: greek .: "hyper" - beyond, "trophos": nutrition
Increase in individual cell size causing overall enlargement of tissue in size/weight

Etiology/ Pathogenesis:
- Myocytes are unable to replicate as a response to increased work demand
- Each myocyte will build more sarcomeres (actin and myosin) and mitochondria due to the increased demand → increase in cell size (hypertrophy) → Myocyte growth signals stimulate local fibroblasts to replicate → fibrosis between myocytes (interstitial fibrosis)
- Physiologic hypertrophy (seen in endurance athletes): Thought to include small vessel proliferation, which supports the increased oxygen demands of the hypertrophied cells
- Pathologic hypertrophy (due to systemic hypertension, valve stenosis, etc.) does not involve increased vasculature, and the increased oxygen demands of the hypertrophied cells are not necessarily met

3 Cellular Adaptation: Hypertrophy, Hyperplasia, Atrophy

Entity: 3.1 Myocardial Hypertrophy
Stain: Hematoxylin - Eosin

Clinical Info: Associated conditions: Systemic hypertension, valvular diseases, COPD, other lung diseases

Types of Hypertrophy		
	Concentric Hypertrophy	**Eccentric Hypertrophy**
Stress:	Increased afterload (working against increased pressure)	Increased preload (working with too much blood volume)
Common Scenarios:	Systemic hypertension, stenotic aortic valve	Mitral valve regurgitation, aortic valve regurgitation
Myocyte Response:	More sarcomeres are added in series (cells get fatter)	More sarcomeres are added in parallel (cells get longer)
Gross Morphology:	Diffuse thickening of the myocardium and decrease in ventricular volume	Variable wall thickening with overall increase in ventricular volume

Consequences:
- Imbalance between oxygen supply and consumption, increased risk of heart failure, myocardial ischemia and/or infarct
- Both types of pathologic hypertrophy can eventually lead to heart failure

Symptoms:

Classification of Heart Failure according to NYHA (New York Heart Association)	
NYHA I	No symptoms with physical activity. Normal functional status.
NYHA II	Mild symptoms with physical activity. Comfortable at rest. Slight limitations of functional status.
NYHA III	Moderate symptoms with physical activity. Comfortable only at rest. Marked limitation of functional status.
NYHA IV	Severe symptoms with even minimal physical activity. Symptoms of heart failure at rest. Severe limitation of functional status.

Heart failure is a clinical diagnosis
Other clinical findings for heart failure:
- Lower extremity edema
- Crackles/rales on lung auscultation
- Shortness of breath, worsened with laying down (orthopnea)
- Jugular venous distension

Diagnostics: ECG, Brain-Natriuretic Peptide (BNP), Troponin (may be elevated in setting of increased demand during acute exacerbation of heart failure), CXR

Echocardiogram with evidence of diastolic dysfunction and/or systolic dysfunction
- Preserved ejection fraction; left ventricular ejection fraction (LVEF): >=50%
- Moderately reduced ejection fraction; LVEF 40-49%
- Reduced ejection fraction: LVEF <40%

Therapy:
- Fluid overload due to heart failure may be treated with diuresis (typically loop diuretics)
- Cardiac hypertrophy treated by optimizing risk factors (e.g. hypertension, hyperlipidemia, contributing lung disease, possible heart valve replacement)

Cellular Adaptation: Hypertrophy, Hyperplasia, Atrophy

Entity:	3.1 Myocardial Hypertrophy
Stain:	Hematoxylin - Eosin

Radiology:

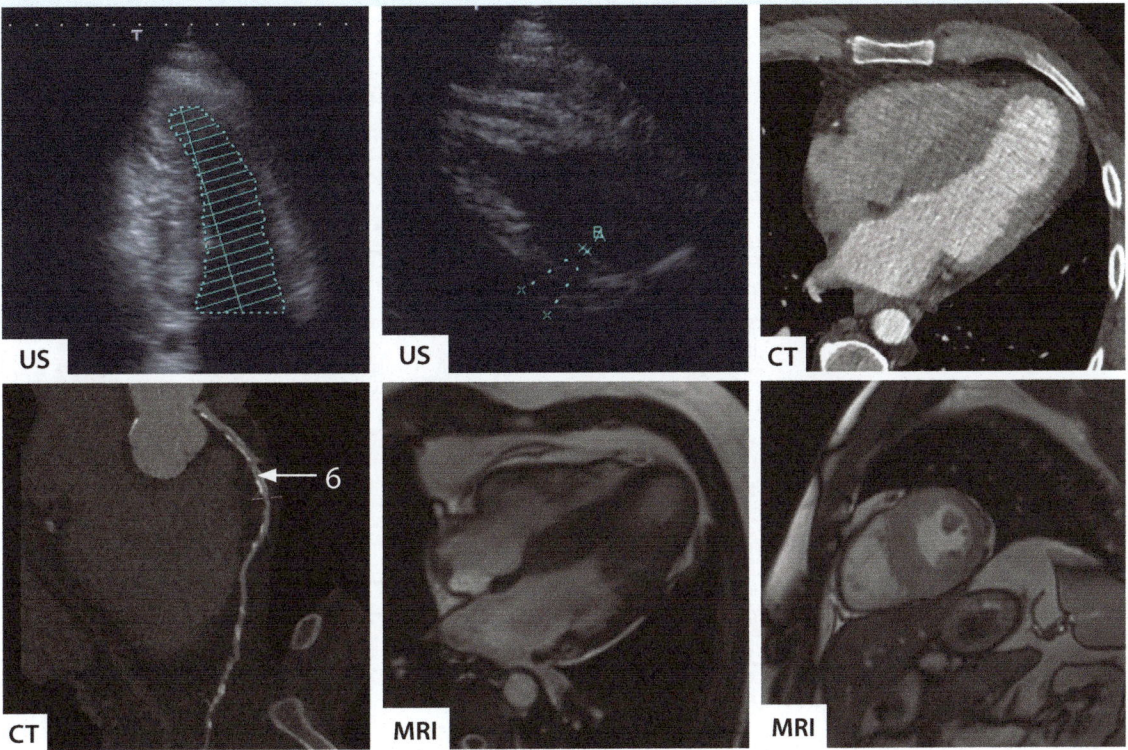

Measurements (always measured end-diastolic):
- Left ventricular (LV) posterior wall thickness and internal diameter: Measured in the parasternal long-axis or short-axis view at or immediately below the level of the mitral valve leaflet tips.
- Relative wall thickness: RWT = 2 × LV posterior wall thickness/LV internal diameter

Left ventricular mass (LVM):
- Myocardial end-diastolic volume: Calculated through geometric formulas (from 2D imaging) or directly measured (3D imaging).
- Conversion of the end-diastolic myocardial volume to mass by multiplying it with the myocardial density (approximately 1.05 g/mL)
- LVM index (LVMi): LVMi = LVM / BSA

LV geometry:
- LVMi and RWT are used to describe the ventricle as normal, concentric remodeled, and concentric or eccentric hypertrophied.

Wall Thickness for Septal and Posterior Wall				
	Normal	Mildly abnormal	Moderately abnormal	Severely abnormal
2DE (men)	6-10 mm	11-13 mm	14-16 mm	> 16 mm
2DE (women)	6-9 mm	10-12 mm	13-15 mm	> 15 mm

US: Used to evaluate left ventricular ejection fraction, wall movement, old muscle defects, valve function

CT: Mainly used for coronary vessel[1] evaluation. Rarely used to evaluate left ventricular ejection fraction, wall movement and muscle defects due to radiation and low contrast.

MRI: Used for complete evaluation of the heart, like ventricular ejection fraction, wall movement, muscle ischemia, old fibrotic muscle defects, diffuse tissue changes and valve function.

3 Cellular Adaptation: Hypertrophy, Hyperplasia, Atrophy

Entity: 3.2 Benign Prostatic Hyperplasia
Stain: Hematoxylin - Eosin

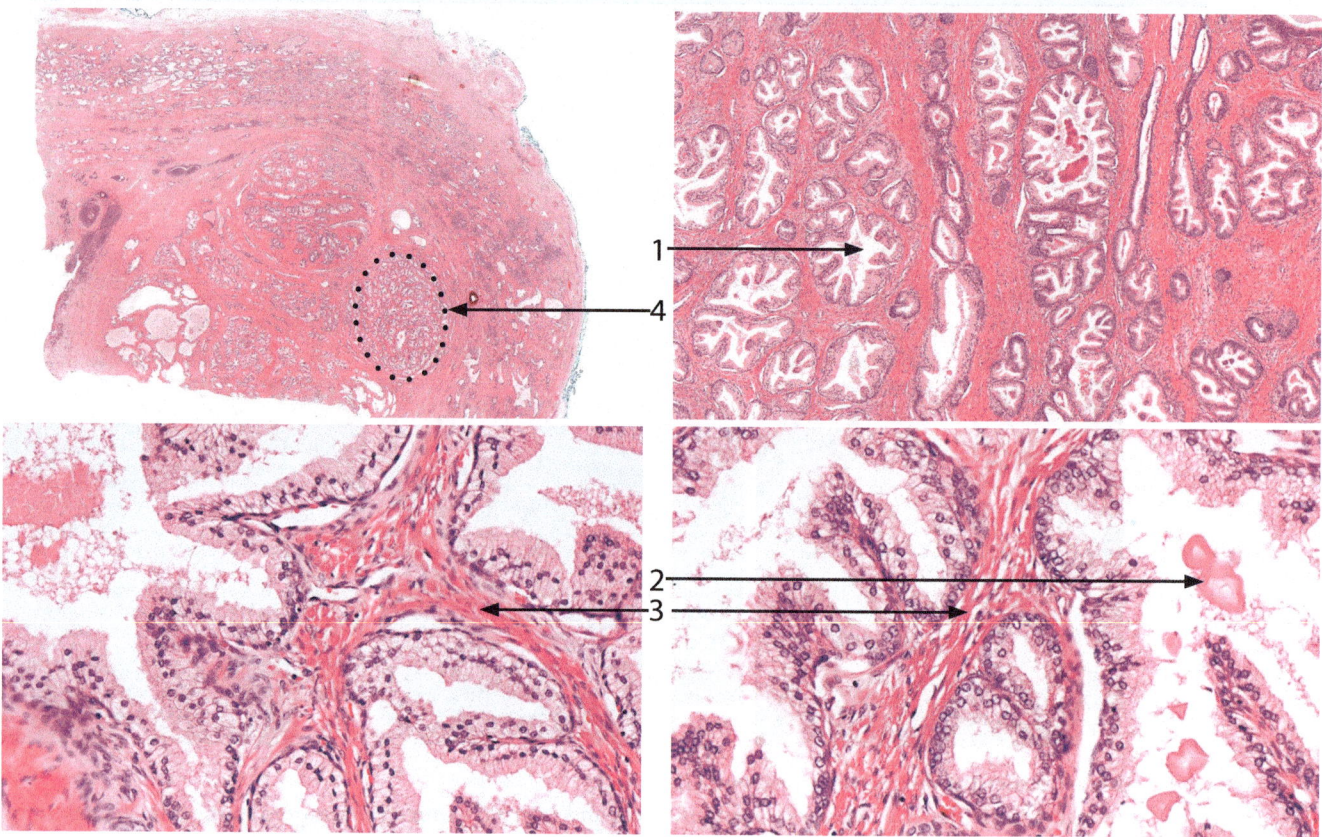

Macroscopy:	Enlarged, nodular prostate, firm consistency
Microscopy:	Tissue/organ: Prostate - Both glandular and stromal components are increased - Hyperplastic secretory glands show lumens with convoluted contours[1] - Congested prostatic secretions[2], possibly calcified - Proliferation of stromal and smooth muscle cells[3] with nodule formation[4] - Possibly ischemic necrosis, with responding inflammation
Definition:	Hyperplasia describes increased numbers (hyperplasia) of cells composing the organ, with overall increased size of the organ
Etiology/ Pathogenesis:	Endocrine-related hyperplasia of all tissue components of the prostate (especially in the transition zone/periurethral tissue) due to age-related hormonal dysregulation, increased response of the cells to androgens, and stimulation by growth factors Common disease, increased incidence with aging (40% of men > 50 years of age)
Clinical Info/ Symptoms:	Benign prostatic hyperplasia (BPH): benign prostatic enlargement (BPE) → compression of prostatic urethra and bladder outlet obstruction (BOO) → lower urinary tract symptoms (LUTS) → umbrella term of benign prostatic syndrome Micturition problems such as increased frequency, nocturia, difficulty initiating urination, weak urine stream, stream stopping and starting, urinary tract infections

Cellular Adaptation: Hypertrophy, Hyperplasia, Atrophy

Entity:	3.2 Benign Prostatic Hyperplasia
Stain:	Hematoxylin - Eosin

Diagnostics:

Important Terminologies	
BPH = benign prostatic hyperplasia	Histomorphologic tissue changes
BPE = Benign prostatic enlargement	Prostate volume > 30 mL
BOO = Bladder outlet obstruction	Urodynamic investigation for dysfunctional bladder emptying
BPO = Benign prostatic obstruction	BOO with underlying BPE
LUTS = Lower urinary tract symptoms	Urination issues

- Digital rectal examination (DRE) recommended to assess size and shape of prostate gland
- BPH is a clinical diagnosis, does not require tissue biopsy unless concerned for malignancy
- Tissue biopsy recommended if 1) asymmetric or nodular gland on DRE or 2) elevated serum prostate-specific antigen (PSA) level

Therapy:

Anti-obstructive drugs:
- Alpha blockers: Alfuzosin, doxazosin, tamsulosin, terazosin
- 5-α-reductase inhibitors: Finasteride Dutasteride
- Phosphodiesterase inhibitors (with concurrent erectile dysfunction): Tadalafil, sildenafil
- Caution: The combination of alpha blockers and phosphodiesterase inhibitors can cause symptomatic hypotension!

Transurethral resection of the prostate (TURP), rarely open surgery/prostatectomy

Radiology:

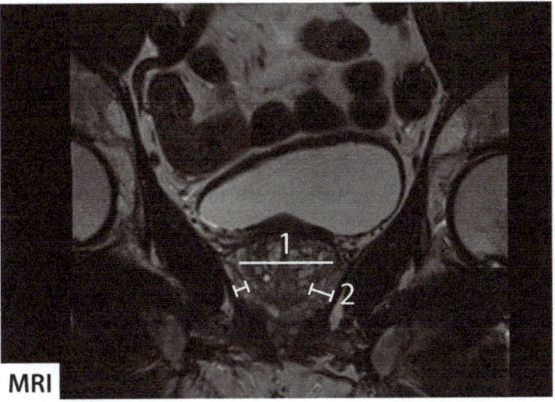
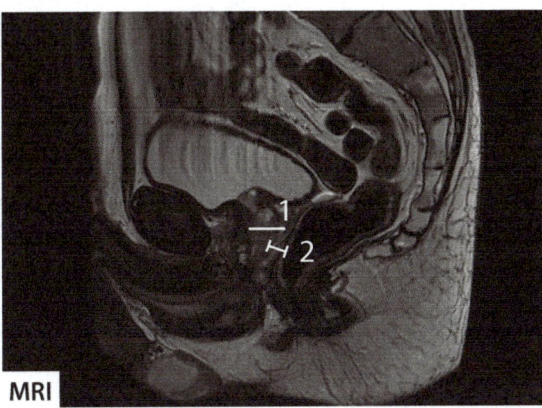

General:
- Prostatic volume > 30 mL (width x height x length x 0.52); often due to an enlarged transitional zone[1].

Ultrasound:
- Transitional zone enlarged, hypoechoic or of mixed echogenicity, may show calcifications. Post-micturition residual volume is measured and is typically elevated. May show hypertrophy of the bladder muscular wall, with trabeculations, due to chronically elevated filling pressures.

MRI:
- Enlarged T2 hyperintense transition zone[1] with heterogeneous signal and intact low signal pseudocapsule. Lesions suspicious for carcinoma are classified according to the PI-RADS classification (e.g. lesions with a high DWI5 and low ADC6 signal in the peripheral zone[2] have a high probability to be cancerous).

3 Cellular Adaptation: Hypertrophy, Hyperplasia, Atrophy

Entity: 3.3 Thyroid Goiter (Hyperplasia)
Stain: Hematoxylin - Eosin

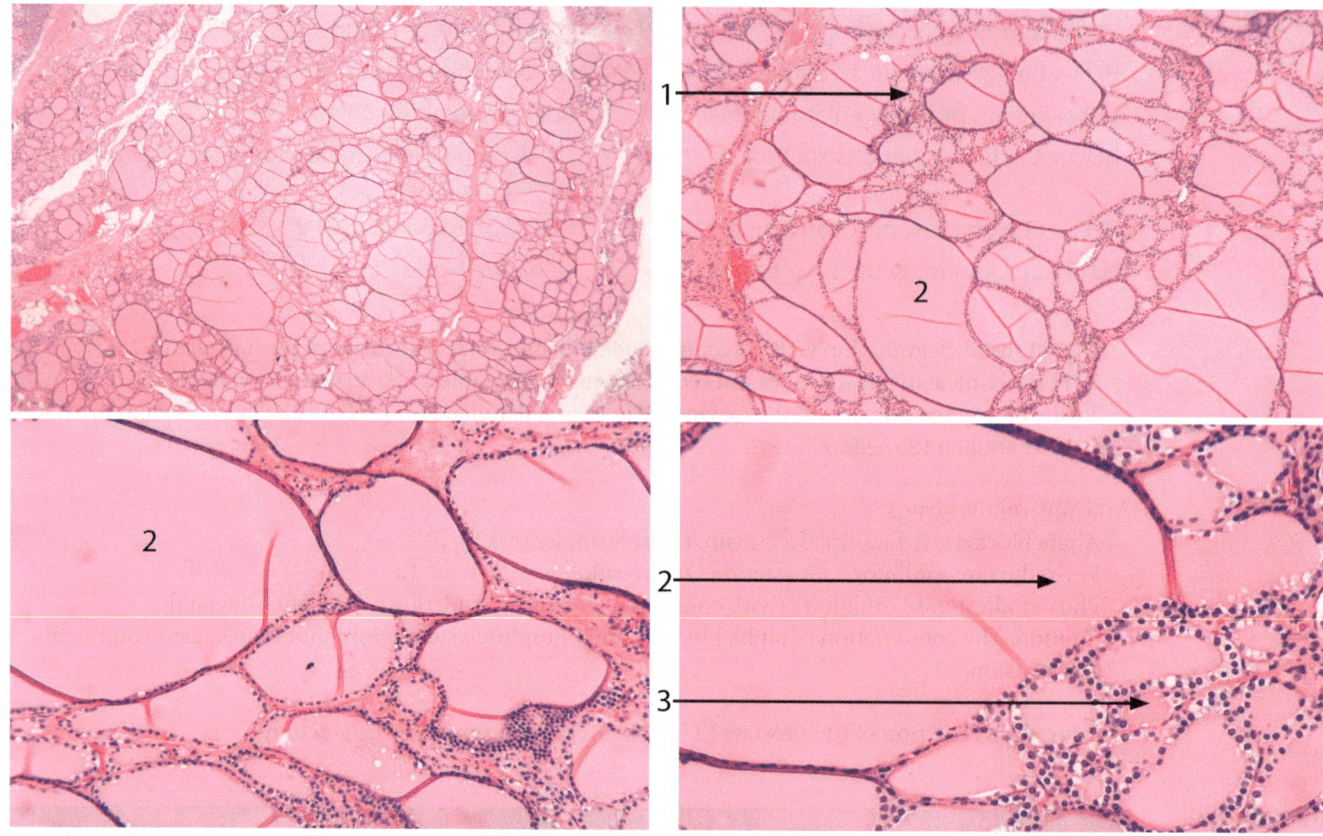

Macroscopy: Nodular (multinodular) enlargement of the thyroid gland

Microscopy: Tissue/organ: Thyroid gland
- Nodular thyroid tissue alternating with compressed atrophic areas[1]
- Nodules composed of increased numbers of cells and follicles:
- Large follicles with abundant colloid (macrofollicles[2])
- Atrophic areas with small compressed follicles with scant colloid (microfollicles[3])

Definition: Thyroid goiter is a clinical description of the enlarged thyroid gland; the increased number (hyperplasia) of cells/follicular structures results in enlarged organ size.

Etiology/ Pathogenesis: Diseases associated with hyperplastic changes: Iodine deficiency, more rarely Hashimoto's thyroiditis, Graves' disease
- Iodine deficiency/endemic goiter occurs in areas with poor iodine intake, and is the most common cause of multinodular goiter worldwide
- Decreased iodine → T3 and T4 deficiency → increased secretion of TSH → increase in the number of follicular epithelium and colloid, in an attempt to respond to the increased TSH
- Sporadic goiter is due to an uneven response to TSH among different areas within the thyroid; this is the most common cause of multinodular goiter in developed countries

Clinical Info/ Symptoms:
- Hypothyroidism: constipation, cold intolerance, weight gain, hyporeflexia, bradycardia, dry skin, hair loss, edema, fatigue
- Hyperthyroidism: diarrhea, heat intolerance, weight loss, hyperreflexia, tachycardia, palpitations, sweating, irritability/anxiety, hyperactivity, hair loss, fatigue
- Goiter: Enlarged thyroid gland on palpation

Cellular Adaptation: Hypertrophy, Hyperplasia, Atrophy

Entity: 3.3 Thyroid Goiter (Hyperplasia)
Stain: Hematoxylin - Eosin

Goiter Classification According to WHO	
Goiter grade 0	Not visibly or palpably enlarged, diagnosed via sonography
Goiter grade 1	Palpable enlargement
Goiter grade 2	Visibly enlarged, palpable without reclining/extending the head
Goiter grade 3	Complications (e.g. respiratory disorder, recurrent palsy, upper influx congestion)

Diagnostics: TSH, Free T4
Thyroid sonography, scintigraphy to determine hot and cold nodules, fine needle aspiration for cold nodules to rule out malignancy

Therapy: Hypothyroidism: Iodine and / or hormone (levothyroxine) supplementation
Hyperthyroidism: Drug suppression (thyrostatic drugs), radioiodine therapy, surgery

Radiology:

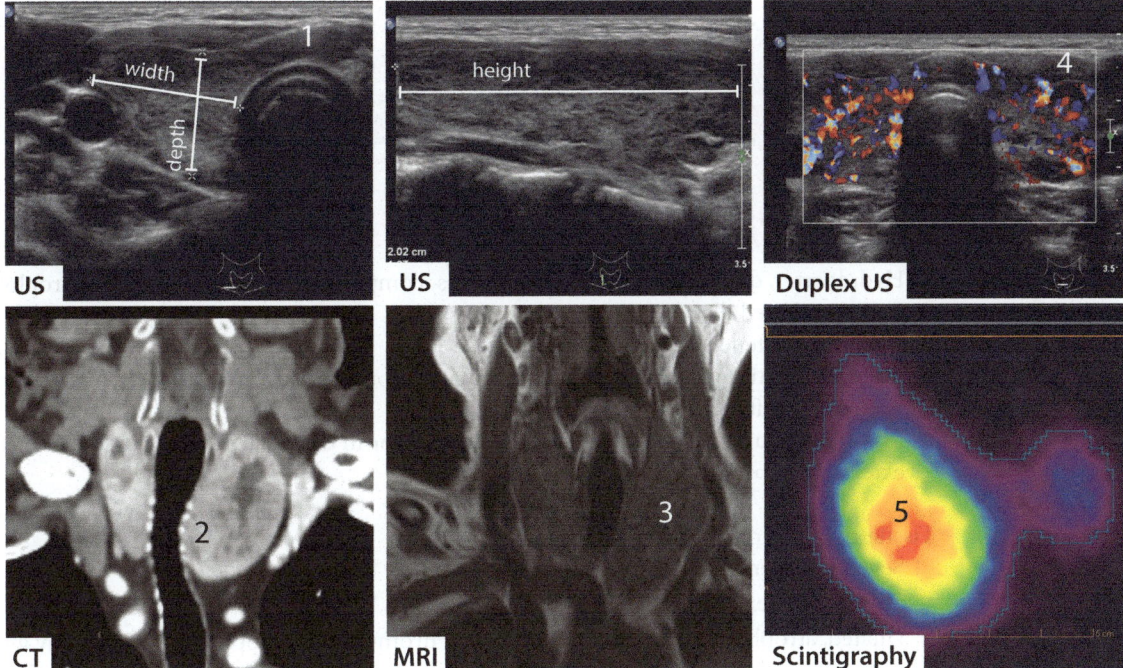

General: Increased thyroid volume (male > 18 ml, female > 15 ml) with thickened isthmus[1] > 0.5 cm. The volume of each lobe can be calculated with: height (cm) x width (cm) x depth (cm) x 0.529

Ultrasound: Increased volume with homogeneous parenchyma. Size may also be measured in the CT[2] or MRI[3], especially if retrosternal component. Graves' disease manifests with heterogeneous echogenicity and enlarged hyper-perfused vessels (thyroid inferno[4]). Thyroid nodules are classified by TIRADS classification. Fine needle aspiration can be performed if concern for malignancy.

Scintigraphy (using radioactive tracers Tc-99m pertechnetate or I-123): Can classify nodules according to their functional status (hot[5] or cold nodules).

3 Cellular Adaptation: Hypertrophy, Hyperplasia, Atrophy

Entity: 3.4 Hydronephrosis (Atrophy)
Stain: Hematoxylin - Eosin

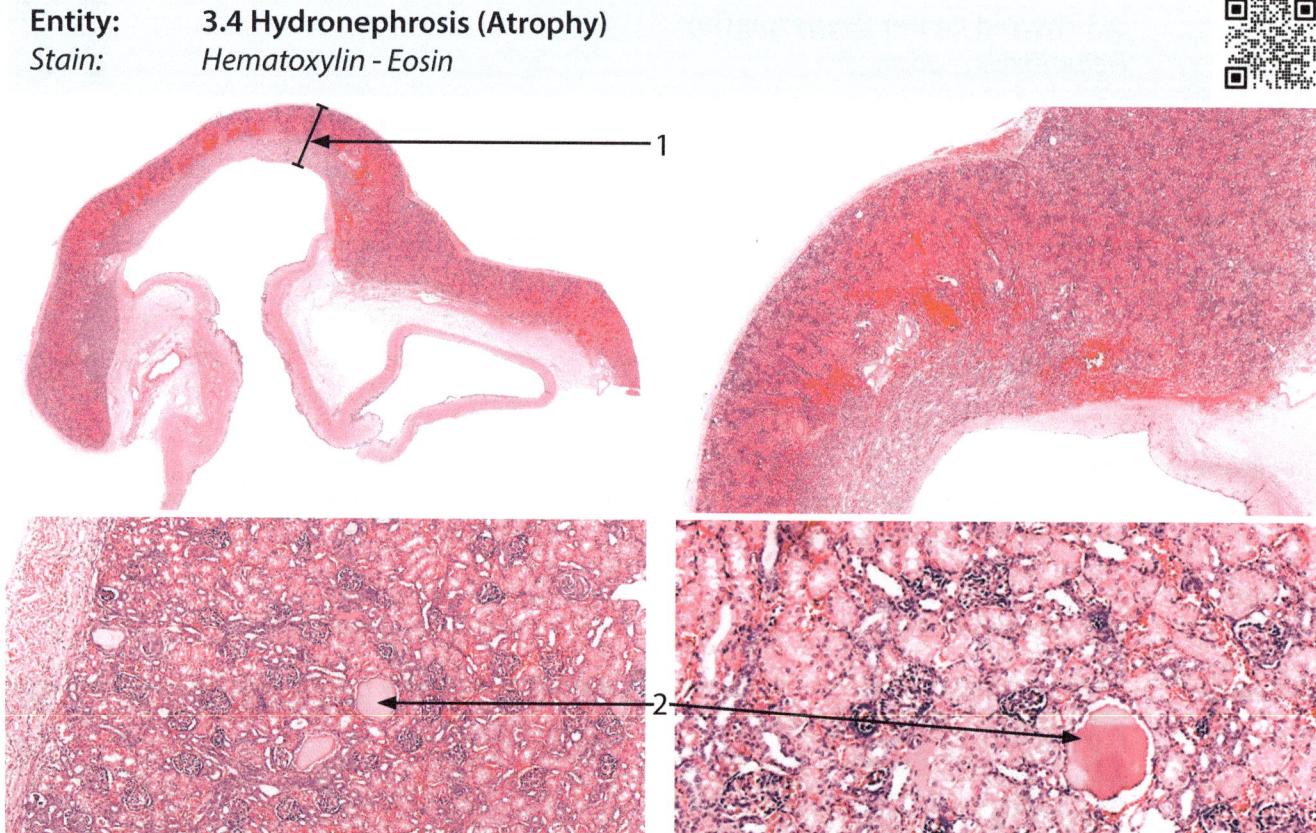

Macroscopy:
- Hydroureter, dilated renal pelvis and calyces, compressive renal parenchymal atrophy (thinned renal cortex and medulla)
- Pyramids flattened, concave in end stage
- End stage: entirely hydronephrotic, very narrow or absent kidney parenchyma (resembles a thin-walled sac), often also with hydroureter
- May be due to impacted stones, scarring, or tumor in the renal pelvis or ureter, sometimes also external compression (see below)

Microscopy:
Tissue/organ: Kidney, atrophic
- Severely flattened renal papillae
- Thinned cortex and medulla[1]
- Dilated, atrophic tubules[2] with intraluminal uromucoid (glycoprotein) casts[2], may give kidney the appearance of thyroid histologically, "thyroidization of the kidney"
- May include interstitial chronic inflammation

End stage:
- Closely spaced atrophic tubules, often with intraluminal glycoprotein casts, histologic appearance of "thyroidization"
- Interstitial chronic inflammation, eventual replacement of tubules by scar

Definition: **Hydronephrosis** is backup of urine with dilatation of the urinary excretory system due to obstruction, causing compressive atrophy of the kidney parenchyma.

Atrophy (Greek: a- not, trophos: nutrition), decrease in tissue size due to decrease in cell size or number.

Cellular Adaptation: Hypertrophy, Hyperplasia, Atrophy

Entity:	3.4 Hydronephrosis (Atrophy)
Stain:	Hematoxylin - Eosin

Etiology/Pathogenesis:
- Acute versus chronic urinary obstruction due to stones, infection, or external compression such as prostatic hyperplasia, tumor, blood clot, or scarring due to prior surgeries
- In children, vesico-ureteral reflux is the most common cause of hydronephrosis; malposition of the ureteral opening in the bladder wall and shortened submucosal course causes backwards flow of the urine and dilatation of the ureter
- In urinary tract disorder with a preserved glomerular filtration → urinary stasis → pressure atrophy → reduced blood flow → chronic parenchymal destruction with fibrous tissue proliferation and often accompanying inflammation
- Chronic renal failure as a possible complication

Clinical Info/Symptoms:
- Divided by location of the obstruction into upper (= supravesical) and lower (= subvesical) urinary tract disorders
- Depending on the cause, may manifest chronically, with few subtle symptoms, or acutely with flank pain
- In acute obstruction by nephrolithiasis, symptoms may include: flank pain, colicky/intermittent episodes of pain, hematuria

Diagnostics:
- Monitoring of kidney function with chemistries (BUN, creatinine)
- In acute obstruction, obtain urinalysis to assess for concomitant urinary tract infection
- Diagnosis and morphological classification usually done by sonography (preferred in children and pregnancy), X-rays, CT (preferred in adults), followed by a timely removal of the obstruction and monitoring of kidney function

If chronically obstructed, may lead to chronic kidney disease:

Stages of Chronic Renal Failure (According to National Kidney Foundation)	GFR (Glomerular Filtration Rate) in mL/minute
I. Kidney damage (as evidenced by albuminuria) with normal kidney function	≥ 90
II Kidney damage with mild loss of kidney function	60 - 89
IIIa. Mild to moderate loss of kidney function	45-59
IIIb. Moderate to severe loss of kidney function	30-44
IV. Severe loss of kidney function	15-29
V. Kidney failure	< 15

Therapy:
Acutely:
- Analgesia with acetaminophen, possibly opioids, avoid NSAIDs in setting of kidney damage
- Remove urinary tract obstruction to avoid further kidney damage
- For urolithiasis, may treat with chemolitholysis via ureterorenoscope (URS), extracorporeal shock wave lithotripsy (ESWL), or percutaneous nephrolithotomy; stones may be submitted for chemical analysis
- Inlay double J catheter or percutaneous nephrostomy (PCN)
- Antibiotic therapy if concern for concurrent urinary tract infection

Treatment of any underlying disease:
- Surgical therapy (risk of symptom recurrence due to postoperative strictures)
- Conservative therapy: Active monitoring, with transition to surgical therapy if kidney function deteriorates

3 Cellular Adaptation: Hypertrophy, Hyperplasia, Atrophy

Entity: 3.4 Hydronephrosis (Atrophy)
Stain: Hematoxylin - Eosin

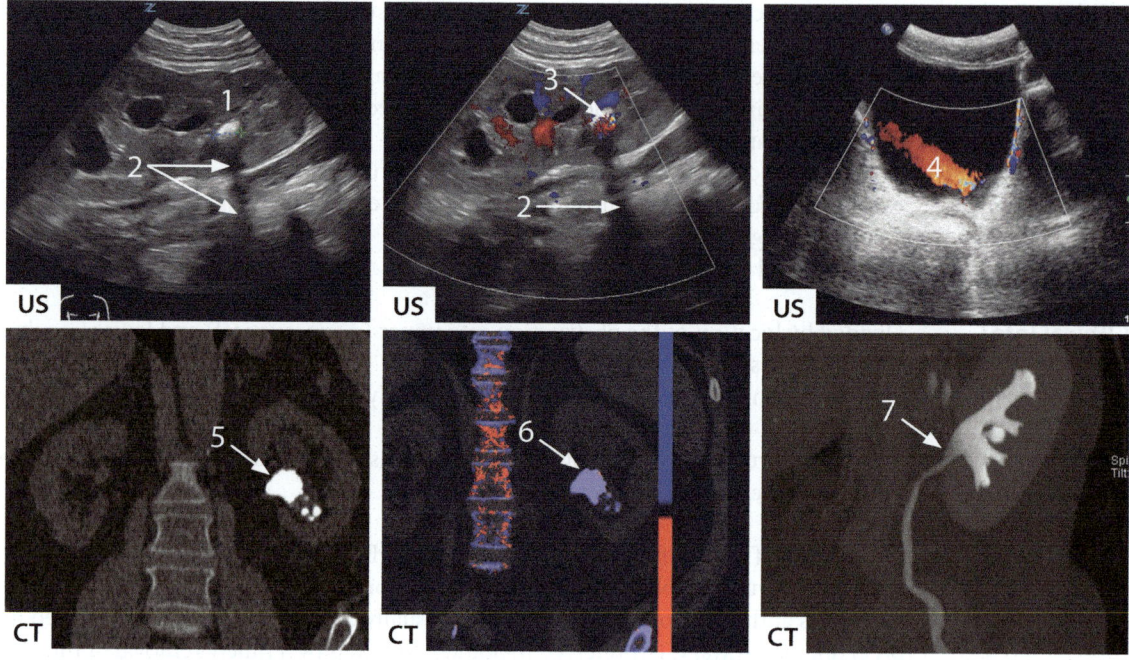

Radiology:

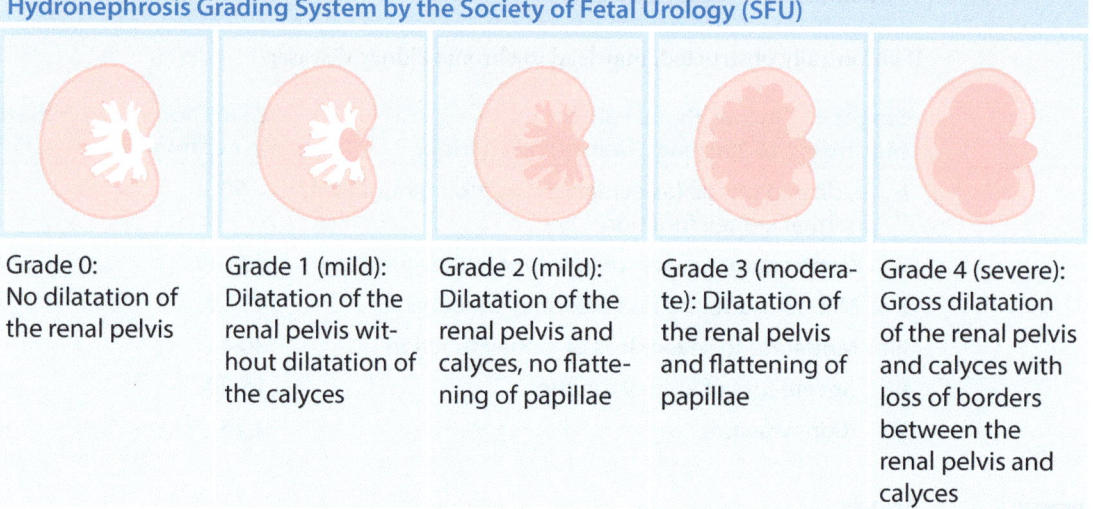

General: Dilatation of the renal pelvis due to obstruction; imaging is used to find the cause of obstruction and for monitoring resolution or progression

Ultrasound: Often used for evaluation of hydronephrosis and search for obstruction. Renal calculi are hyperechoic[1] with acoustic shadows[2] and twinkling artifact[3]. Duplex is used to search for urine jets[4] indicating a still working urine drainage.

CT: Unenhanced scans can show any hyperdense urinary tract calculi[5]; calculi can be further analyzed by dual energy CT[6]. Contrast-enhanced scans in the portal venous phase can help to determine other causes of hydronephrosis, such as retroperitoneal fibrosis or pelvic malignancies. Delayed phase contrast[7] is useful to evaluate ureteral strictures or carcinomas, bladder malignancies and non-calcified stones.

SPECT: Tc-99m MAG3 is used to evaluate the kidney function and evaluate for pre-renal, renal or post-renal problems; MRI used in pediatric population children to avoid radiation exposure

Cellular Adaptation: Hypertrophy, Hyperplasia, Atrophy

Entity:	3.5 Pulmonary Emphysema
Stain:	Hematoxylin - Eosin

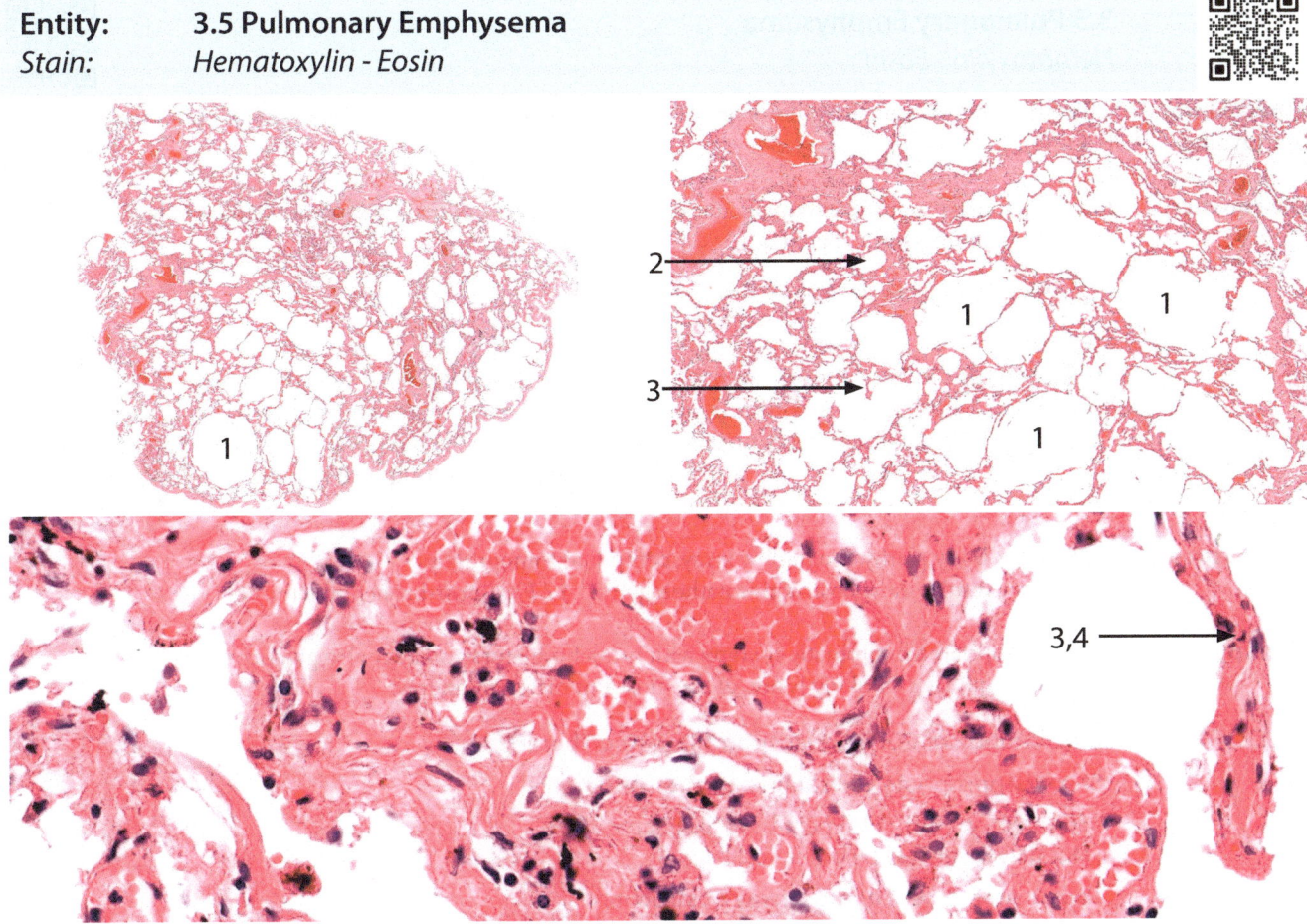

Macroscopy:	– Grossly over-inflated; sectioning shows large, grossly visible alveolar spaces
	– Marked alveolar space enlargement > 1cm in size = "bullae"
	– Softer parenchyma, reflects loss of alveolar septae; loss of septal capillaries gives the parenchyma a pale gray, "anemic" coloration

Microscopy:	Tissue/organ: Lungs
	– Increased volume of alveolar space[1], decreased surface area for gas exchange as compared to normal alveoli[2] (functionally atrophic)
	– Fragmented[3] and shortened "stubby"[4] alveolar septa/walls; no fibrosis seen
	– Additional finding, independent of the emphysema: macrophages containing black pigment ("dust cells") = anthracosis[5] due to air pollution/smoking

Definition:	Lung emphysema is a chronic lung disease and a type of COPD, characterized by loss of alveoli and decreased area for gas exchange; most common cause is insult from smoking

Etiology/ Pathogenesis:	– Smoking destroys alveolar septae, causing permanent enlargement of the alveolar spaces and gas entrapment; tissue destruction is mediated by inflammation, oxidative stress and proteinase/antiproteinase imbalance; the loss of alveolar septae causes reduction in surface area for gas exchange
	– Other exogenous causes: Recurrent infections/inflammatory processes of the respiratory tract (e.g. tuberculosis, silicosis, asbestosis)
	– Endogenous causes of emphysema: Alpha-1 antitrypsin deficiency, ciliary dyskinesia (Kartagener's syndrome)
	– Obstructive emphysema is due to functional stenosis of the bronchi (e.g., mucus overproduction due to chronic stimuli such as smoking) → air trapping → expansion of the alveoli, possible inflammation and scarring → emphysema

3 Cellular Adaptation: Hypertrophy, Hyperplasia, Atrophy

Entity:	3.5 Pulmonary Emphysema
Stain:	*Hematoxylin - Eosin*

Clinical Info/ Symptoms: Clinically and functionally, pulmonary emphysema is one of the chronic obstructive pulmonary diseases (COPD)

Diagnostics: Key symptoms: progressive dyspnea due to reduced alveolar diffusion area and inefficient breathing mechanics (flattening of the diaphragm)

Types of Patients with Chronic Emphysema	
Pink Puffer	**Blue Bloater**
Body habitus slim to lean - Emphysema with minor bronchitis, mild pulmonary hypertension, no cor pulmonale, limited signs of hypoxia	Body habitus overweight to obese - Emphysema with severe bronchitis, severe pulmonary hypertension, cor pulmonale with right heart failure, pronounced signs of hypoxia

Diagnostics: Spirometry, body plethysmography, x-ray, computed tomography
Spirometry results show obstructive pathology FEV1 / FVC post-bronchodilator <0.7

Therapy: Stage-appropriate symptomatic therapy with bronchodilators and later also glucocorticoids
For COPD, quitting smoking is one of the most important measures!

Classification of COPD Severity and Targeted Therapy

Step 1: Appropriate clinical history and spirometry
- Spirometry: FEV1 / FVC post-bronchodilator <0.7
- Not fully reversible by bronchodilator

Step 2: Assessment of the airway obstruction

Classification	FEV1 (% of target)
GOLD 1	≥ 80
GOLD 2	50 - 79
GOLD 3	30 - 49
GOLD 4	< 30

Step 3: ABCD classification according to symptom burden using the mMRC or CAT questionnaire

Previous exacerbations	Symptoms	
	mMRC 0-1 or CAT <10	mMRC ≥ 2 or CAT ≥ 10
0 or 1 without hospital admission	A	B
≥ 2 or ≥ 1 with hospitalization	C	D

Step 4: Therapy according to the group scheme

Group A:
- SAMA or SABA
- LAMA or LABA
- Medication rotation/change

Group B:
- LAMA or LABA
- 2-person combination LAMA + LABA

Group C:
- LAMA
- Combination of 2: LAMA + LABA
- Combination of 2: LABA + ICS

Group D:
- Combination of 2: LAMA + LABA
- 3-drug combination: LAMA + LABA + ICS
- Roflumilast in addition, if FEV1 <50% target

Cellular Adaptation: Hypertrophy, Hyperplasia, Atrophy

Entity:	3.5 Pulmonary Emphysema
Stain:	Hematoxylin - Eosin

SABA:	Inhaled short-acting beta agonists: salbutamol, fenoterol
SAMA:	Inhaled short-acting muscarinic antagonists: ipratropium bromide
LABA:	Inhaled long-acting beta agonists: salmeterol, formoterol, indacaterol
LAMA:	Inhaled long-acting muscarinic antagonists: tiotropium bromide
ICS:	Inhaled corticosteroids: budesonide, fluticasone, beclometasone
PDE-4 inhibitors:	Phosphodiesterase-4 inhibitors: roflumilast

Radiology:

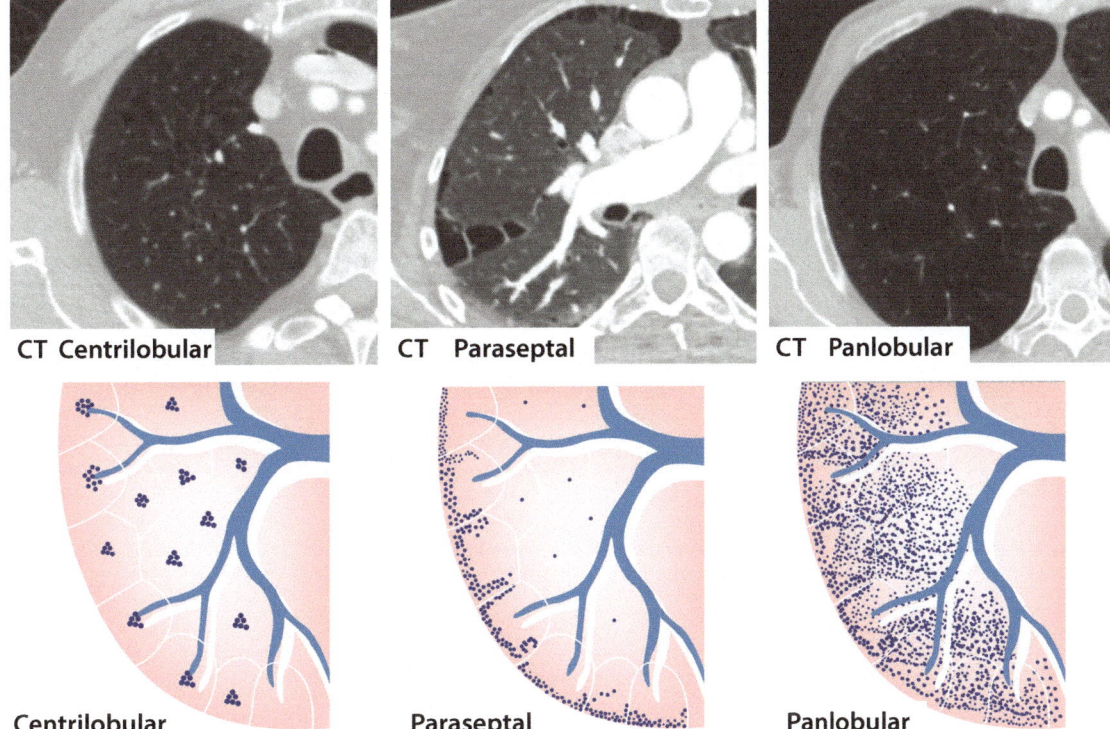

CT Centrilobular | CT Paraseptal | CT Panlobular

Centrilobular | Paraseptal | Panlobular

General: Divided in morphological subtypes according to the location:
- Centrilobular emphysema (most frequent) affects proximal respiratory bronchioles of the secondary pulmonary lobule, is pronounced in the upper zones. Strong dose-dependent association with smoking.
- Paraseptal emphysema affects peripheral parts of the secondary pulmonary lobule, usually adjacent to pleural surfaces; associated with spontaneous pneumothorax.
- Panlobular emphysema affects the entire secondary pulmonary lobule and is pronounced in the lower zones; seen in alpha-1-antitrypsin deficiency or I.V. Ritalin use.

X-Ray:
- Emphysema only indirectly observed and suggested by signs like flattened hemidiaphragms, increased lung radiolucency, widely spaced ribs.

CT:
- Best method to directly observe, evaluate, and quantify emphysematous change, and determine overall reduction in lung volume

Cell Death: Necrosis, Apoptosis

Mariana Canepa, Ann Ding, Carsten Fechner

4.1 Coagulation Necrosis (Kidney Infarction)

4.2 Liquefactive Necrosis (Encephalomalacia)

4.3 Caseous Necrosis (Tuberculosis)

4.4 Fat Necrosis (Acute Pancreatitis)

4.5 Gangrenous Necrosis (Wet Gangrene, Peripheral Arterial Disease)

4 Cell Death: Necrosis, Apoptosis

Necrosis is a term for tissue or cell death due to pathologic insult. The most common cause of tissue necrosis is lack of adequate oxygenation of the tissue, or ischemia. Ischemia is often focal, due to a localized vascular occlusion by a thrombus or embolus that obstructs the vascular lumen, although widespread ischemia may occur in the setting of extreme hypotension or shock, with failure of oxygenation across many tissues of the body. Cell death by necrosis is pathologic, and is distinct from cell death by apoptosis, which is a programmed, organized cell death.

Necrotic tissue can take several different gross/microscopic forms, depending on the tissue involved. The most commonly seen form of necrosis is coagulative necrosis, and is seen in many different organs; we will discuss kidney, although similar changes would be seen in infarcts of the heart, spleen, intestine, etc. Less common types of necrosis are liquefactive (seen in the central nervous system), caseous necrosis (tuberculosis), fat necrosis (adipose tissue), and wet and dry gangrene (often the distal extremities, such as the toes and feet). The bulk of this chapter will focus on the varied forms of necrosis seen in the body.

Apoptosis is another manner of cell death, often referred to as "programmed cell death," where the cell is triggered to dismantle itself in an organized fashion. This trigger to apoptose can arise within the cell (intrinsic/mitochondrial pathway) or can be conveyed from another cell such as a T-lymphocyte (extrinsic pathway). In contrast to necrosis, which is always pathologic, apoptosis can be physiologic or pathologic.

The intrinsic apoptotic pathway is moderated by the Bcl-2 family of proteins. Bcl-2 protein itself is the main anti-apoptotic member, and BAX is the main pro-apoptotic member; other proteins in the family act in an anti- or pro-apoptotic manner, or serve as "sensing" proteins that monitor the health of the cell. During usual cell function, there is more bcl-2 than BAX in the cell, and apoptosis will not occur. If BAX becomes increased in relation to bcl-2, however, BAX travels to the mitochondria and damages its membrane, spilling cytochrome c and activating the caspase cascade. Things that can lead to increased BAX include deprivation of growth signal (e.g. in breast tissue once lactation has finished (physiologic)), endoplasmic reticulum stress (e.g. numerous unfolded viral proteins overwhelming the ER (pathologic)), and errors of DNA replication that cannot be repaired (physiologic).

The extrinsic apoptotic pathway involves another cell, often a cytotoxic T-cell, that sends a message to the cell to apoptose; the classic example of this pathway involves FAS. FAS-receptor is found on many cell types, and FAS ligand (FAS-L) is expressed on the T-cells. If the T-cell recognizes, for example, viral proteins displayed on a cell, it will bind FAS-receptor on that cell. This triggers an assembly of "death domains" that activates the caspase cascade.

The caspase cascade is triggered via both intrinsic and extrinsic pathways. Caspases activate numerous enzymes that break down cell constituents in an organized fashion, and cell membranes are used to repackage the cell contents into small, dense apoptotic bodies that attract macrophages, but do not elicit a full immune response. Apoptotic cells are usually seen singly and scattered within a tissue.

	Necrosis	Apoptosis
	Always pathologic	**Physiologic or pathologic**
Common setting	Lack of blood flow/oxygenation	Withdrawal of growth hormone Viral proteins accumulating in ER Viral proteins displayed on plasma membranes Others
Cellular changes	Fading of nuclei, clumping of cytoplasmic contents, loss of cell borders, dissolution	Condensation of cell contents, fragmentation into discrete dense bodies (apoptotic bodies)
Pathways	None; results from cell irreversible injury due to variety of insults; common terminal events are cell membrane failure and flooding by calcium	Two pathways: Intrinsic/mitochondrial (BAX>bcl2) Extrinsic (FAS receptor/FAS-Ligand
Enzymes involved	None specific; all enzymes within cell are spilled	Both pathways converge on caspase cascade, which acts to dismantle cell into apoptotic bodies
Immune cell response	Neutrophils and macrophages	Macrophages only

Cell Death: Necrosis, Apoptosis

Entity:	4.1 Coagulation Necrosis (Kidney Infarction)
Stain:	Hematoxylin - Eosin

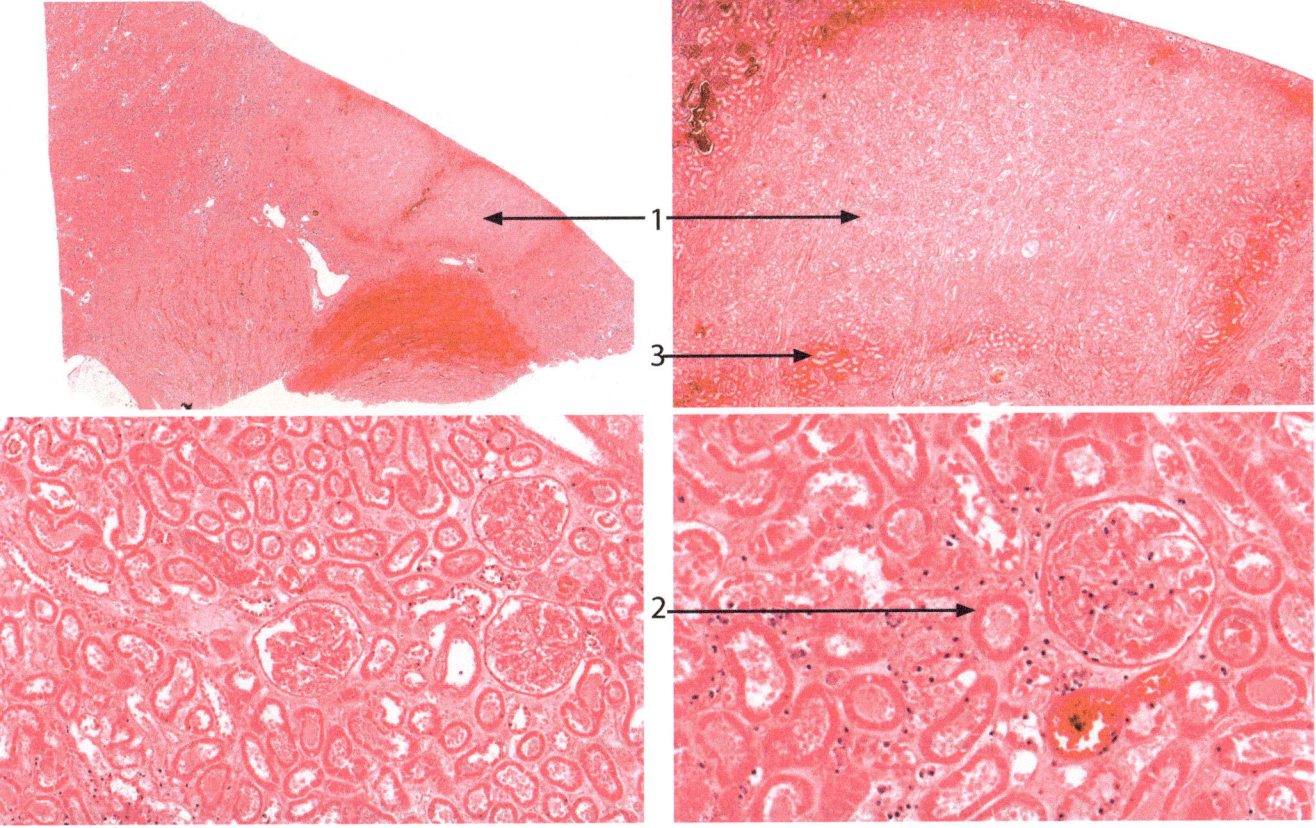

Macroscopy:
- Wedge-shaped area of pale discoloration, representing coagulative necrosis, extending from the capsular surface into the medulla; later it will appear brown/yellow due to migration of leukocytes and macrophages
- Infarct of entire kidney (via occlusion of the renal artery) is very rare

Microscopy: Tissue/organ: Kidney parenchyma (glomeruli and tubule profiles recognizable, cortical and medullary zones may still be defined)
- Renal parenchyma:
- Wedge-shaped infarction area[1], homogeneous and eosinophilic at low power
- Higher-power shows outlines of residual microarchitecture (glomeruli, tubules)
- Highest power shows drop-out of cell nuclei in necrotic cells, cell outlines may still be visible →
  Ghost cells[2] ("ghost cells"), clumpy eosinophilic cytoplasm
- Borders of the infarction area appear hemorrhagic[3], with granulocyte response and signs of resorption (macrophages)
- Represents ischemic infarct, due to embolic or thrombotic blockage of vessel (e.g. local vessel with plaque and superimposed thrombus, thromboembolism originating from left heart, rarely a septic thrombus from valve vegetations in endocarditis)

Definition: Kidney infarction is death of the renal parenchyma due to loss of blood supply. The histomorphologic change is coagulation necrosis, where the cells are necrotic, but the microarchitecture of the tissue is preserved. This will eventually be replaced by fibrous scar (in contrast to liquefactive necrosis).

Etiology/Pathogenesis:

Coagulation necrosis caused by:
- Lack of oxygen delivery to tissue (ischemia), can be caused by multiple clinical conditions including thromboembolism or hypotension
- Thromboembolism is often due to atrial fibrillation; less often due to mitral valve defects, aneurysms, endocarditis, venous thrombosis in cases of right ventricular failure or tumor compression

4 Cell Death: Necrosis, Apoptosis

Entity: 4.1 Coagulation Necrosis (Kidney Infarction)
Stain: *Hematoxylin - Eosin*

Coagulation necrosis: solidified necrotic area (in contrast to liquefactive necrosis)
- Early phase: macroscopically pale (gray-white) due to loss of blood flow, microscopically eosinophilic (H&E stain) as exposed intracellular proteins bind eosin
- Later phase: macroscopically yellow-brown, due to numerous white blood cells and macrophages, and proteolysis (yellow infarct)

Clinical Info/ Symptoms:

Symptoms of atrial fibrillation: often few symptoms, may have palpitations, dizziness

Systemic embolization in atrial fibrillation:
- Most affected organ is the brain (stroke) (see 3.2 liquefactive necrosis section), but also can affect kidneys (kidney infarct), spleen (splenic infarct), intestines (mesenteric ischemia with intestinal infarct)

Diagnostics:

For kidney infarction:
- Duplex sonography of renal vessels

Analysis of arrhythmia to assess for atrial fibrillation:
- Resting ECG, long-term ECG, event recorder

Therapy:

For renal artery stenosis:
- Consider percutaneous transluminal angioplasty (PTLA)

For atrial fibrillation:
- Anticoagulation, cardioversion, and antiarrhythmic therapy

Risk-benefit tools to decide on anticoagulation in the setting of atrial fibrillation, risk of thromboembolism vs risk of bleed:

Risk Stratification of the Risk of Thromboembolism in Atrial Fibrillation Using the CHA2DS2VASc Scores from the Guidelines of the European Society of Cardiology (2016)	
CHA2DS2-VASc Risk Factor	**Points**
Chronic heart failure: Characteristics / symptoms of heart failure or objective evidence for a reduced left ventricular ejection fraction	+1
Hypertension: Blood pressure at rest> 130/80 mmHg on at least two measurement events or during antihypertensive therapy	+1
Age 75 years or older	+2
Age 65-74 years	+1
Diabetes mellitus: Fasting glucose value> 125 mg/dl, HbA1C >/=6.5%, or treatment with oral antidiabetic and / or insulin	+1
Stroke / transient ischemic attack or thromboembolism event	+2
Vas**c**ular disease: previous myocardial infarction (MI), peripheral arterial occlusive disease (PAD), aortic plaque	+1
Sex **c**ategory (female)	+1
Indication of thromboembolism prophylaxis/anticoagulation: 0 points: "Low" risk, no need for anticoagulation 1 point: "Low-moderate" risk, could consider antiplatelet or anticoagulation but not necessary ≥ 2 points: "Moderate-high" risk, recommended to start anticoagulation	

Cell Death: Necrosis, Apoptosis

Entity: 4.1 Coagulation Necrosis (Kidney Infarction)
Stain: Hematoxylin - Eosin

Risk Stratification of the Risk of Bleeding in Patients with Atrial Fibrillation Using the HAS-BLED Score	
HAS-BLED Risk factor	**Points**
H: Hypertension	+1
A: Abnormal kidney or liver function (1 point each)	Max +2
S: Stroke	+1
B: History of bleeding	+1
L: Unstable INR	+1
E: Elderly (age> 65 years)	+1
D: Drugs or alcohol (1 point each)	Max +2
3 or more points = high risk of bleeding, alternatives to anticoagulation should be considered	

Radiology:

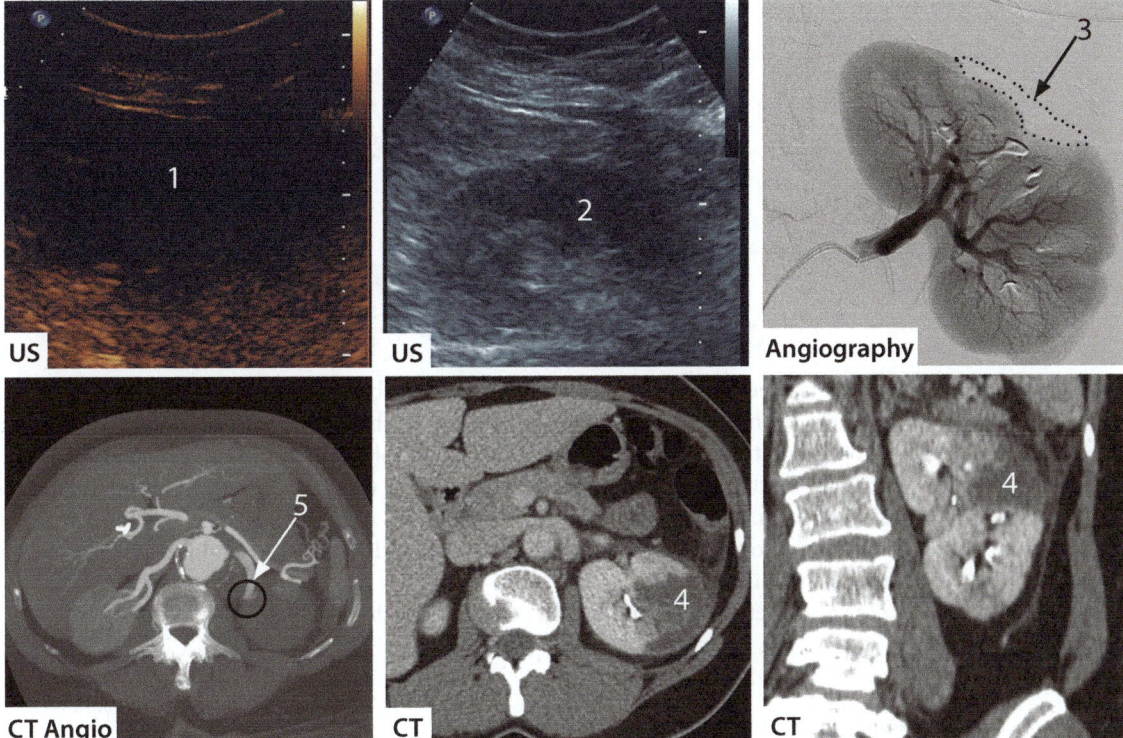

General: Interruption of blood flow to part of (rarely entire) kidney; initially results in a wedge shaped infarct/necrosis, later forms a retracted scar.

Ultrasound: Lack of regional flow in duplex or contrast-enriched ultrasound[1]. In early images, there is no change in echogenecity. Resulting edema[2] can be hyperechogenic, with cortical volume loss.

Angiography: Lack of contrast in the occluded vessel or infarcted area[3]. In early occlusion a thrombectomy may be performed to save tissue at risk.

CT: On post-contrast images, infarctions are seen as hypodense wedge-shaped areas[4] lacking enhancement. If the renal artery[5] is occluded, the entire kidney fails to enhance. After 8 hours post-infarction, a thin rim of cortex continues to enhance, due to collateral capsular perfusion (cortical rim sign).

MRI: Diffusion restriction, with high signal in DWI and low on ADC. High T2 (FS) signal due to edema within the infarct.

4 Cell Death: Necrosis, Apoptosis

Entity: 4.2 Liquefactive Necrosis (Encephalomalacia)
Stain: Hematoxylin - Eosin

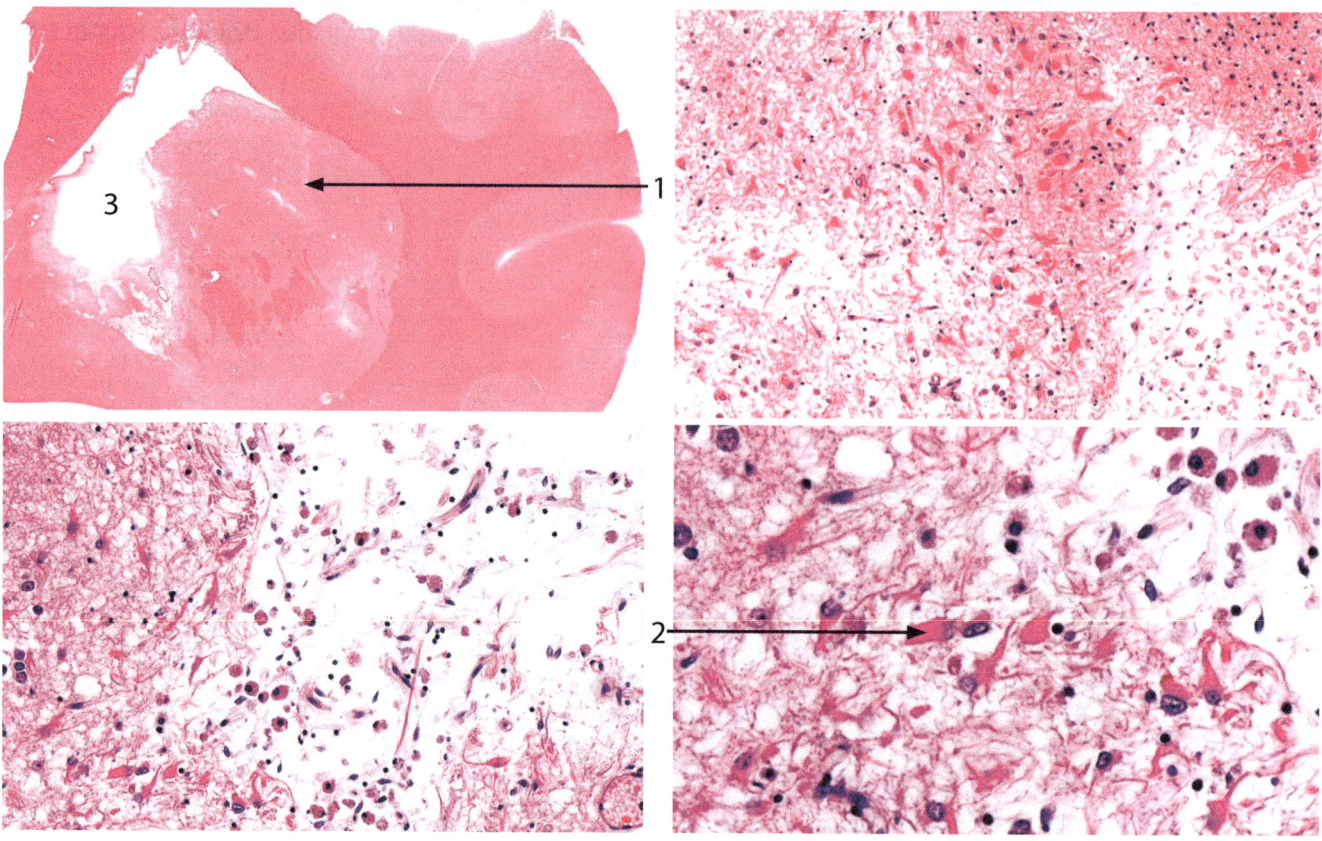

Macroscopy: Severe cerebral edema with associated flattened cerebral sulci:
- 1st stage (fresh necrosis): Visible after approx. 12 h - 3 days, infarct may show raised cut surface, blurred border between gray and white matter, possibly hemorrhagic
- 2nd stage (softening / liquefaction): Approx. 2 - 3 days to several weeks, infarct area increasingly whitish-yellowish, softer, liquefies
- 3rd stage (resorption and organization): Approx. 1 week to several weeks, over years will form a permanent cyst-like defect
- Transitions between the individual stages are gradual, not entirely distinct

Microscopy:
- Tissue/organ: Brain cortex

Stages of Liquefactive Necrosis	
Stage	**Histologic Changes**
1st stage (fresh necrosis):	- Days 0-3, depending on the size of the tissue - Swelling and softening of affected tissue, edema - Arrival of inflammatory cells (macrophages and neutrophils) via a damaged blood-brain barrier
2nd stage (softening, liquefaction):	- Day 2-3 - Loss of tissue architecture, replacement by amorphous material[1] - Dead neurons appear eosinophilic/pink ("red neurons"[2]) with lack of nuclei - Macrophages phagocytize liquefied tissue, acquiring clear cytoplasmic vacuoles containing myelin - Dissolved tissue eventually entirely removed by macrophages, leaving a cyst-like space[3] with permanent loss of parenchyma (neurons cannot regenerate)

Cell Death: Necrosis, Apoptosis

Entity:	4.2 Liquefactive Necrosis (Encephalomalacia)
Stain:	Hematoxylin - Eosin

Stages of Liquefactive Necrosis	
Stage	Histologic Changes
3rd stage (organization, pseudocyst formation):	After 4-8 weeks Proliferation of vessels and glial tissue (reactive gliosis) at the margins of the infarct, in attempt to heal the defec
Permanent cystic defects may remain Individual stages of liquefactive necrosis are not discrete but gradual	

Definition: **Liquefactive necrosis:** liquefaction of the necrotic tissue = grossly seen as malacia
- Predominantly occurs in lipid-rich tissues (CNS) or with bacterial colonization, presumably a consequence of autolytic or heterolytic enzyme activity
- Autolysis: digestion by the body's own enzymes
- Heterolysis: degradation by bacterial enzymes

Etiology/Pathogenesis: Liquefactive necrosis is due to: Hypoxia/ischemia (most common), trauma, infection
- Ischemia of the brain can be a consequence of:
- Thromboembolic occlusion of arteries (atherosclerosis, arrhythmias, etc)
- Fibromuscular dysplasia of the vessels
- Global cerebral ischemia (due to, for example, cardiac or respiratory arrest, shock, status epilepticus, drowning, or anesthesia side effect)

In brain and other tissues, liquefactive necrosis can be due to bacterial or fungal infections; in these cases, tissue degradation is due to heterolysis (bacterial enzymes) and autolysis (the body's own enzymes, spilled from necrotic cells or discharged by inflammatory cells)

Clinical Info/Symptoms: Stroke
- Regional lack of cerebral perfusion due to thromboembolic events or bleeding

Symptoms: depending on the damaged brain area (Remember "FAST")
- **F:** Facial expression: asymmetric facial expression, such as one corner of the mouth drooping
- **A:** Arm weakness: inability to hold one arm up, when attempting to hold up both arms
- **S:** Speech difficulties: slurred speech, impaired speech understanding (Wernicke), or impaired speech production (Broca)
- **T:** Time is Brain: if one of the above criteria applies, arrange for immediate transport to emergency department

Diagnostics:
- Acute diagnostics: Quick clinical examination for gross deficits, CT brain, CT angiography to assess for large vessel occlusion; MRI brain often done later
- Later diagnostics: Find and address cause, to avoid recurrences and optimize risk factors; lipid panel, A1C, ECG, echocardiogram with bubble study (to assess for patent foramen ovale), Doppler / duplex sonography of the cerebral vessels, CT brain, MRI, digital subtraction angiography

NIHSS for Standardized Initial and Course Assessment of Neurological Deficits in a Stroke	
National Institute of Health Stroke Scale (NIHSS): Severity Classification of the Apoplexy	
1. Level of consciousness	2. Horizontal eye movements (gaze)
3. Visual fields	4. Facial palsy
5. Arm motor skills	6. Leg motor skills
7. Limb ataxia	8. Sensory
9. Language	10. Dysarthria
11. Extinction and inattention	

4 Cell Death: Necrosis, Apoptosis

Entity: 4.2 Liquefactive Necrosis (Encephalomalacia)
Stain: Hematoxylin - Eosin

Therapy: Acute therapy
- Within 4.5 hrs from symptom onset: Thrombolysis with alteplase (recombinant tissue-specific plasminogen activator), after 4.5 hrs high risk of cerebral bleeding due to tissue necrosis
- Within 6h of symptom onset: Thrombectomy (in select patients may be extended to 24h from onset)

Exclusion criteria for thrombolysis with alteplase:
- Ischemic stroke or severe head trauma in the past three months
- Any prior intracranial hemorrhage
- Intracranial neoplasm, or GI malignancy
- GI bleed in the past three weeks
- Intracranial or intraspinal surgery in the past three months
- Symptoms suggestive of subarachnoid hemorrhage, infective endocarditis, or aortic arch dissection
- Acute bleeding diathesis
- Persistent systolic BP ≥ 185 mmHg or diastolic BP ≥ 110 mmHg
- Active internal bleeding
- Platelet <100K
- Anticoagulant use with INR>1.7, PT>15, or aPTT>40
- Therapeutic dose of low molecular weight heparin in prior 24 hours
- Use of direct thrombin inhibitor or direct Xa inhibitor in prior 48 hours

Radiology:

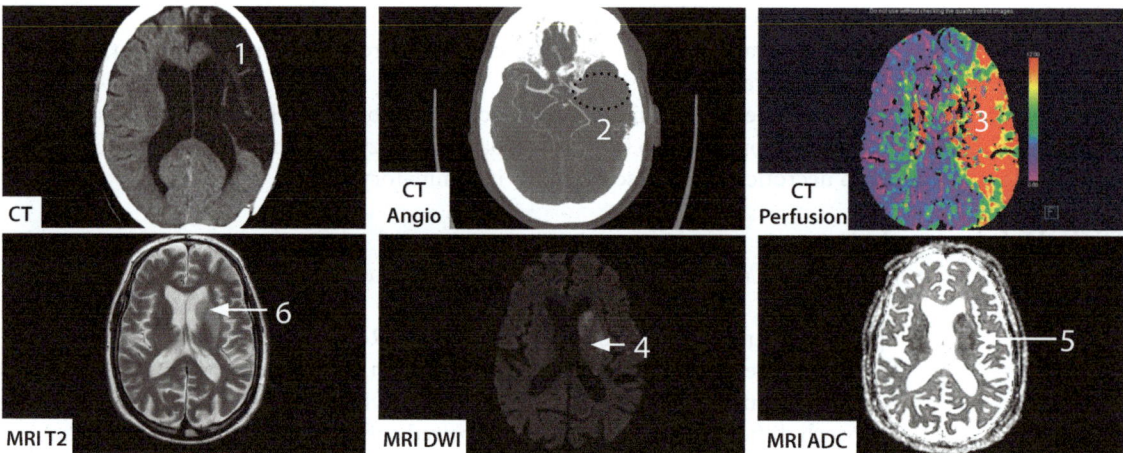

General: Cortical infarctions often result from occlusion of arterial blood vessels, veins, or direct trauma. Oxygen-deprived cells swell and die, resulting in liquefactive necrosis.

CT native: Use to exclude intracranial hemorrhage (hyperdense) which permits thrombolytic therapy, or to visualize hypodense, irreversibly injured necrotic tissue[1]. A hyperdense thrombus inside the occluded vessel (hyperdense artery sign) can sometimes be seen immediately. Hypoattenuation of deep nuclei can be seen as early as one hour after occlusion. Hypodense parenchymal swelling and loss of gray-white differentiation can be observed after several hours.

CT angiography: May see complete vessel occlusion[2], hypoattenuating intravascular thrombus, or arterial stenosis.

CT perfusion: Repetitive post-contrast cranial scan directly after contrast injection (e.g every second for a duration of 40 seconds) allows calculation of blood flow (CBF), cerebral blood volume (CBV) and the time for blood to reach the tissue (Tmax[3]). Can delineate irreversibly injured tissue from reversibly injury.

Angiography: May identify occluded vessel and open it with thrombectomy and intra-arterial lysis
MRI: Infarction typically shows high DWI[4] and low ADC[5] signal; later the ADC normalizes and the T2 signal increases[6].

Cell Death: Necrosis, Apoptosis

Entity:	4.3 Caseous Necrosis (Tuberculosis)
Stain:	Hematoxylin - Eosin

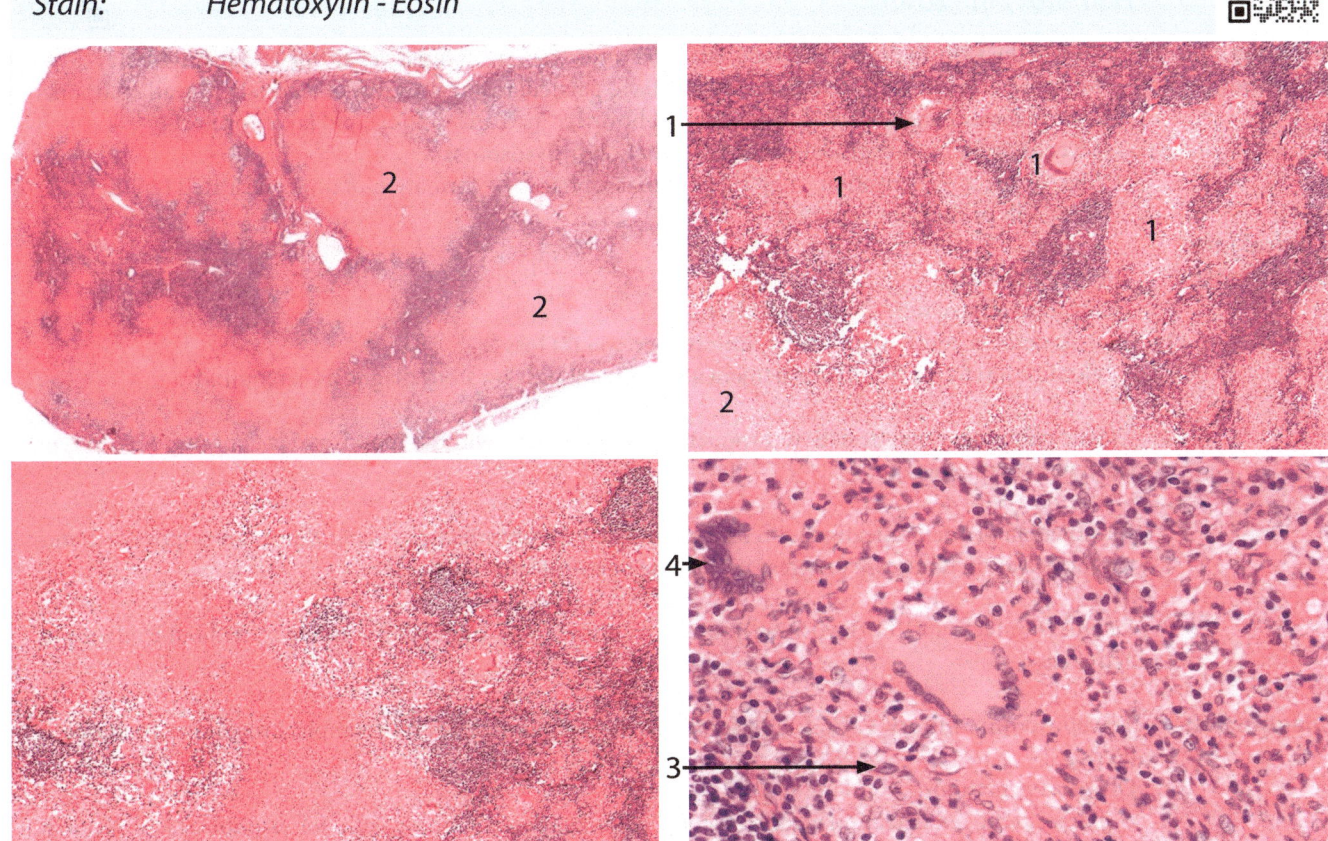

Macroscopy: Geographic, whitish, cheesy (cream cheese-like) or crumbly (feta cheese-like) areas on the cut surface of involved lung parenchyma or lymph node
- In nodes, capsules may be distended by coalescence of granulomas
- Complications include involvement of neighboring structures, fistula formation to skin surface or to bronchus

Microscopy: Tissue/organ: Lymph nodes
- **Granulomas[1]:** Palisade-like aggregates of activated macrophages with occasional multinucleated giant cells, with rim of lymphocytes
- **Caseating/necrotizing[2] granulomas:** Granulomas with central eosinophilic/pink acellular necrotic debris (lysed cells); seen in tuberculosis and certain fungal infections
- **Activated macrophages[3]** have elongated nuclei (like the sole of a shoe) and may resemble epithelial cells ("epithelioid") due to abundant granular pink cytoplasm
- **Multinucleated giant cells[4]** are multiple macrophages fused together; nuclei may be arranged like a horseshoe along the periphery of the giant cell, called a Langhans-type giant cell (as seen in tuberculosis). In contrast, a foreign body-type giant cell has the multiple nuclei are arranged randomly
- **Mycobacteria** are not visible with routine H&E stain; and requires special stains such as Auramine-Rhodamine or Ziehl-Neelsen

Definition: **Caseous necrosis:** Type of necrosis in which tissue is grossly white and crumbly, microscopically the cell outlines are lost, typically seen with caseating granulomas in tuberculosis infection

4 Cell Death: Necrosis, Apoptosis

Entity:	**4.3 Caseous Necrosis (Tuberculosis)**
Stain:	*Hematoxylin - Eosin*

Etiology/Pathogenesis:
- 30% of the world's population have latent TB infection, most often via airborne transmission
- Mycobacteria induce T-cell mediated reaction, particularly against mycobacterial cell wall components
- Macrophages phagocytize M. tuberculosis, however its Cord factor (Lipid layer) protects Mycobacteria from degradation and destruction by lysosomes
- Macrophages → activation → epithelioid macrophages → formation of multinucleated (epithelioid) giant cells of the Langhans type

Clinical Info/Symptoms:

Tuberculosis (TB):
- Mycobacterium tuberculosis infection
- B-symptoms: fever, night sweats, unintended weight loss
- Notification to the health department after clinical or laboratory diagnosis is required

Classic pulmonary manifestation: Productive cough with or without blood, and lack of response to typical symptomatic therapy

Reactivation of latent infection with extrapulmonary involvement can occur if immunosuppressed; mutual acceleration of disease progress in the case of co-infection with HIV

Latent TB Infection (LTBI): Positive immune response to M. tuberculosis antigens, without evidence of active disease

Diagnostics:
Travel/exposure history, CXR, γ-interferon test, tuberculin test, sputum sample, bronchoscopy, tissue biopsy
Diagnostic methods:
- Direct pathogen detection via microscopy, requires special staining with, for example, Ziehl-Neelsen stain on tissue section
- Cultivation on Löwenstein-Jensen agar
- Mycobacteria DNA detection using polymerase chain reaction (PCR)

Therapy:
Active TB:
- Rifampin, Isoniazid, Pyrazinamide, Ethambutol (RIPE) x 6 months total*
- Alternate therapy: Isoniazid, Rifapentine, Moxifloxacin, Pyrazinamide x 4 months

Latent TB:
- Rifampin monotherapy x 4 months
- Isoniazid and rifampin x 3 months
- Isoniazid monotherapy x 6-9 months

Drug-resistant TB strains require protracted combination therapies

First-line Therapy for Active TB
*RIPE - 2 months of intensive phase with RIPE, 4 months of continuous phase with Rifampin and Isoniazid

Active Ingredients	Side Effects	Duration of Therapy
Isoniazid	Hepatotoxicity, neurotoxicity (Vit B6 supplementation may improve this), optic neuritis, polyneuropathy, hemolysis / aplastic anemia	6 months
Rifampin	Hepatotoxicity, red discoloration of body fluids / urine, hemolysis	6 months
Ethambutol	Optic neuritis, hyperuricemia	2 months
Pyrazinamide	Hepatotoxicity, arthralgia, myopathies, hyperuricemia	2 months

Cell Death: Necrosis, Apoptosis

Entity: 4.3 Caseous Necrosis (Tuberculosis)
Stain: Hematoxylin - Eosin

Radiology:

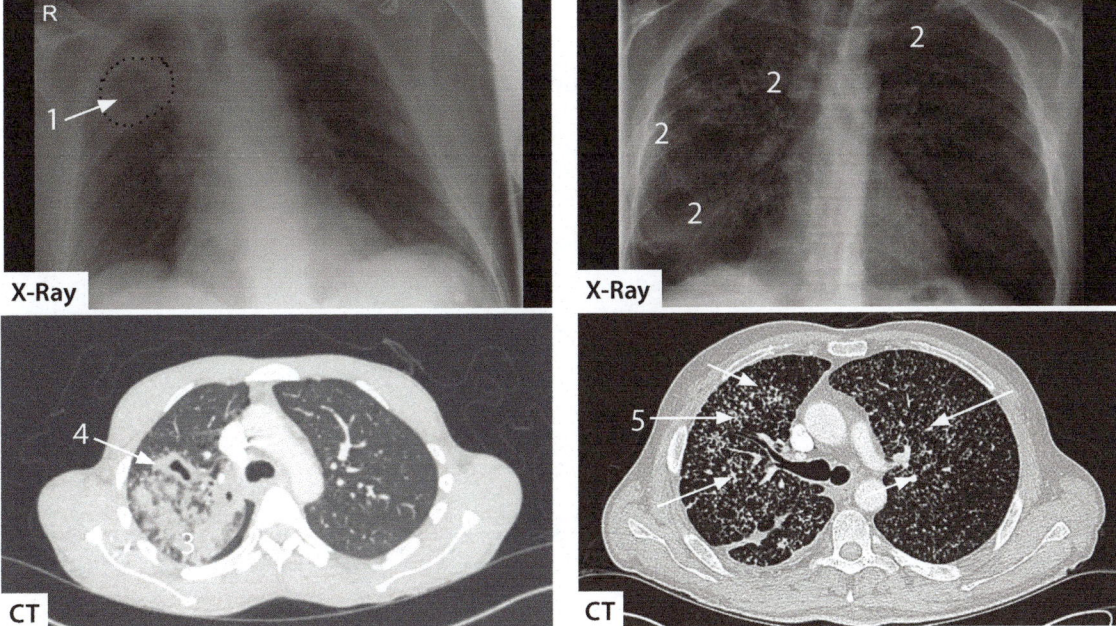

General:
- Primary infection may be in any area of the lung, ranges from not visible to lobar consolidation
- Upon resolution, may leave large residual and often calcified granuloma
- May reactivate if immunosuppressed, manifesting as a post-primary infection in the upper lobes (these lesions tend to cavitate[1])
- Miliary tuberculosis (see X-ray): Disseminated infection, with hematogenous spread and granulomas diffusely[2] scattered across the entire lung
- Can affect every organ, particularly in immunocompromised patients

CT:
- Primary pulmonary tuberculosis: Non-specific appearance, ranging from no lesion to patchy areas of consolidation[3] to lobar consolidation[3]. Cavitation[4] is uncommon. Consolidation resolves to a calcifying granuloma (tuberculoma) called a "Ghon lesion." A Ghon lesion + calcified lymph node = "Ranke complex". In children, may see hilar lymphadenopathy with a hypodense center and rim enhancement.
- Post-primary pulmonary tuberculosis: Typically patchy consolidations[3], poorly defined linear or nodular opacities in upper lobes. Frequent cavitations. Fistular communication with the airway may be indicated by air-fluid levels, or endobronchial spread along nearby airways, with well-defined nodules or tree-in-bud sign lesions.
- Miliary pulmonary tuberculosis: Disseminated 1-3 mm diameter nodules[5]

Differential Diagnosis:

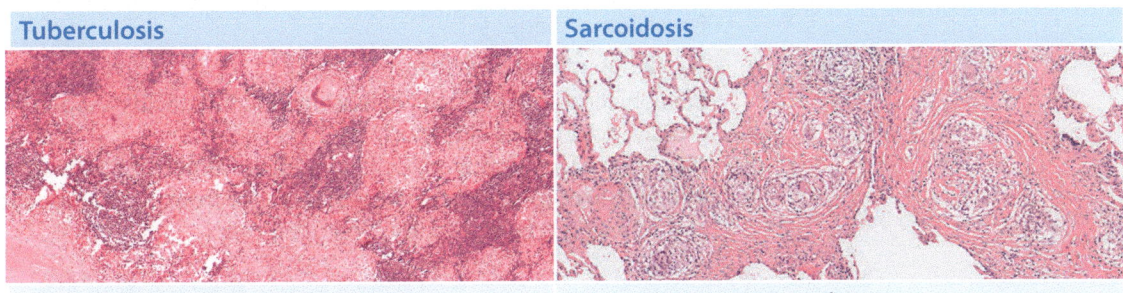

Tuberculosis
- Caseating/necrotizing granulomas
- Etiology: M. tuberculosis infection

Sarcoidosis
- Non-necrotizing granulomas
- Etiology: Unknown
- Associated Syndromes: Lofgren syndrome, Heerfordt syndrome, Jüngling's disease

4

Cell Death: Necrosis, Apoptosis

Entity: 4.4 Fat Necrosis (Acute Pancreatitis)
Stain: Hematoxylin - Eosin

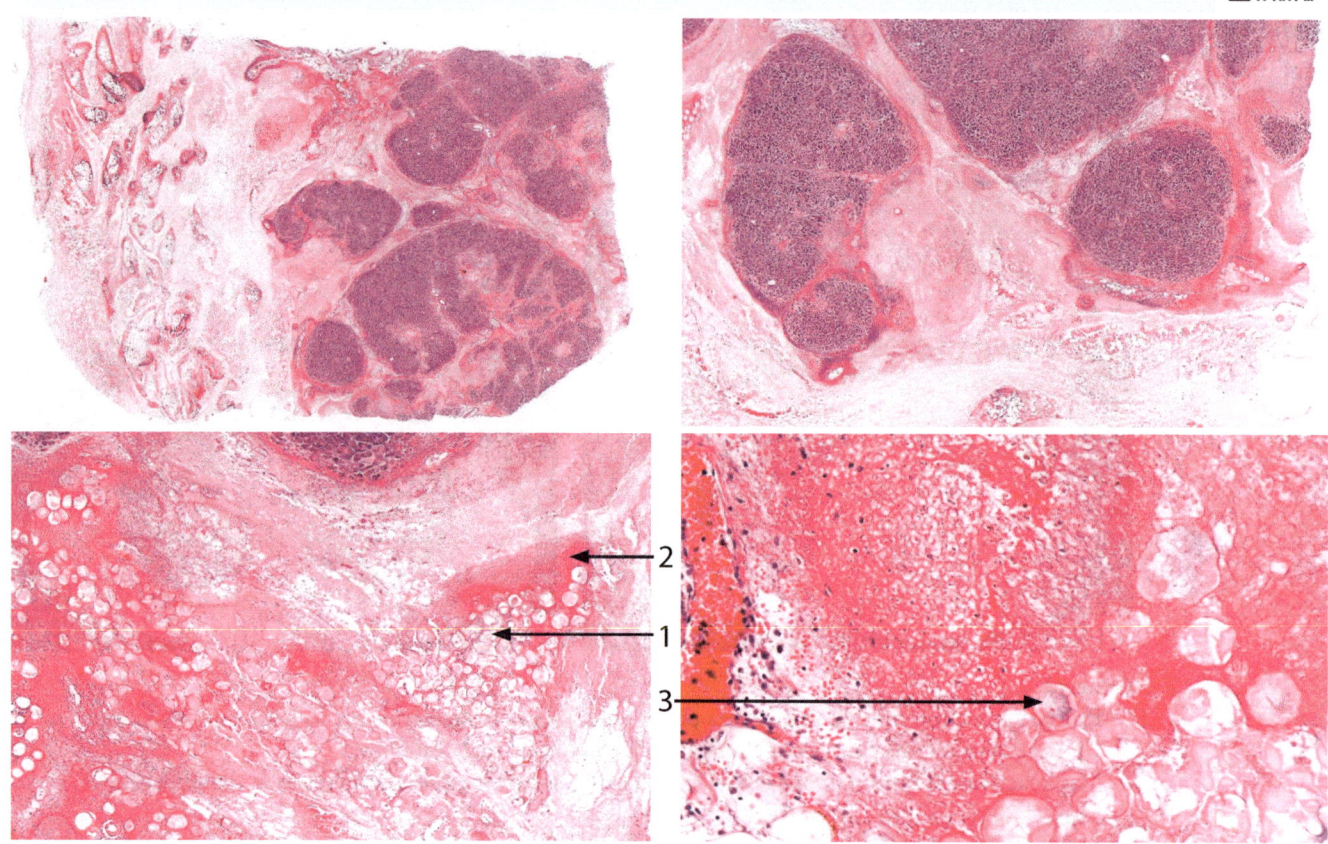

Macroscopy: Severe form of acute pancreatitis with necrosis of associated adipose tissue, and edematous pancreatic parenchyma

Microscopy:
- Bright yellow, small nodules or masses with well-demarcated edges; older lesions may show pseudocystic formation with oily contents, chalky white calcifications, firm gray scarring
- May also see "lime splatter-like" involvement of retroperitoneal fatty tissue and greater omentum, with ascites (possibly bloody)

Tissue/organ: Background pancreatic tissue at the margins, with viable exocrine and endocrine components seen; necrotic tissue appearance varies across time:

Stage	Histologic Changes
Early stage	- Necrotic adipocytes: Fading/loss of adipocyte nuclei, pink finely vacuolated cytoplasm[1] (instead of the normal large single clear lipid vacuole), decrease in cell size, and cell dropout - Focal hemorrhage[2]
Later stage	- Formation of cystic cavities - Basophilic/purple deposits of calcium and fatty acids[3] (saponification that grossly looks like calcification) - Migration of inflammatory cells, including numerous lipid-laden foamy macrophages (phagocytized lipids released from dead adipocytes), and multinucleated foreign-body type giant cells

Definition: **Fat necrosis** refers to death of adipocytes, often affecting peripancreatic, omental, and peritoneal fat in the context of a severe acute pancreatitis

Cell Death: Necrosis, Apoptosis

Entity:	**4.4 Fat Necrosis (Acute Pancreatitis)**
Stain:	*Hematoxylin - Eosin*

Etiology/Pathogenesis:
Acute pancreatitis: 45% obstructive biliary causes (gallstones, carcinomas, etc.), followed by 35% alcohol-induced, and 15% idiopathic/unknown, others are infection, trauma, ischemia
- Autodigestion of the organ by spilling of digestive enzymes, with vasodilation, edema formation, bleeding
- If severe: Necrosis of parenchymal and local fat cells, with release of fatty acids and soap formation with calcium ions (saponification)
- Fat necrosis: A special form of necrosis, can also occur post-surgery or post-trauma (e.g. in the breast following contact with steering wheel in motor vehicle accident)

Clinical Info/Symptoms:
Symptoms of acute pancreatitis: Acute, persistent, severe epigastric pain radiating to the back, nausea/vomiting; if hemorrhagic pancreatitis, possible clinical signs are Gray-Turner, Cullen, and Fox signs

Diagnostics:
Diagnosis of acute pancreatitis requires two of three following criteria:
- Acute onset of severe epigastric pain, typically radiating to back
- Elevation in serum lipase or amylase (three times the upper limit of normal)
- Evidence of pancreatitis on imaging (stranding, edema)

Laboratory:
- Elevated serum lipase, amylase, CRP, ALT, calcium (correlates with severity)
- Assess for underlying etiologies: serum triglycerides, ethanol
- Imaging: abdominal ultrasound, CT with contrast, MRI with contrast

Therapy:
IV fluids: typically lactated ringers or normal saline at 1.5x to 2x maintenance rate, analgesia, antiemetics, elimination of the cause (e.g. ERCP for obstructing stone), trialing diet when patient tolerates

Radiology:

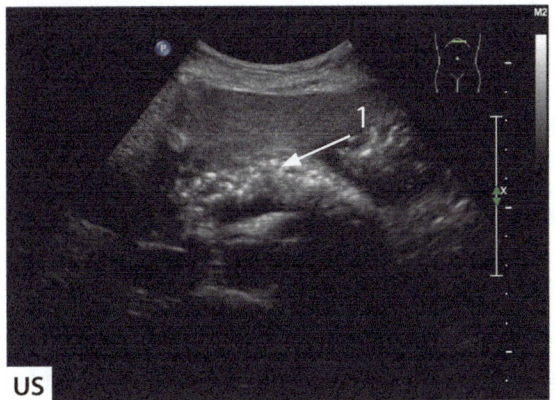
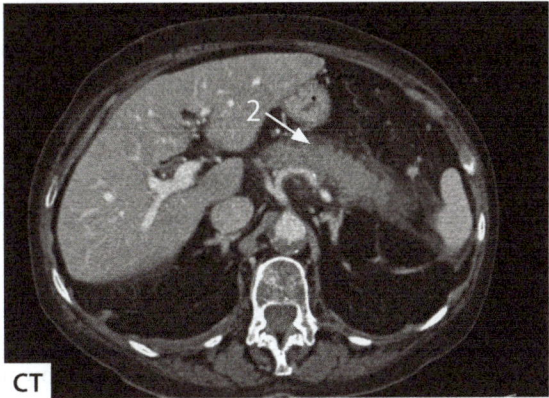

General: Acute pancreatitis often shows edema (edematous interstitial pancreatitis (EIP)), can progress to necrosis of pancreas and surrounding fat (necrotizing pancreatitis). Post-acute phase, may transition to a chronic inflammatory pancreatitis with tissue fibrosis, calcifications[1] and atrophy.

Ultrasound: May identify hyperechoic gallstones, particularly cholesterol stones which may not show on CT. Inflammation and edema give a hypoechoic appearance to the pancreas, with increased transverse thickness of the head. Areas of necrosis appear hypoechoic. Hypoechoic fluid surrounding the pancreas may be seen. In chronic pancreatitis hyperechoic spotty calcifications[1] and tissue atrophy are seen.

CT: Changes may not appear in the first three days post-symptom onset. Once visible, post-contrast CT shows indistinct pancreatic margins with hypodense edema and surrounding fat stranding[2] and fluid collections. Pancreatic necrosis is seen as hypodense, non-enhancing tissue. Air may indicate infection. In chronic pancreatitis hyperdense spotty calcifications and tissue atrophy are seen.

MRI: Edema has a high T2 (FS) signal. T1 fat signal of the tissue is decreased. Gadolinium uptake is decreased in necrotic parenchyma with hypointense signal in T1 FS.

4 Cell Death: Necrosis, Apoptosis

Entity: 4.5 Gangrenous Necrosis (Wet Gangrene, Peripheral Arterial Disease)
Stain: Hematoxylin - Eosin

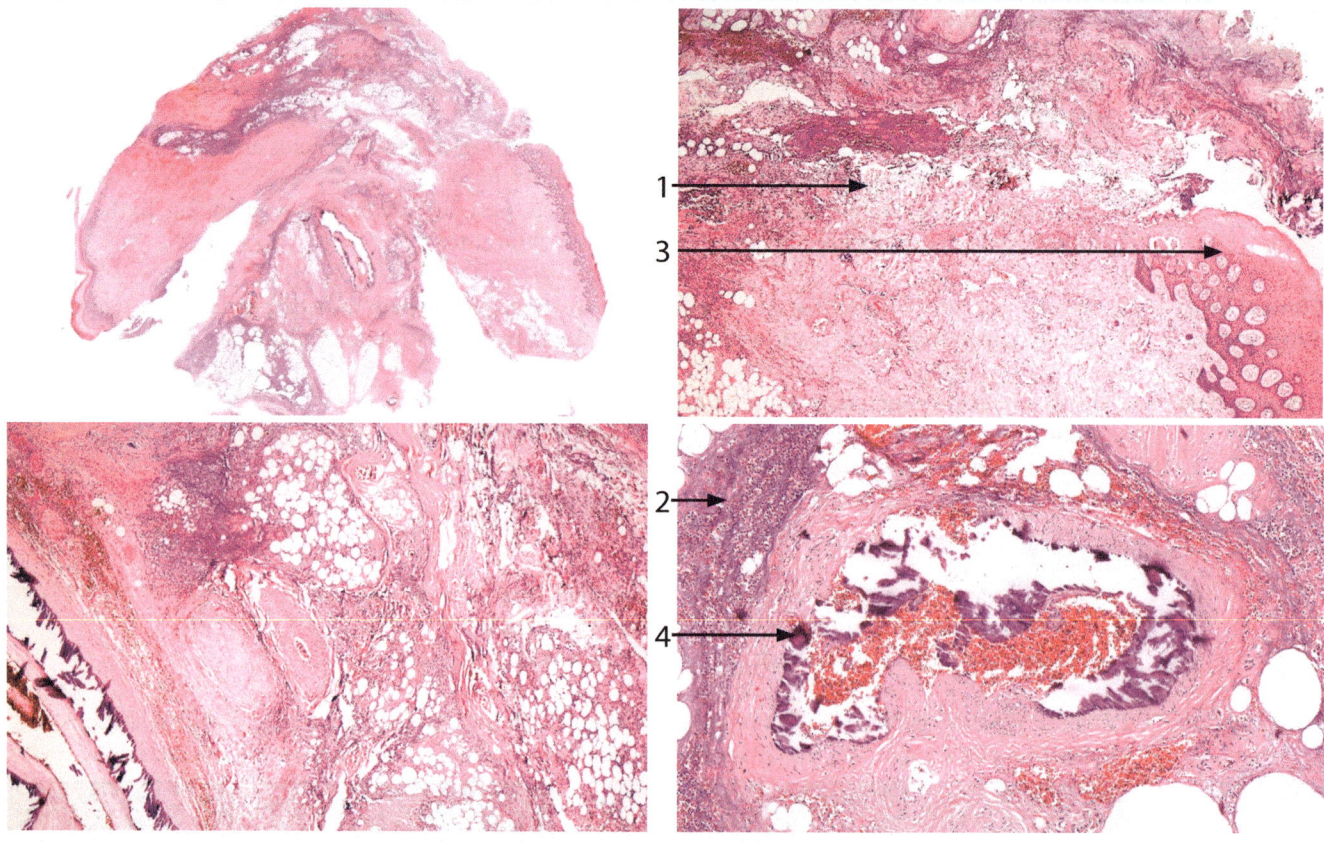

Macroscopy: A distinction is made between dry gangrene and wet gangrene
- **Dry gangrene:** Coagulative necrosis due to prolonged ischemia with desiccated/mummified extremity; the tissue appears burnt black

Microscopy:
- **Wet gangrene:** Ulcer with pus (dead neutrophils and putrefactive/anaerobic bacteria), reddened and swollen adjacent skin, due to infection superimposed on the ischemic tissues

Tissue/organ: Skin, subcutaneous tissue, bone
Dry gangrene:
- Coagulative necrosis with preserved architecture of the tissue
- Dead cells appear as shadows or ghosts: darker pink, with intact cell outlines, but lacking intact cell nuclei

Wet gangrene:
- Skin defect/ulceration[1] with deep acute inflammation, and necrosis of the subcutaneous fat
- Bacterial colonies[2] on tissue gram stain
- Reactive epidermal hyperplasia/acanthosis around the edge of the ulcer[3]
- Calcific arteriosclerosis[4]

Definition: Gangrenous necrosis is not a specific pattern of cell death, but a description of ischemic necrosis of the distal lower extremities

Etiology/Pathogenesis:
Gangrene is a special form of coagulation necrosis
- Causes: Often peripheral vascular disease due to arteriosclerosis; an uncommon cause is thromboangiitis obliterans (Bürger's disease)
- Dry gangrene: Coagulation necrosis + desiccation (mummification)
- Wet/moist gangrene: Coagulation necrosis + secondary colonization by putrefactive agents (anaerobes), with tissue digestion and liquefaction

Cell Death: Necrosis, Apoptosis

Entity: 4.5 Gangrenous Necrosis (Wet Gangrene, Peripheral Arterial Disease)
Stain: Hematoxylin - Eosin

Clinical Info/Symptoms: Peripheral Arterial Disease (PAD)
- Common causes: Arteriosclerosis, smoking, diabetes
- Chronic disease with reduced peripheral arterial perfusion due to vascular stenosis or occlusion; chronic low-grade ischemia of tissues
- Frequent locations: Lower extremities (buttock, thigh, calf, forefoot)
- Clinically manifests as intermittent claudication, induced by exercise and relieved by rest, affected area feels cold and weak
- In advanced stages: Gangrene

Diagnostics: Duplex sonography, angiography, ankle-brachial index, exercise testing
- Ankle-Brachial-Index (ABI) to evaluate the severity of the PAD

ABI Value	PAD Severity
> 1.3	Falsely high values (suspected noncompressible calcified vessels)
0.9-1.3	Normal findings
0.7-0.9	Slight PAD
0.4-0.7	Moderate PAD
< 0.4	Severe PAD

Therapy:
- Smoking cessation, exercise therapy
- Cilostazol (PDE inhibitor), ASA or clopidogrel, statins
- Consider percutaneous or surgical intervention, if significantly impacting quality of life or inadequate response to pharmacologic/exercise therapy
- stent, balloon, vein grafts, or other prosthetic material
- Fontaine and Rutherford classifications used for risk stratification

Fontaine Classification		Rutherford Categories		
Stage	Clinic	Grade	Category	Clinic
I	Freedom from complaints	0	0	Asymptomatic
IIa:	Mild pain with walking distance > 200m	I	1	Slight intermittent claudication
IIb	Mild pain with walking distance <200m	I	2	Moderate intermittent claudication
		I	3	Severe intermittent claudication
III	Ischemic pain at rest	II	4	Ischemic pain at rest
IV	Ulcer/gangrene	III	5	Small area necrosis
		III	6	Extensive necrosis

Circulatory Diseases and Disorders
Katelyn Dannheim, Ann Ding, Carsten Fechner

5.1 Arterial Thromboembolism (White/Precipitation Thrombus)

5.2 Venous Thromboembolism (Red/Coagulation Thrombus)

5.3 Hyaline Microthrombi

5.4 Pulmonary Embolism

5 Circulatory Diseases and Disorders

A thrombus is formed by the aggregation of platelets, blood cells, fibrin, and other coagulation cascade components that collectively adhere to the vessel wall and occlude the lumen. Arterial (case 5.1) or venous (case 5.2) thrombi that are formed in pathophysiological states can lead to embolic events in which a portion of a thrombus detaches, relocates, and obstructs blood flow in a different part of the vasculature. Both thrombi and emboli can, in severe cases of vascular blockage, lead to ischemic tissue injury and organ damage. In certain clinical contexts (e.g. sepsis, pregnancy, cancer), intravascular microthrombus formation (case 5.3) can lead to disseminated intravascular coagulation and subsequent organ failure and uncontrolled hemorrhage.

Predisposition to venous thrombosis includes risk factors such as hypercoagulability, endothelial injury, and stasis, which have been referred to as "Virchow's triad." In the venous circulation, stasis of blood flow in the lower extremities can increase the risk of deep venous thrombosis, which can embolize to the pulmonary circulation, potentially leading to a life-threatening pulmonary embolism (case 5.4). The formation of arterial thrombi secondary to vascular diseases such as atherosclerosis can (with or without embolism) lead to infarction and ischemic necrosis in any organ, including the lung (case 5.5), heart, brain, and kidney.

Entity: 5.1 Arterial Thromboembolism (White/Precipitation Thrombus)
Stain: Hematoxylin - Eosin

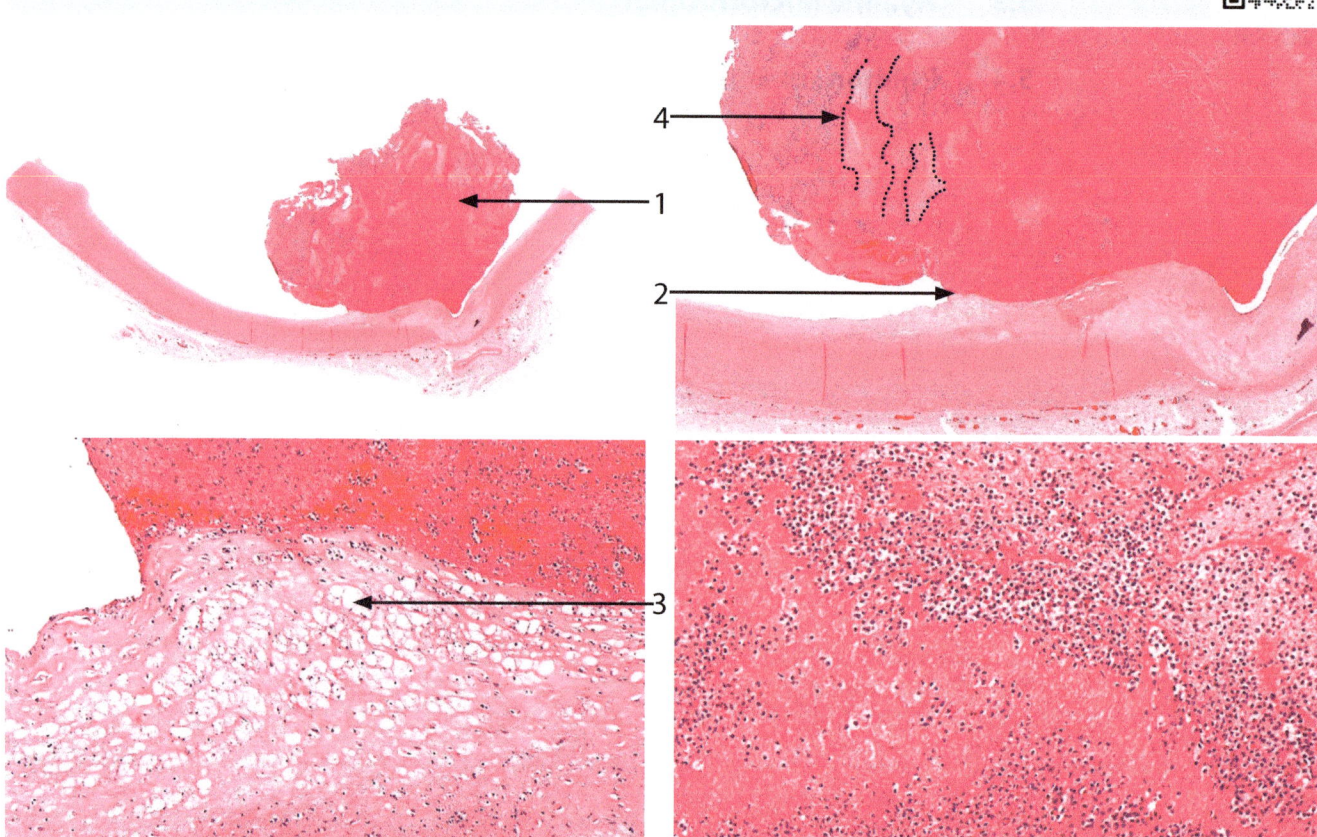

Macroscopy: Gray-white, brittle, ridged surface, holds shape of vessel in which it formed

Microscopy: Tissue/Organ: Artery
Arterial section with thrombus[1] partially adherent to the endothelium (attached to vessel wall)[2]
Histiocytes (tissue macrophages)[3] found at the border between the thrombus and tunica intima
Subendothelial fibrosis → increase in fibroblasts and capillary sprouting
Alternating layers of platelets, leukocytes, few erythrocytes, and fibrin ("Lines of Zahn")[4]
Aggregates of platelets form a homogeneous mass

Definition: **White thrombus:** Blood clot rich in fibrin/platelets layered with leukocytes/erythrocytes ("Lines of Zahn") formed within the vascular system as a result of vascular injury
Thromboembolus: Thrombus traveling in the circulation away from the location where it was formed

83

Circulatory Diseases and Disorders

Entity:	**5.1 Arterial Thromboembolism (White/Precipitation Thrombus)**
Stain:	*Hematoxylin - Eosin*

Etiology/Pathogenesis: Develops secondary to damage of the vessel wall/endothelium (e.g. arteriosclerosis/atherosclerosis), in the setting of active blood flow.
- Thrombocyte activation and accumulation (aggregation) on the endothelium secondary to vascular damage → activation of the coagulation system with fibrin formation → active blood flow results in layering/organization of platelets/fibrin with leukocytes/erythrocytes → white thrombus formation (rich in fibrin and platelets)
- May develop within the arterial system or heart ventricles/ auricles-atrial appendages

Clinical Info/Symptoms: Vascular occlusion resulting in downstream ischemia may present as pain (e.g. limb ischemia → claudication, or mesenteric ischemia → abdominal pain) or organ infarction (e.g. coronary artery thrombosis → myocardial infarction, or pulmonary thromboembolism → pulmonary infarct)

Diagnostics: Angiography (CT, MR, catheterization), type of angiography depends on affected organs; Lactate to assess organ damage secondary to ischemia

Therapy:
- Thrombectomy (surgical removal of thrombus)
- Thrombolysis (disruption of thromboemboli using medication)
- Prophylaxis, such as platelet aggregation inhibitors (ASA, clopidogrel)

5 Circulatory Diseases and Disorders

Entity: 5.2 Venous Thromboembolism (Red/Coagulation Thrombus)
Stain: Hematoxylin - Eosin

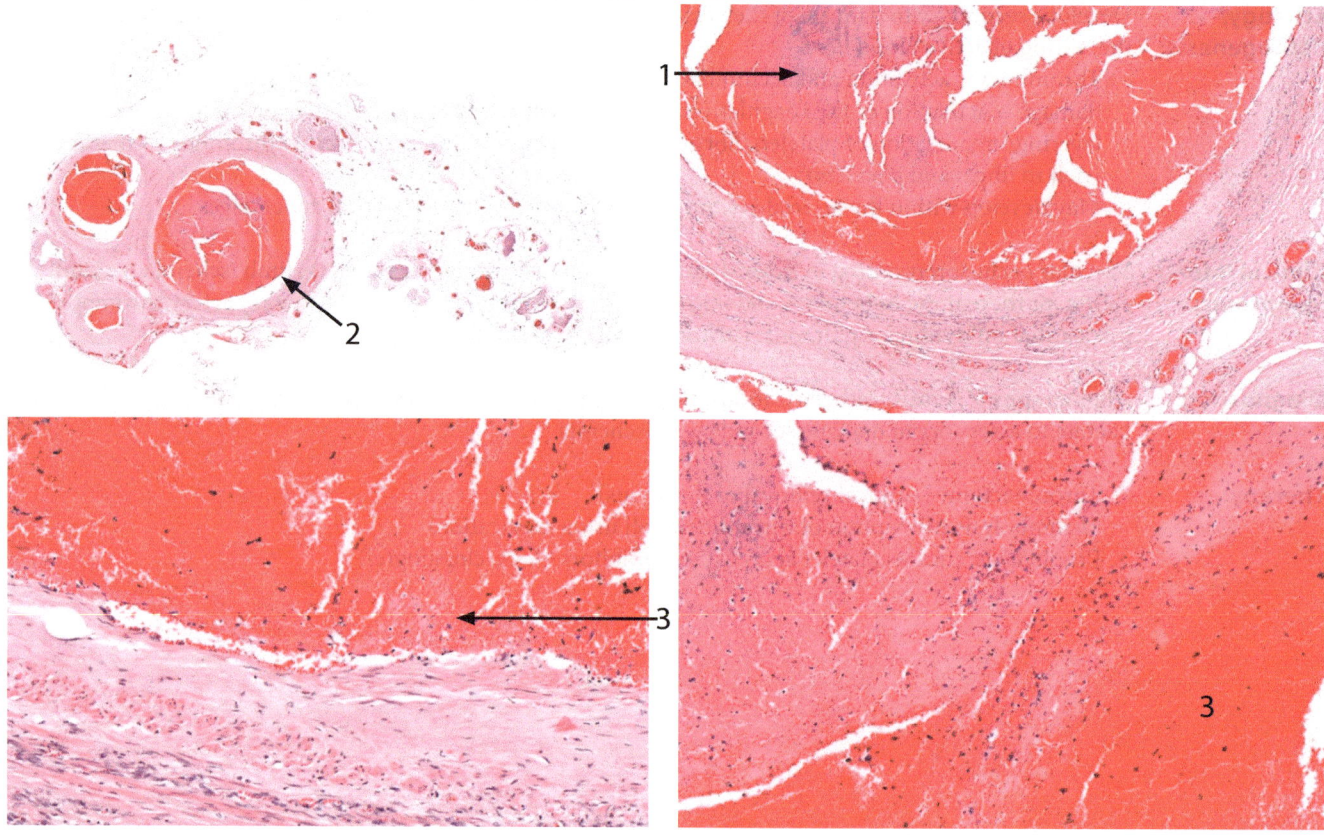

Macroscopy: Dark red, smooth surface; minimal adhesion to the vessel wall

Microscopy: Tissue/organ: Vein
- Blood clot rich in erythrocytes with layers of fibrin[1]
- Obstruction of the entire lumen
- No connection to the vessel wall or endothelial disruption[2]
- Erythrocytes no longer distinguishable from one another → eosinophilic red homogeneous mass[3], with few admixed leukocytes

Definition: Solidified blood clot rich in erythrocytes with layers of fibrin, arising secondary to coagulopathic environment (e.g. blood stasis, coagulation activation) without significant attachment to the vessel wall

Etiology/Pathogenesis: Vascular occlusion most commonly secondary to reduced blood flow (stasis) and subsequent activation of the coagulation cascade
- No attachment to the vessel wall-endothelium
- Mostly in the venous system

Phlebothrombosis (deep vein thrombosis) occurs as part of the Virchow triad:
1. Vascular wall damage
2. Change in blood circulation (reduced flow velocity/ stasis)
3. Hypercoagulability

Clinical Info/Symptoms: Deep Vein Thrombosis (DVT) Symptoms:
Swelling / increase in circumference, erythema with warmth, tenderness (e.g. tumor, rubor, calor, dolor)

Circulatory Diseases and Disorders

Entity:	5.2 Venous Thromboembolism (Red/Coagulation Thrombus)
Stain:	Hematoxylin - Eosin

Diagnostics: Color duplex compression sonography is the gold standard; D-dimer is very sensitive, but not specific to site (obtain in patients with low probability of DVT)

Clinical Signs	
Tests	**Findings**
Homans sign	Calf pain with dorsiflexion of the foot
Meyer sign	Calf compression pain along the Meyer pressure points
Leg circumferences	Side difference of > 3 cm

Wells' Criteria for DVT (Wells et al. 1995)	
Clinical Risk Factor	**Score**
Active tumor disease (ongoing or palliative treatment in the last 6 months)	+1
Paralysis, paresis, or recent lower limb immobilization	+1
Bed rest for > 3 days and/or major surgery within 12 weeks	+1
Localized pain / induration along the deep leg vein distribution	+1
Entire leg swollen	+1
Calf swelling > 3cm to the opposite side (10 cm measured below the tibial tuberosity)	+1
Pitting edema on the affected leg	+1
Superficial unilateral collateral veins	+1
DVT history	+1
Alternative diagnosis at least as likely as DVT	-2

0 points: Low probability of DVT
1-2 points: Moderate probability of DVT
3+ points: High probability of DVT

Therapy:
- Anticoagulation with low molecular weight heparin, fondaparinux, or direct oral anticoagulants (rivaroxaban, apixaban); duration of anticoagulation minimum 3 months, depends on provoking factors
- Surgical or interventional thrombectomy and thrombolytic therapy reserved for those who fail anticoagulation

5 Circulatory Diseases and Disorders

Entity: 5.3 Hyaline Microthrombi
Stain: Hematoxylin - Eosin

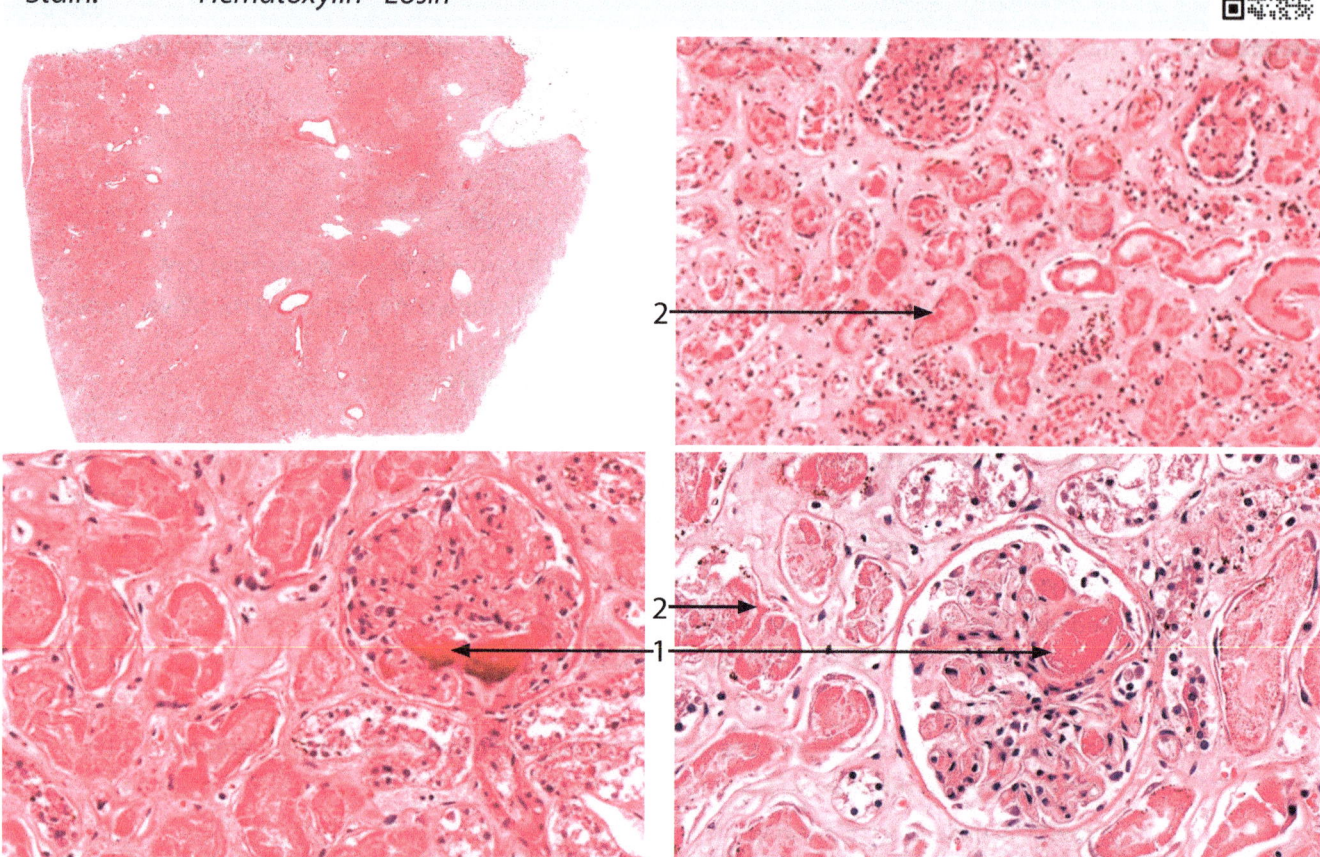

Macroscopy:	No specific gross findings in kidneys; possibly signs of shock with pale renal cortex and blood-rich, dark red renal medulla
Microscopy:	Tissue/organ: Kidney Round or oval eosinophilic bodies with hyaline appearance (2-3 um), found predominantly in small vessels (frequently in the glomerular capillaries[1]) Homogeneous mass of platelets and fibrin filling capillary lumen From Greek "hyalinos" = "glass" → homogeneously eosinophilic In kidney: Frequent background tubular necrosis (renal tubules show loss of nuclear basophilia[2])
Definition:	Homogenous capillary thrombus consisting of balanced proportions of fibrin and platelet; also known as hyaline microthrombi
Etiology/ Pathogenesis:	Develop in the context of a disseminated intravascular coagulation (DIC) or thrombotic microangiopathy (TMA) (e.g. thrombotic thrombocytic purpura, hemolytic uremic syndrome)
Clinical Info/ Symptoms:	**Disseminated Intravascular Coagulopathy (DIC)** Causes: Sepsis, trauma, malignancy, obstetric complications, intravascular hemolysis Release of factor II activators (Prothrombin) → Formation of microthrombi through activation of the coagulation system → Consumption of the coagulation factors → Simultaneous bleeding and clotting tendency

Circulatory Diseases and Disorders

Entity:	5.3 Hyaline Microthrombi
Stain:	*Hematoxylin - Eosin*

Thrombotic microangiopathy (TMA):
1. **Thrombotic thrombocytopenic purpura (TTP)**
   - Causes: can be hereditary or acquired (e.g. autoimmune, drug-related); results from ADAMTS13 deficiency; ADAMTS13 is protease responsible for cleaving large multimers of von Willebrand factor, which are more thrombogenic
   - Presents with fever, neurologic signs/symptoms, renal compromise, microangiopathic hemolytic anemia and thrombocytopenia
2. **Hemolytic uremic syndrome (HUS)**
   - Causes: often infection related (e.g. E. coli, shiga toxin-mediated)
   - Presents with watery diarrhea, fever, renal insufficiency/acute renal failure

Diagnostics: Clinical presentation of simultaneous bleeding (e.g. bruising, petechiae, oozing) and thrombosis (e.g. venous or arterial)

Lab markers:
- Elevated D-dimer
- Decreased fibrinogen from consumption (though may be normal, as fibrinogen can be elevated in inflammatory states)
- Elevated PT, aPTT, INR
- Decreased platelets (a.k.a. thrombocytopenia)

Therapy:
- Treatment of underlying/inciting disease
- Supportive care
- No prophylactic anticoagulation, but standard treatment for thrombosis with anticoagulation
- Platelet transfusions and substitution of coagulation factors (e.g. FFP, cryoprecipitate) for those with serious bleeding

Radiology: **General:** Only indirect results of the DIC are observed like thrombosis with infarction or hemorrhage / bleeding e.g. resulting in renal infarction, pulmonary embolism or abdominal bleeding.

5 Circulatory Diseases and Disorders

Entity: 5.4 Pulmonary Embolism
Stain: Hematoxylin - Eosin

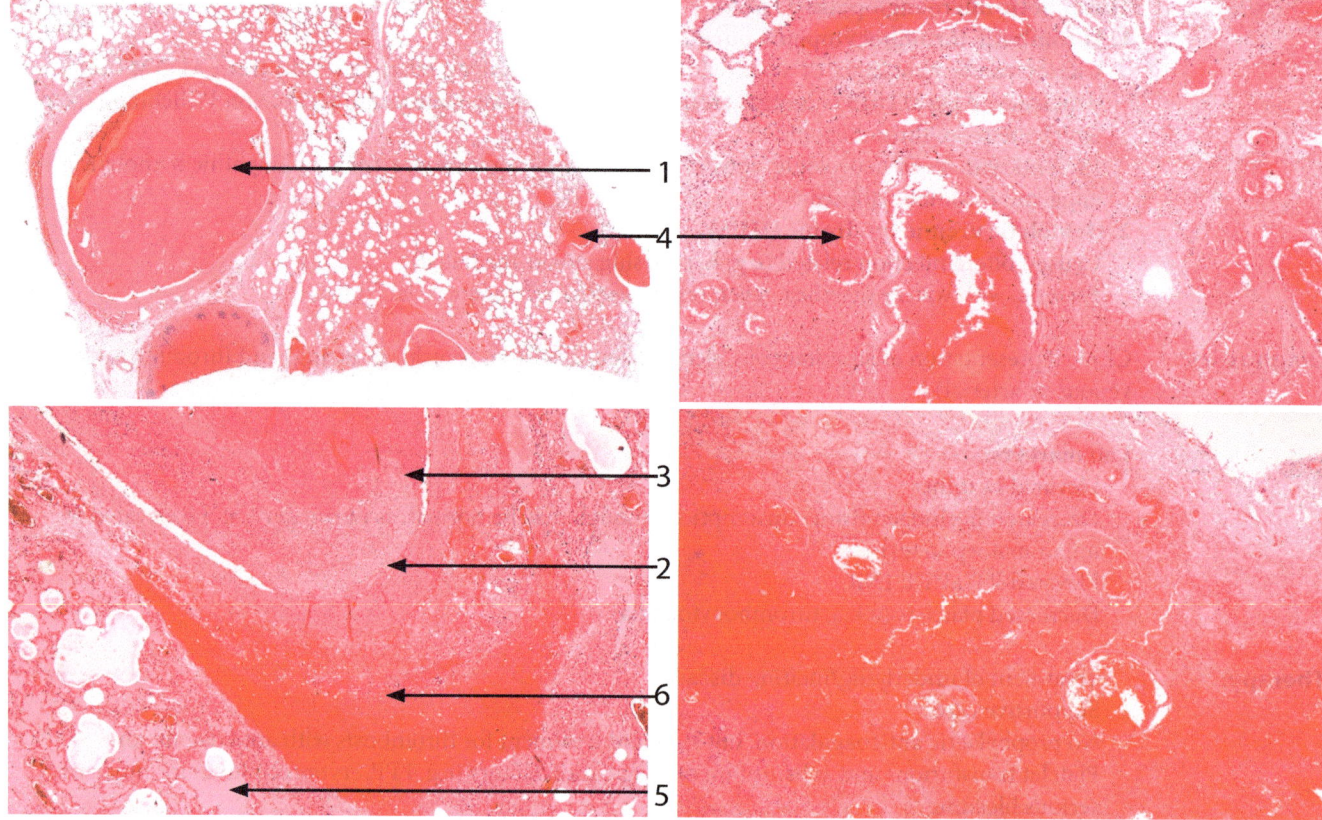

Macroscopy:
- Tan and red-brown, firm blood clot within pulmonary arteries of variable size
- Peripheral pulmonary thromboembolism: occludes peripheral lobe or segmental arteries
- Central pulmonary thromboembolism: occludes pulmonary trunk or both main branches
- When chronic, can undergo recanalization

Microscopy:
- Tissue/organ: Lungs
- Lung parenchyma with pulmonary artery and intravascular thrombus[1]
- Thromboembolus attached to the vessel wall/endothelium[2]
- Organization/layering of fibrin, platelets, erythrocytes, and leukocytes[3]
- Other findings: Dilated alveolar spaces, vascular congestion[4], pulmonary edema[5], and sometimes infarction (hemorrhagic infarction[6] due to dual blood supply; see below)

Definition:
Occlusion of one or more of the main arterial branches in the lungs by thromboembolism

Etiology/Pathogenesis:
- Often secondary to deep vein thrombosis (DVT), bone marrow embolism (released into circulation after bone fractures), bone cement during orthopedic surgeries, fat embolism
- Less often septic embolism, air embolism, tumor embolism, etc.

Dual vascular supply of the lungs:
- Bronchial arteries (branches of aorta responsible for supplying oxygenated blood to lung parenchyma)
- Pulmonary arteries (deoxygenated blood from the heart, traveling through the pulmonary circulation to be reoxygenated)
- Thromboemboli enter pulmonary arteries from upstream (e.g. DVT), while bronchial arteries maintain oxygenation of the lung parenchyma
- Infarction does not occur unless there is simultaneous left heart failure (usually secondary to congestion of the pulmonary vein in the setting of large PE), leading to ischemia, necrosis, and oozing from the bronchial arteries

Circulatory Diseases and Disorders

Entity:	5.4 Pulmonary Embolism
Stain:	Hematoxylin - Eosin

Clinical Info/Symptoms:
- Tachycardia, dyspnea, tachypnea, chest pain (acute or insidious), hemoptysis
- Concomitant symptoms of DVT (unilateral leg swelling, tenderness, erythema)
- Possible to be asymptomatic

Risk factors: Immobilization, hypercoagulable states (e.g. malignancy, DIC), hormonal therapy

Diagnostics:
- Abnormal vital signs (tachycardia is a common presenting sign, may have hypotension in setting of obstructive shock, hypoxia)
- ECG demonstrating signs of right heart strain (e.g. S1Q3T3, right bundle branch block, P pulmonary, T-negatives, ST-segment changes)
- Elevated D-dimer
- Elevated Troponin-T and BNP due to heart strain
- CT angiography demonstrating flow defects
- Echocardiography in those with concern for right heart strain

Risk Stratification of Pulmonary Embolism Using the Wells Score (Wells et al. 1998)

Clinical Risk Factor	Original	Score (Simplified)
Clinical signs of DVT	+3	+1
PE is most likely or equally likely diagnosis	+3	+1
Tachycardia with HR > 100 beats/min	+1.5	+1
Recent surgery in the last 4 weeks or immobilization for at least 3 days	+1.5	+1
Previous DVT or PE	+1.5	+1
Hemoptysis	+1	+1
Malignancy with treatment in last 6 months or palliation	+1	+1
0 - 4 points (original) / 0 - 1 points (simplified):	PE unlikely	
≥ 5 points (original) / ≥ 2 points (simplified):	PE is likely	

Therapy:

Symptomatic management:
- Oxygen administration under pulse oximetry control
- Anxiolysis and analgesia, e.g. with opioids or diazepam

Radiology:

Treatment:
- Anticoagulation: unfractionated heparin, low molecular weight heparin, fondaparinux, Direct Oral Anticoagulants (DOAC such as rivaroxaban, apixaban)

Differentiation based on hemodynamic stability:
- Mild PE with hemodynamic stability:
- Therapeutic anticoagulation for at least 3 months with Vitamin-K antagonists (warfarin) or direct oral anticoagulants (rivaroxaban, apixaban)
- Submassive PE with evidence of right heart strain on imaging but hemodynamic stability
- Similar management to mild PE with hemodynamic stability
- Monitor hemodynamics carefully in case of progressing to massive PE
- Caution with inferior vena cava filter so as not to cause RV overload
- Massive PE with hemodynamic instability:
- Recanalizing measures with systemic thrombolysis (alteplase) or local catheter lysis or interventional thrombectomy
- Pressors (e.g. norepinephrine)

5 Circulatory Diseases and Disorders

Entity: 5.4 Pulmonary Embolism
Stain: Hematoxylin - Eosin

Radiology:

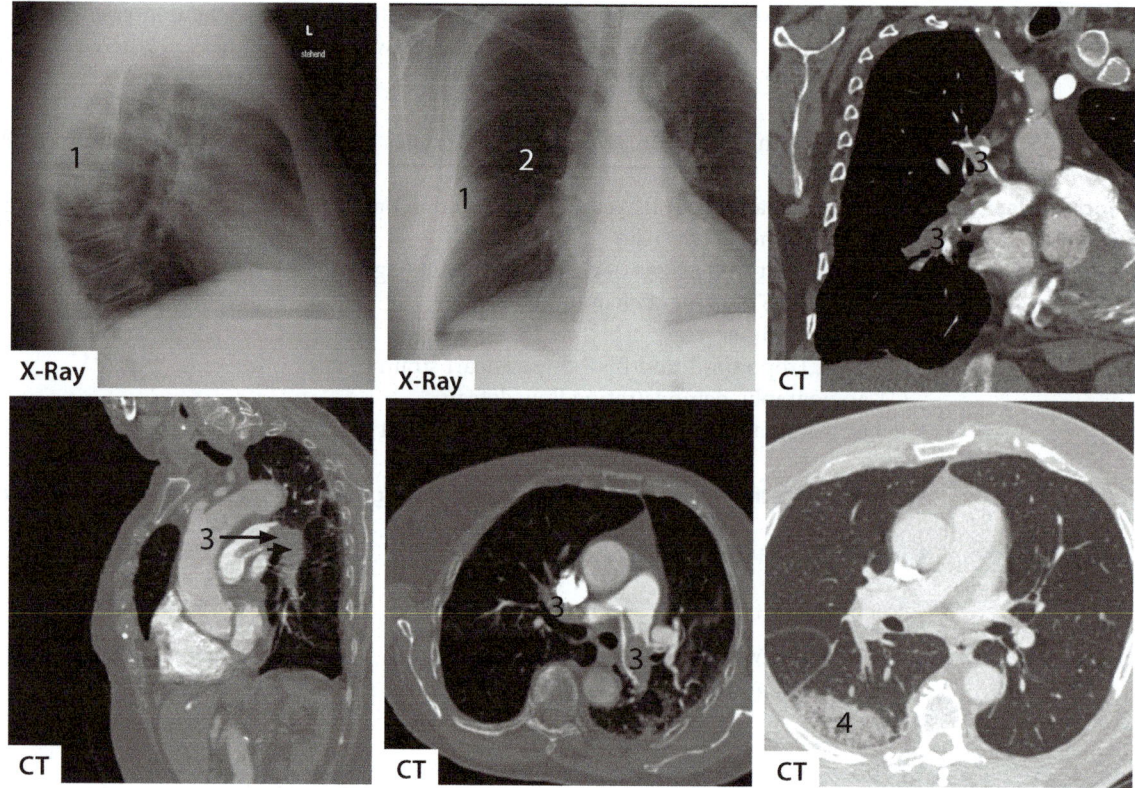

General:
- Embolic occlusion of the pulmonary arteries often due to venous blood clots originating from the legs
- Other possible embolic materials: gas, fat, tumor, amniotic fluid or bone cement
- Lung infarction also occurs when bronchial arteries are compromised

X-Ray:
- Unspecific
- Wedge shaped dense infarction in the pulmonary periphery is called Hampton hump[1]
- A thrombus occluded dense pulmonary artery with adjacent hypoperfusion is called Westermark sign[2]

CT:
- Pulmonary angiography is used for finding thrombotic filling defects[3] in the branches of the pulmonary arteries
- Thrombus location can be differentiated in saddle/central, paracentral, lobar, segmental and subsegmental
- Signs of right ventricular strain like a flattened interventricular septum should be evaluated
- Wedge shaped pulmonary infarction[4] can be seen as consolidation adjacent to to the occluded vessels

Ventilation/perfusion scan:
- Performed when CT is contraindicated (pregnancy)
- Pulmonary embolism is shown where areas of the lung are ventilated but not perfused

Vascular Pathology and Myocardial Infarction

Katelyn Dannheim, Ann Ding, Carsten Fechner

6.1 Atherosclerosis (Aorta)

6.2 Atherosclerosis (Coronary Artery Disease)

6.3 Cystic Medial Degeneration/Necrosis

6.4 Myocardial Infarction

6 Vascular Pathology and Myocardial Infarction

Entity: 6.1 Atherosclerosis (Aorta)
Stain: Hematoxylin - Eosin

Vascular pathology is a leading cause of disease in developed countries, largely due to a preponderance of fatty and processed foods. Atherosclerosis, or "hardening of the arteries" is often due to deposition of excess lipids and cholesterol with plaque development and subsequent changes to the vessel wall. Atherosclerosis can occur in any size vessel; here we will review this process in a large vessel (aorta), as well as its role in the development of aortic aneurysms. We will also discuss atherosclerosis of a smaller vessel (coronary artery), and myocardial infarction, which most often directly results from coronary artery disease.

Another important though less common form of vascular pathology is cystic medial degeneration, which is a misnomer (no true cysts are formed), but which does involve a degenerative change of the tunica media, resulting in a weakened vessel wall. When occurring in the aorta, it may be associated with the catastrophic sequelae of aortic dissection. This topic is also addressed in the cases that follow.

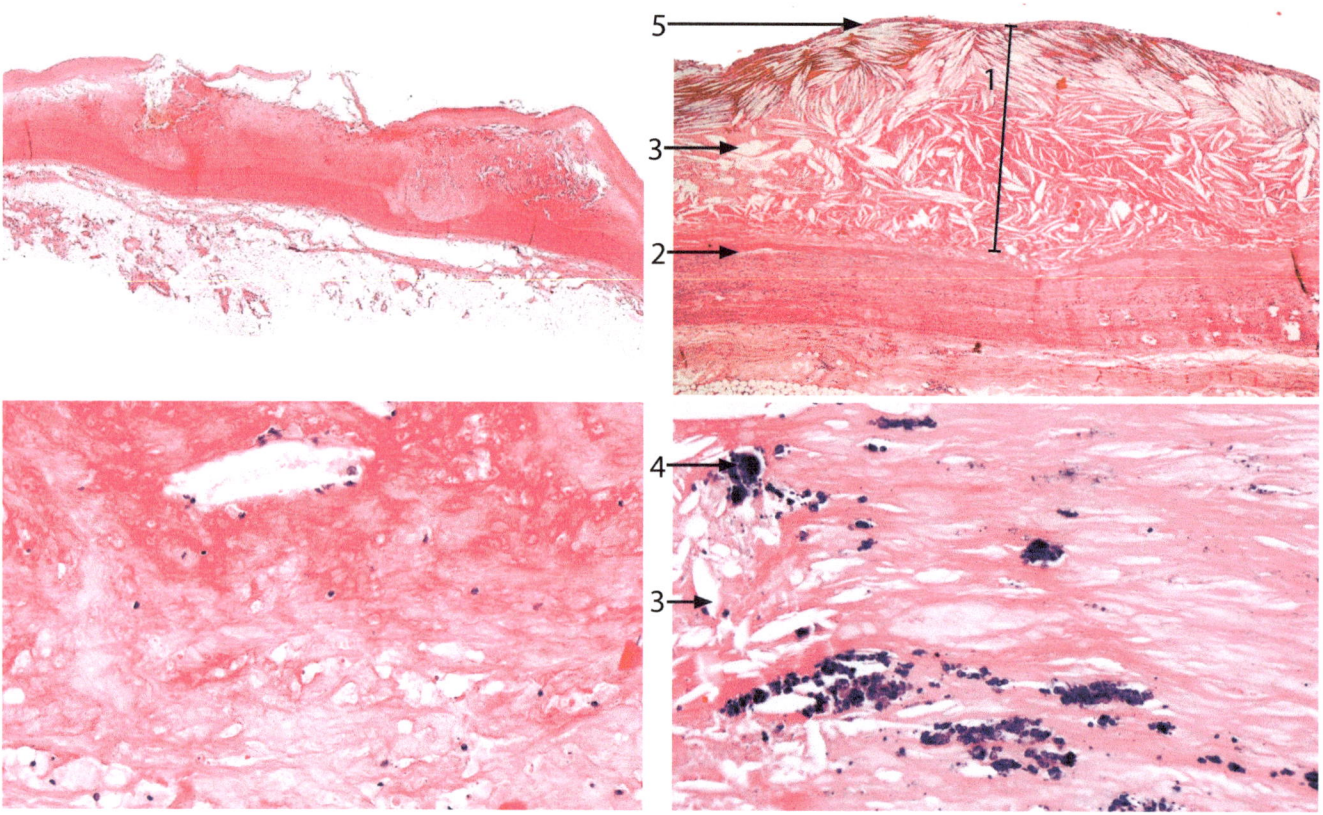

Macroscopy: Aorta with atherosclerotic plaques (raised yellow-tan stripes and spots), as well as ulcerated and / or calcified atheroma beds and induration (sclerosis) of the affected vascular segment
- Fatty streaks: early lesion from yellowish, striped or nodular fat deposits
- Atherosclerotic plaque: intimal thickening with lipid accumulation in foam cells
- Ruptured plaque: fibrous cap covering lipids ruptures, with exposure of the subendothelial lipid core and connective tissue → extremely thrombogenic

Microscopy: Tissue/organ: Aorta
- Thickened intima[1] with fibrosis of the subendothelial layer[2]
- Cholesterol crystals (needle shaped) and lipids embedded in the subendothelial connective tissue[3] correspond to the lipid core (atheroma) of the plaque
- Foam cells[3] (lipid-laden macrophages) often seen around edges of lipid core
- Lipid core may show calcifications[4] or blood/hemosiderin (if plaque previously disrupted)
- Fibrous cap[5] covers the lipid-laden core (the thinner the cap, the greater the risk of plaque rupture)
- Over time, plaque can grow in size, with thinning of the underlying tunica media; extreme cases can cause a weakened wall and aneurysmal dilatation

Vascular Pathology and Myocardial Infarction

Entity:	6.1 Atherosclerosis (Aorta)
Stain:	Hematoxylin - Eosin

Definition: **Atherosclerosis:** Intravascular intimal deposition of cholesterol and lipids, with macrophages, smooth muscle cell proliferation, and extracellular matrix formation; grossly described as a "plaque."

Etiology/Pathogenesis: Formation of atherosclerotic plaques in the "response to injury" model
- Lipids and cholesterol deposit in intima and macrophages respond
- Intimal connective tissue responds with increased extracellular matrix formation, leads to hardening of the artery (arteriosclerosis) and loss of elastic fibers
- Increasing plaque size may erode and thin the underlying tunica media
- Risk factors: smoking, obesity/metabolic syndrome, diabetes, dyslipidemia esp. hypercholesterolemia, hypertension, inactivity, depression, family history (male <55 years, female < 65 years)
- Consequences: Coronary artery disease, myocardial infarction, aneurysm
- Very large plaques in the aorta can cause aneurysmal dilatation

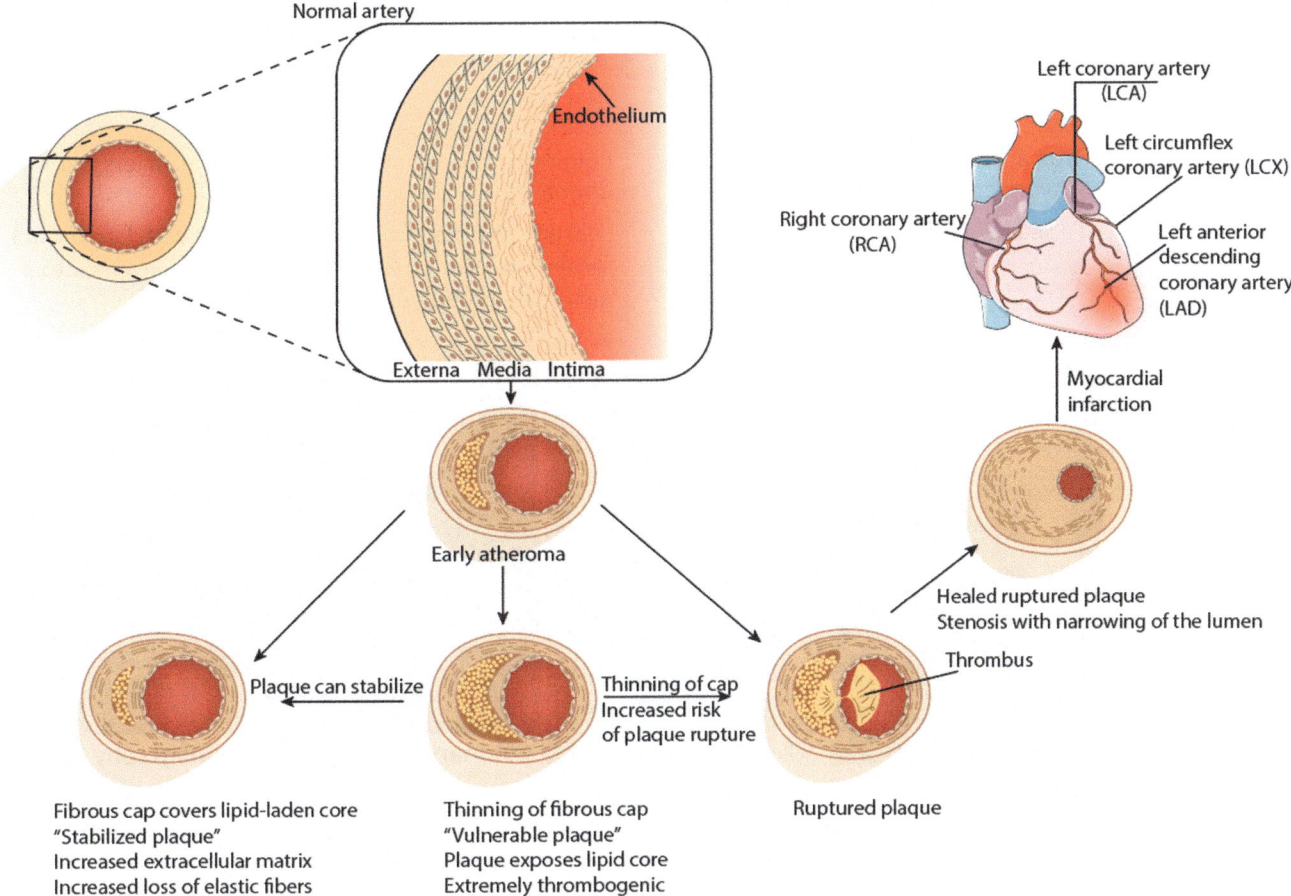

Clinical Info/Symptoms: Atherosclerotic vascular disease (ASCVD): One of the leading causes of death for adults

Prevention: Risk factor reduction
- Quit smoking, lower blood pressure, weight reduction, change in diet, exercise, stress reduction

Aortic aneurysm formation:
- Usually abdominal (abdominal aortic aneurysm or AAA), most often below the level of the renal arteries (increased turbulences), may result in decreased perfusion of lower extremities, may embolize plaque fragments downstream

6 Vascular Pathology and Myocardial Infarction

Entity: 6.1 Atherosclerosis (Aorta)
Stain: Hematoxylin - Eosin

Diagnostics: Perform clinical risk assessment for ASCVD:
- LDL-Cholesterol (normal: < 100 mg/dl)
- HbA1c (Diabetes mellitus)

Radiology: Ultrasound of the carotid arteries, screening for aortic aneurysm, abdominal sonography recommended for men with smoking history, age 65-75

Therapy:
- Lifestyle changes (diet, exercise, weight loss)
- Blood pressure control, antihypertensive therapy if needed
- Blood sugar control (HbA1C > 6.5% = T2DM)
- Statin therapy
- Aspirin therapy (75-100mg/day for high risk patients, 40-75 years of age)

None for routine aortic plaques, continue risk factor reduction
If aneurysm develops; vascular surgery if aneurysm is symptomatic, >5.5 cm diameter, or increased size >0.5 cm in six months

Aneurysm Classification by Shape	
True aneurysm - Two shapes: Saccular and fusiform	Bulging of the entire vessel wall with all layers (tunica intima, media and adventitia)
False aneurysm	Leakage of blood from a vascular leak with hematoma formation, later organization of this hematoma into a new false lumen next to that vessel

Radiology:

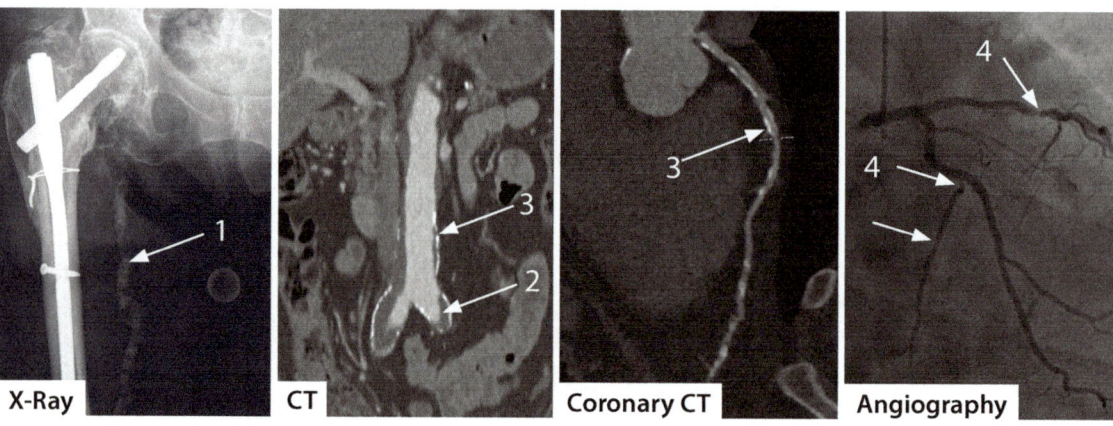

X-Ray | CT | Coronary CT | Angiography

General: Plaques can be classified by composition, degree of stenosis and morphology. The plaque may be calcified (>130 HU), partially calcified, or noncalcified, and the plaque surface can be smooth, ulcerated or ruptured. Stenosis is classified according to the percentage of luminal narrowing.

Ultrasound: For evaluation of plaque and measurement of blood flow. Lipids are seen as hypoechoic or isoechoic tissue changes; calcifications are hyperechoic.

X-Ray: Calcified plaques[1] can be observed as dense tubular tissues.

CT angiography: For evaluation of stenosis, search for occlusion, and search for collateral blood supply. Lipid rich plaques are more hypodense <30 HU than thrombotic plaques[2], while calcifications[3] are hyperdense; arteries tend to be stenotic or aneurysmal.

MRI: Can be used for plaque characterization and stenosis assessment, but yields lower resolution.

Angiography: Identification of stenosis[4] and treatment via angioplasty, with or without stenting.

Vascular Pathology and Myocardial Infarction

Entity: 6.2 Atherosclerosis (Coronary Artery Disease)
Stain: Hematoxylin - Eosin

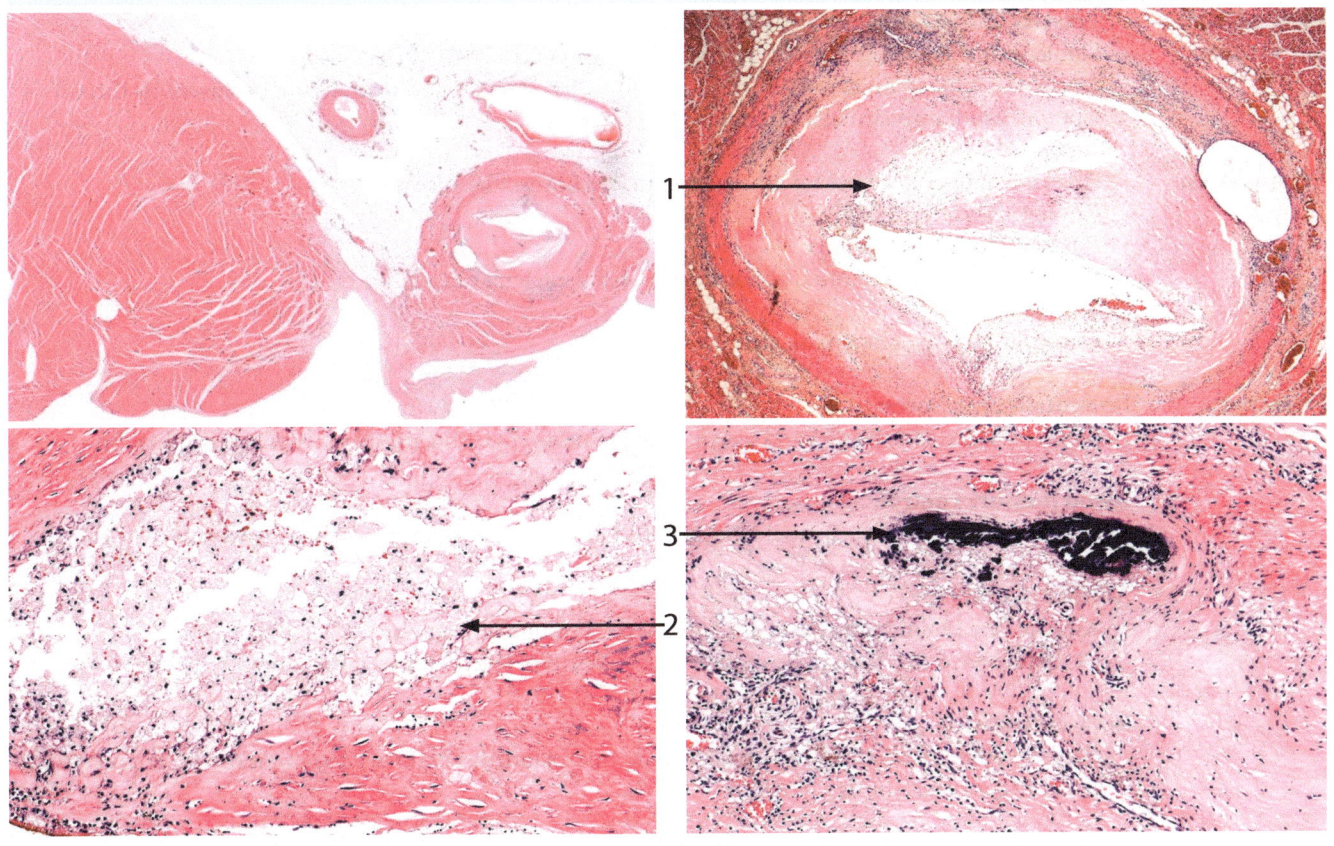

Macroscopy: Coronary artery with fixed narrowing of the lumen (stenosis)

Microscopy: Tissue/organ: Coronary arteries
- Lumen narrowed, rarely can be totally occluded[1]
- Microscopic findings of plaque, with thickened intima, fibrous cap overlying lipid core.
- Coronary sclerosis: Focal lipoid plaques that can be detected over shorter or longer distances with foam cells[2], Atheroma beds, possibly with ulceration and possibly additional thrombosis, fibrosis roses, calcifications[3]
- concentric or eccentric coronary sclerosis
- If in association with myocardial infarct, may see plaque with overlying thrombus → complete occlusion

Definition: **Coronary artery disease (CAD):** A subsequent process of narrowing with later on occlusion of the coronary arteries most often related to atherosclerotic changes

Etiology/Pathogenesis: See aortic chapter above regarding lipid deposition and plaque formation
- As stenosis increases, blood flow decreases, may yield symptoms of ischemia (angina, myocardial infarction)
- 70-75% stenosis considered a "critical stenosis" with risk to the myocardium
- 50% narrowing of the left main is a also a significant stenosis
- Rupture of plaque exposes lipid core → extremely thrombogenic

Clinical Info/Symptoms:
- Myocardial ischemia may cause:
- Discomfort in chest, epigastrium, jaw, shoulder
- Symptoms of ischemia can occur during rest or stress/exercise
- Symptoms may be aggravated with increased levels of stress (physical)
- Symptoms rapidly subside when returning to rest

6 Vascular Pathology and Myocardial Infarction

Entity: 6.2 Atherosclerosis (Coronary Artery Disease)
Stain: Hematoxylin - Eosin

Clinical Info/Symptoms:
- Less than 70-75% stenosis likely asymptomatic
- Stable/typical angina (pain with activity): corresponds to 70-90% stenosis
- Unstable angina (pain at rest): corresponds to >90% stenosis and/or transient occlusion by thrombus
- Complication: myocardial infarction

Diagnostics:
- Assessment of risk factors for atherosclerotic cardiovascular disease
- Resting and exercise ECG
- Pharmacological stress tests
- ECHO (regional wall motion abnormalities, left ventricular function)
- CT angiography
- Coronary angiography if indicated

Therapy:

Preventative measures:
- Blood pressure control, diet and weight loss, smoking cessation, exercise, cardiac rehabilitation

Blood pressure control:
- Beta-blockers, Calcium channel blockers, ACE inhibitors, nitrates for angina symptoms

Antiplatelet therapy:
- Aspirin, P2Y12 inhibitors (such as Clopidogrel, Prasugrel, ticagrelor)
- Dyslipidemia: Statin therapy to reduce LDL cholesterol levels (simvastatin, atorvastatin etc.)

Revascularization:
- Cardiac catheterization with stent placement = percutaneous coronary intervention (PCI), coronary artery bypass graft surgery (CABG)

Radiology:

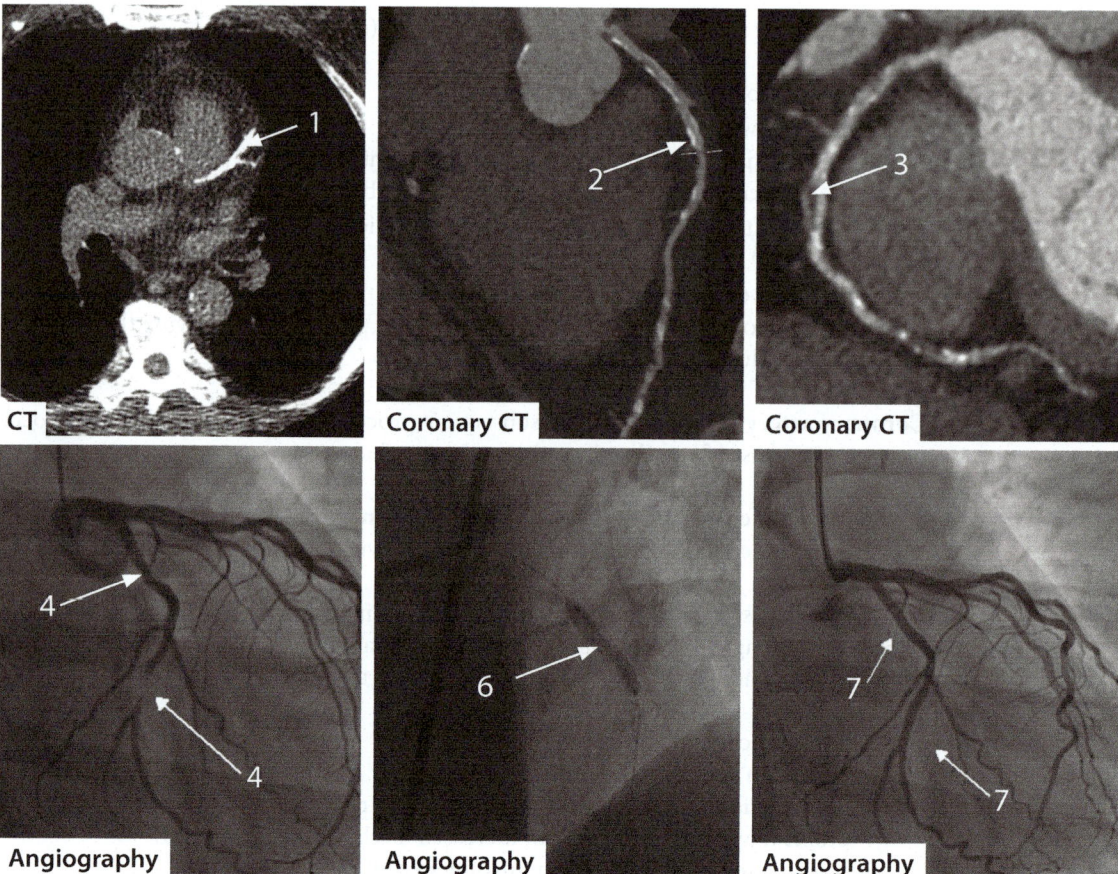

CT | Coronary CT | Coronary CT
Angiography | Angiography | Angiography

Vascular Pathology and Myocardial Infarction

Entity: 6.2 Atherosclerosis (Coronary Artery Disease)
Stain: Hematoxylin - Eosin

CT angiography: Identifies vascular calcifications[1], calcified[2] or non-calcified plaques[3], and stenosis[4].

Coronary Angiography: Enables identification of coronary artery stenosis[5], treatment of the stenotic vessels (thrombectomy, angioplasty[6], stenting), and post-interventional visualization of the treated vessels[7]

Coronary Artery Disease-Reporting and Data System (Cad-Rads) Classification:
Plaque types: Calcified (>130 HU on non-enhanced CT), partially calcified, non-calcified

Scoring degree of stenosis:
- Cad-Rads 0: No stenosis
- Cad-Rads 1: 1-24% stenosis, or plaque without stenosis
- Cad-Rads 2: 25-49% stenosis
- Cad-Rads 3: 50-69% stenosis
- Cad-Rads 4A: 70-99% stenosis
- Cad-Rads 4B: >50% of left main, or three vessels >70%
- Cad-Rads 5: 100% stenosis/total occlusion
- Cad-Rads N: Non-diagnostic study

Modifiers:
- N: not all segments >1.5 mm are diagnostic
- S: presence of stents
- G: coronary artery bypass grafts
- V: if two or more vulnerable features are present

Vulnerable plaque features:
- Low-attenuation3: Density <30 HU
- Remodeling present: Outward distension of the vessel wall at plaque site with preservation of lumen
- Spotty calcification: calcifications < 3 mm
- Napkin-ring sign: High-risk plaque feature; central low-attenuation area adjacent to lumen with higher "ring-like" attenuation surrounding it

6 Vascular Pathology and Myocardial Infarction

Entity: 6.3 Cystic Medial Degeneration/Necrosis
Stain: Hematoxylin - Eosin

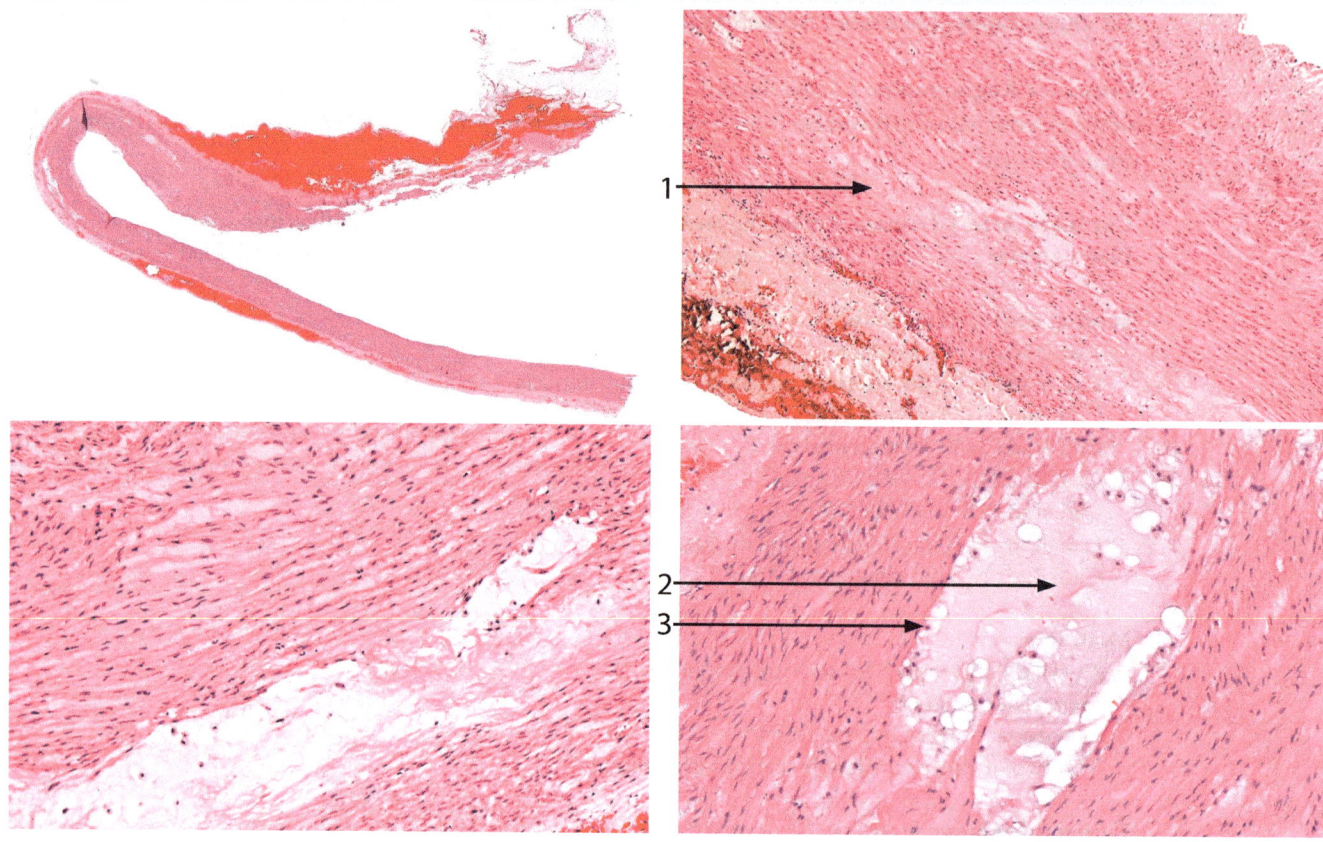

Macroscopy: Subtle change; may be widened lumen

Microscopy: Tissue/organ: Aorta
- Disorder of the tunica media with tissue degeneration[1]
- Some dropout of muscle cells with increased matrix material[2]
- May see foam cells (lipid-laden macrophages)[3]
- Fragmentation of elastic fibers on elastic stain
- No inflammation

Definition: **Cystic medial degeneration** (a misnomer, not technically cystic): Fragmentation of elastic fibers and smooth muscle of the tunica media in large arteries; aorta often affected

Etiology/Pathogenesis:
Causes of cystic medial degeneration: Most often idiopathic, but also connective tissue disorders such as Marfan's or Ehlers-Danlos syndromes
Cause of aortic dissection: Presence of precursor vascular abnormality (cystic medial degeneration or connective tissue disorder); blood enters wall via nick in the intima, enters weakened media and dissects longitudinally along it; aided by hypertension

Clinical Info:
Aortic dissection as a complication:
- Risk factors: Systemic hypertension (the #1 risk factor for dissection), cystic medial degeneration and/or connective tissue disease (Marfan's syndrome, Ehlers-Danlos syndrome), also arteriosclerosis, aortitis, vasculitis, trauma,
- Most often found in ascending aorta (65% of cases), descending (20%), abdominal (10%), aortic arch (5%)
- Dissection may extend backwards into pericardial sac, resulting in tamponade

Vascular Pathology and Myocardial Infarction

Entity:	6.3 Cystic Medial Degeneration/Necrosis
Stain:	Hematoxylin - Eosin

Classification of Dissection According to Location		
DeBakey I (60%)	Stanford A	Both ascending and descending aorta
DeBakey II (15%)	Stanford A	Ascending aorta only
DeBakey III (25%)	Stanford B	Descending aorta only
Mnemonic for DeBakey classification: BAD B: Both ascending and descending aorta (type I) A: Ascending aorta (type II) D: Descending aorta (type III)		

Symptoms: Sudden tearing pain in chest/back, abdominal pain
Pain may migrate as dissection extends along vessel

Diagnostics: Computer tomography (CT), Magnetic resonance imaging (MRI), Transthoracic echocardiography (TTE), Transesophagea echocardiography (TEE), Abdominal ultrasound, Intravascular ultrasound

Therapy: Blood pressure management, control hemodynamics, surgical or endovascular stent-graft repair

Radiology:

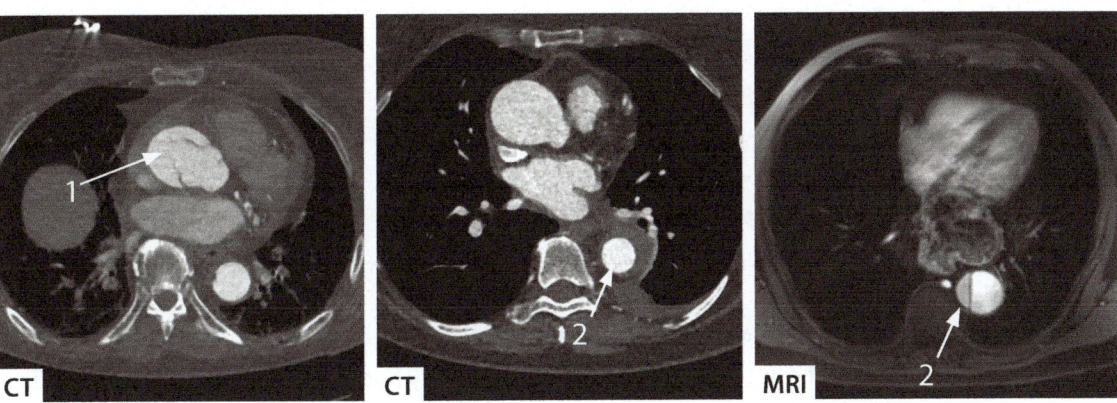

General: Aneurysms can be devided in three groups.
- Aneurysma Verum (True Aneurysm): Outpouching or dilatation of all three layers of an artery. The resulting arterial shape is mostly fusiform or saccular.
- Aneurysma Dissecans (Dissecting Aneurysm): The intimal layer is dissected from the other layers due to an arterial wall defect or trauma. A distinctive double lumen appearance is seen when contrast is applied. In the process of dissection sometimes a hyperdense wall hematoma is seen.
- Aneurysma Spurium (False Aneurysm): Resulting from a defect in the arterial wall, blood escapes into surrounding tissues but is confined by perivascular tissue. Continuous flow between the artery and the pseudoaneurysm prevents the blood or hematoma from clotting.

CT: Preferred modality, CT scans with arterial contrast phase effectively detect and categorize aneurysms. Dissecting aneurysms, characterized by a distinctive double lumen and floating membrane, are classified using Stanford and DeBakey criteria based on their origin (aortic root, ascending aorta[1], aortic arch, or descending aorta[2]). CT scans provide insights into the extent of dissection, organ perfusion, and guide surgical decisions. Control CTs for size measurement of aneurysms can be done with or without contrast.

MRI: Primarily used for assessing arterial walls, particularly in conditions like vasculitis. Additionally, MRI serves as a radiation-free alternative.

6 Vascular Pathology and Myocardial Infarction

Entity: 6.4 Myocardial Infarction
Stain: Hematoxylin - Eosin

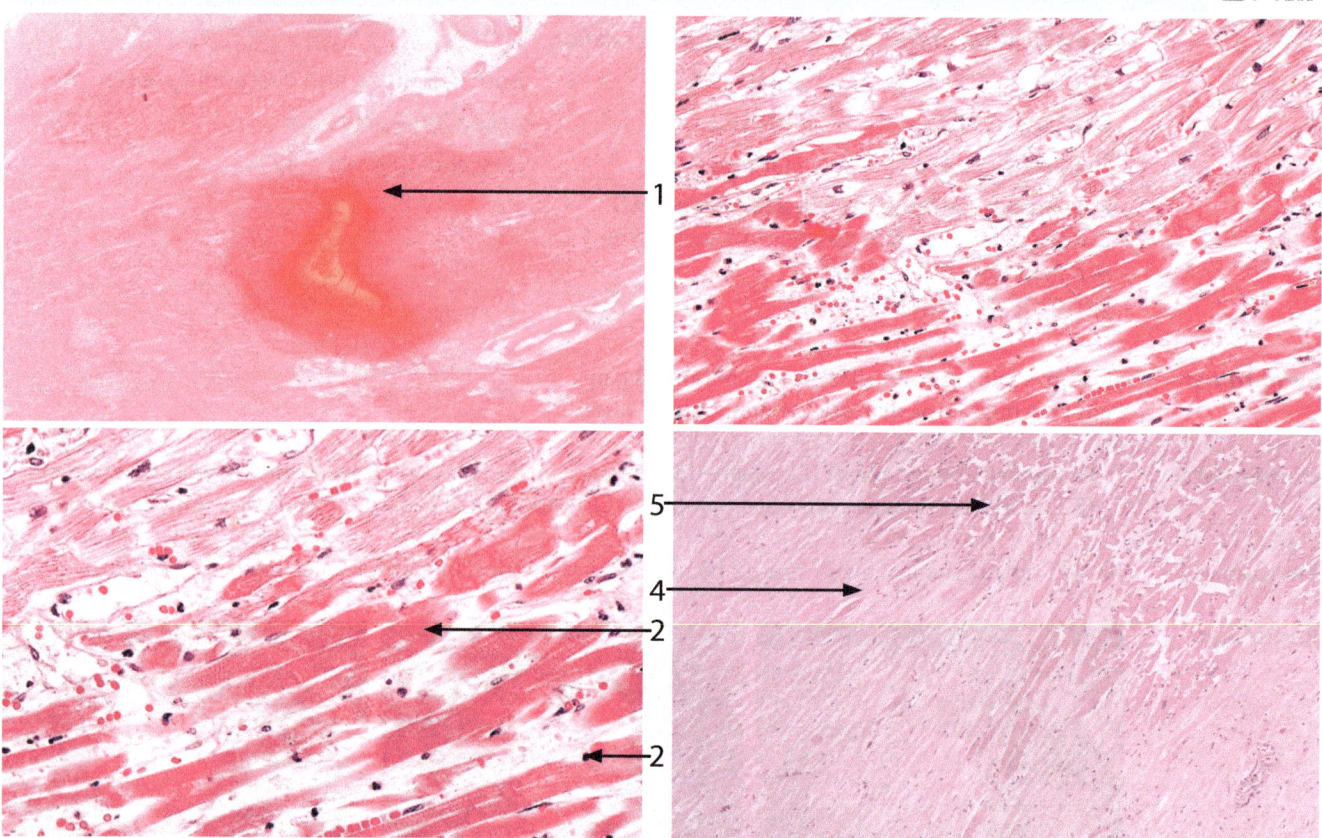

Macroscopy: Initially soft and red, then very soft and yellow-tan with red borders, eventual fibrous scar

Time Since Infarct	Gross Findings
Up to 12 hours	No gross findings (may find occluded coronary artery)
12-48 hours	Reddened, soft, or bruised in region of infarct
2 days - 7 days	Increasing yellow tinge to infarct, with hyperemic (red) edges. Around 6-7 days maximally yellow-tan, very soft
1 week - 1 month	Increasingly white-tan with fibrous texture
1 month - decades	Mature white-tan scar formed, is permanent and inert

Microscopy: Organ/tissue: Heart/myocardium

Acute Phase:
- Area of infarct hemorrhagic and brightly eosinophilic[1]
- Cardiac myocytes undergo coagulative necrosis, show total loss of cytoplasmic striations[2], nuclei faded and lost, cytoplasm eosinophilic with homogenous texture
- Neutrophils[3] (small cells with dark, segmented nuclei) infiltrate the area of infarct

Healed/Scar:
- Collagen/fibrous connective tissue[4] (area of prior infarct)
- Residual viable cardiomyocytes[5]

Vascular Pathology and Myocardial Infarction

Entity:	6.4 Myocardial Infarction
Stain:	Hematoxylin - Eosin

Interval post-MI	Histopathologic Changes
1 hour	Subtle myocardial edema
4 hours	Early coagulative necrosis of the myocardium; myocytes show loss of cytoplasmic striations, homogenous eosinophilic cytoplasm, faded nuclei
4-8 hours	Early infiltration by neutrophils, coagulative necrosis continues
24 hours	Extensive coagulative necrosis, full infiltration by neutrophils
3 days to 1 week	Numerous macrophages, early vascular proliferation/granulation tissue
1 week - months	Progressive fibrosis with scar formation

Definition: Obstructed blood supply, with ischemic insult and necrosis of affected myocardium

Etiology/Pathogenesis:
- Lack of blood flow is most often due to coronary artery atherosclerosis
- Acute event is plaque rupture and development of occluding thrombus
- May evolve from unstable angina
- Involvement of regions containing the conduction system may result in arrhythmias
- Full-thickness myocardial wall infarct → STEMI (ST-elevation myocardial infarction)
- Partial-thickness infarct → NSTEMI (non-ST-elevation myocardial infarction)

Clinical Info/Symptoms: Chest tightness, chest pain with referral (retrosternal > left chest > left arm > left shoulder > neck, jaw, back > epigastric region), dyspnea, diaphoresis, or "atypical symptoms" of nausea/vomiting, heartburn/indigestion (atypical symptoms frequently seen in women)

Diagnostics: ECG, Troponin, CK-MB/total CK ratio, ECHO, coronary angiography, cardiac CT

Therapy: MONA-LYSE (Morphine, Oxygen, Nitroglycerin, Aspirin, Lysis/stent)
Dual antiplatelet therapy (DAPT) after stent placement with a combination of aspirin + P2Y12 inhibitor (Clopidogrel, ticagrelor, prasugrel)

Radiology:

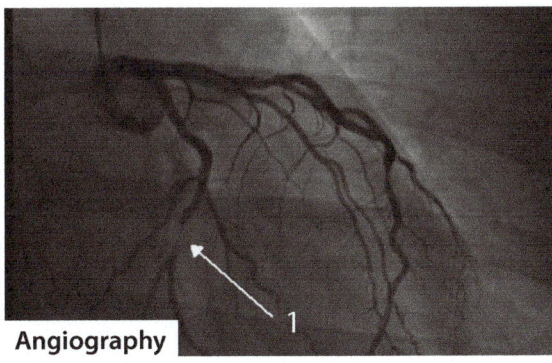
Angiography

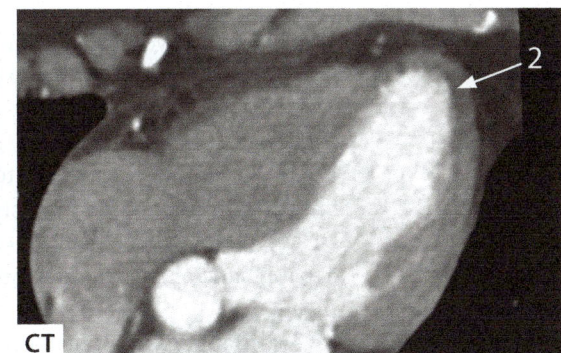
CT

6 Vascular Pathology and Myocardial Infarction

Entity: **6.4 Myocardial Infarction**
Stain: *Hematoxylin - Eosin*

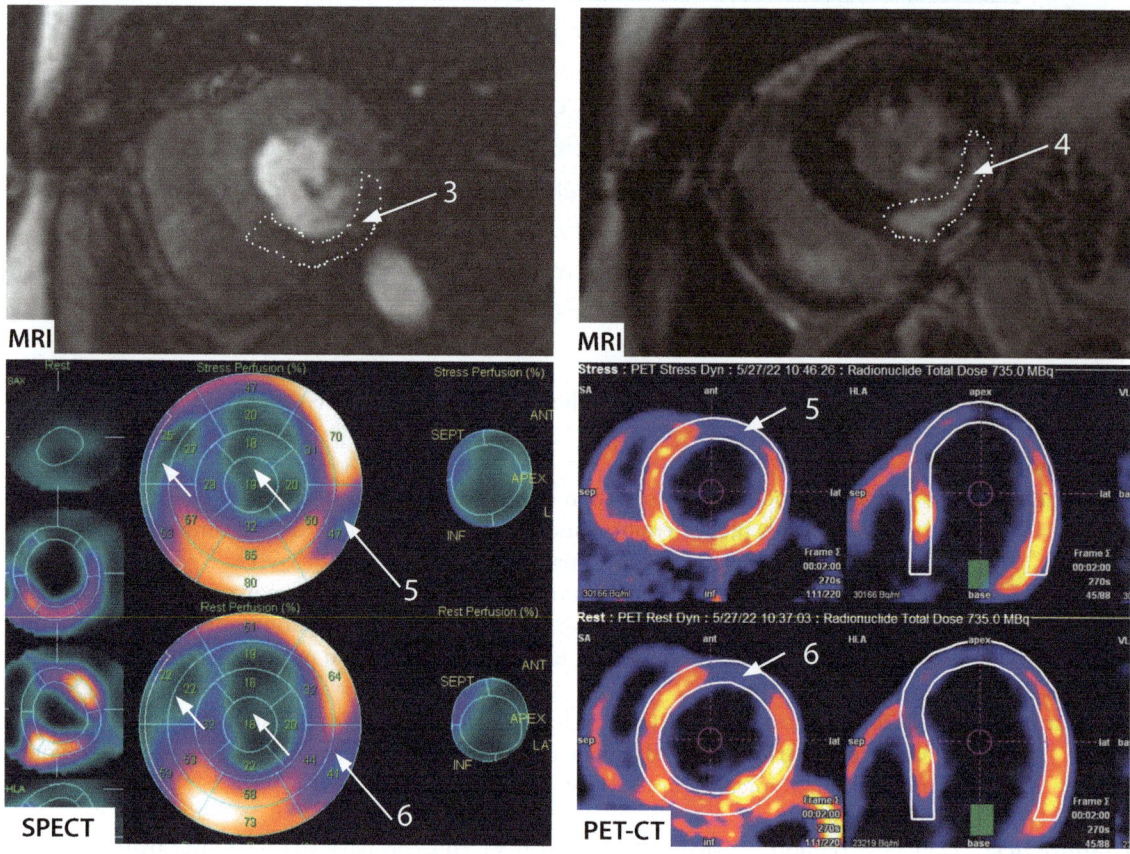

General: Patients with risk factors and atypical symptoms are often evaluated using non invasive techniques like CT, MRI, SPECT or PET-CT. In acute STEMI, minimally invasive angiography is often used to spot the occluded or stenosed vessel and treat the vessel by angioplasty (and stenting).

Angiography: Method of choice in the diagnosis and treatment of acute STEMI or elective in other stenosis. Stenosis[1] is best assessed using multiple angles of the c-arm.

CT: Dynamic myocardial perfusion imaging can be used to quantify myocardial perfusion but is quite dose intensive and rather rarely used. Sometimes hypodense subendocardial hypoperfusion[2] can be seen in standard CT.

MRI: Cine sequences are used to evaluate myocardial motion. T1 perfusion imaging (first-pass images) while contrast administration shows hypoperfused myocardium[3] as hypoenhancing areas. Delayed myocardial enhancement imaging 10 minutes after gadolinium contrast administration shows hyperenhancing myocardial fibrosis[4] with loss of volume.

Myocardial SPECT: Evaluation of myocardial perfusion and viability
Stunned myocardium: Wall dysfunction but normal perfusion (resting and stress)
Myocardial ischemia: Decreased stress perfusion but normal rest perfusion. These patients will benefit from treatment.
Hibernating myocardium: Decreased rest and stress perfusion. Myocytes are still viable and will benefit from revascularization.
Myocardial infarction: Absence of stress[5] and rest[6] perfusion. No benefit from revascularization.

PET-CT: Rubidium-82 (Rb-82) is used for evaluation of myocardial perfusion and viability like myocardial SPECT. Its unique feature is the measurement of the coronary flow reserve.

Immunopathology

Nora Lamp, Annette Zimpfer, Jao Ou, Samantha Scetta, Ricky Grisson, Andreas Erbersdobler

7.1 **Bronchial Asthma**

7.2 **Rheumatic Myocarditis**

7.3 **Lymphocytic Thyroiditis (Hashimoto's Thyroiditis)**

7.4 **Graves' Disease**

7.5 **Temporal/Giant Cell Arteritis**

7.6 **Vascular Rejection of Kidney Transplant**

7 Immunopathology

Innate and adaptive immunity are two broad categories of immune response against infection. Innate immunity generates an inflammatory response, triggered by activation of cellular receptors (e.g. Toll-like receptors) against microorganisms and cell injury byproducts, leading to downstream biochemical cascades of cytokine release, complement activation, and interferon release (the latter in response to viral infections). Innate immunity also provides activating signals to the adaptive immune system, which has the capacity to develop memory and specificity against new foreign antigens.

Two types of adaptive immunity involve B lymphocytes (humoral immunity with soluble antibody production) and T lymphocytes (cellular immunity that activates direct killing or phagocytosis). Circulating antibodies are produced by B lymphocyte-derived plasma cells and consist of a four-chain immunoglobulin molecule (see Figure "Immunglobulin Structure") containing two identical heavy (H) chains and two identical light (L) chains. An antibody's function and immunoglobulin isotype is determined by the combination of light chains (kappa or lambda) and heavy chains (five types: IgA, IgD, IgE, IgG, IgM, see table below for summary of structure and function). Antigens bind at unique antigen–binding sites in the variable (V) regions of the Fab portion of an antibody, which allows for combinatorial diversity and target specificity. The subsequent functionality of an antibody is dependent on the Fc region which interacts with cell surface receptors or complement protein (e.g. C1q) to ultimately trigger "effector" functions ranging from antibody-dependent cell-mediated cytotoxicity and antibody-dependent cellular phagocytosis to immune modulation and direct viral neutralization.

In contrast, T lymphocytes generate specificity to foreign antigens through two types of T cell receptors (TCRs) which associate with transmembrane proteins to form a TCR complex that is needed for MHC antigen recognition. Different types of T cells recognize different MHC antigens; cytotoxic T cells recognize MHC Class I, while helper T cells recognize MHC Class II. Helper T cells also contribute to humoral immunity by helping to activate plasma cells for antibody production.

Immunoglobulin Overview

Immunoglobulin (Ig) Type	Structure	Location	Function	Clinical Relevance
IgM	Pentamer	Predominately in blood and lymph	Evidence of recent infection First Ig to be formed	- Blood group antibodies - Early immune reaction - Waldenstrom's macroglobulinemia
IgG	Monomer	Most abundant Ig in blood Can cross the placenta	Delayed formation during infection Fixes complement Opsonization of bacteria	- Rhesus antibodies - Late immune reaction - Hypersensitivity: Type II/Type III
IgA	Monomer/Dimer	Mucosal surfaces and in body fluids, most abundant Ig in tissues	Prevents pathogens from binding to mucus membranes	- Celiac disease - IgA deficiency - Peyer's patches
IgE	Monomer	Lungs, skin, mucus membrane	Binds to mast cells and releases histamine Binds to basophils	- Type I hypersensitivity reaction mediator - Recruits eosinophils
IgD	Monomer	Small amounts in blood	Not completely understood	Not completely understood

Immunopathology

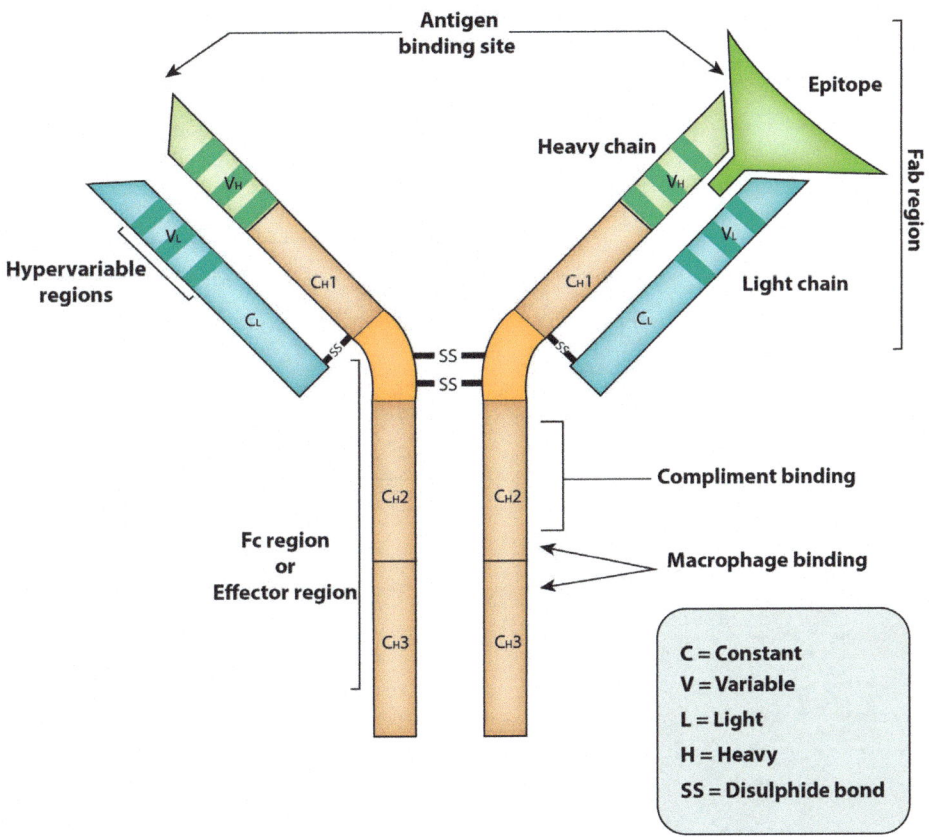

Hypersensitivity Reaction			
Immunological Mediator	Autoantigen	Mechanism	Associated Syndromes
Type I Hypersensitivity			
IgE	Soluble antigen	Mast cell degranulation Histamine release Inflammatory mediators	- Anaphylaxis - Hay Fever - Food & Drug allergies - Asthma
Type II Hypersensitivity			
IgG, IgM, Complement	Cell bound antigen	Cell destruction mediated by antibody and complement leading to epitope spreading	- Autoimmune hemolytic anemia - Autoimmune thrombocytopenic purpura - Acute rheumatic fever - Grave's disease - Myasthenia gravis
Type III Hypersensitivity			
IgG	Soluble antigen	Antigen-Antibody complexes are deposited in tissues, activating complement chain, and resulting in inflammatory response	- Mixed essential cryoglobulinemia - Systemic lupus erythematosus
Type IV Hypersensitivity			
T Cells	Cell bound/ Soluble antigen	Antigen presenting cells activate cytotoxic T cells, recruiting macrophages and releasing inflammatory cytokines	- Rheumatoid arthritis - Multiples sclerosis - Hashimoto's disease - Insulin-dependent diabetes mellitus

7 Immunopathology

Entity: 7.1 Bronchial Asthma
Stain: Hematoxylin - Eosin

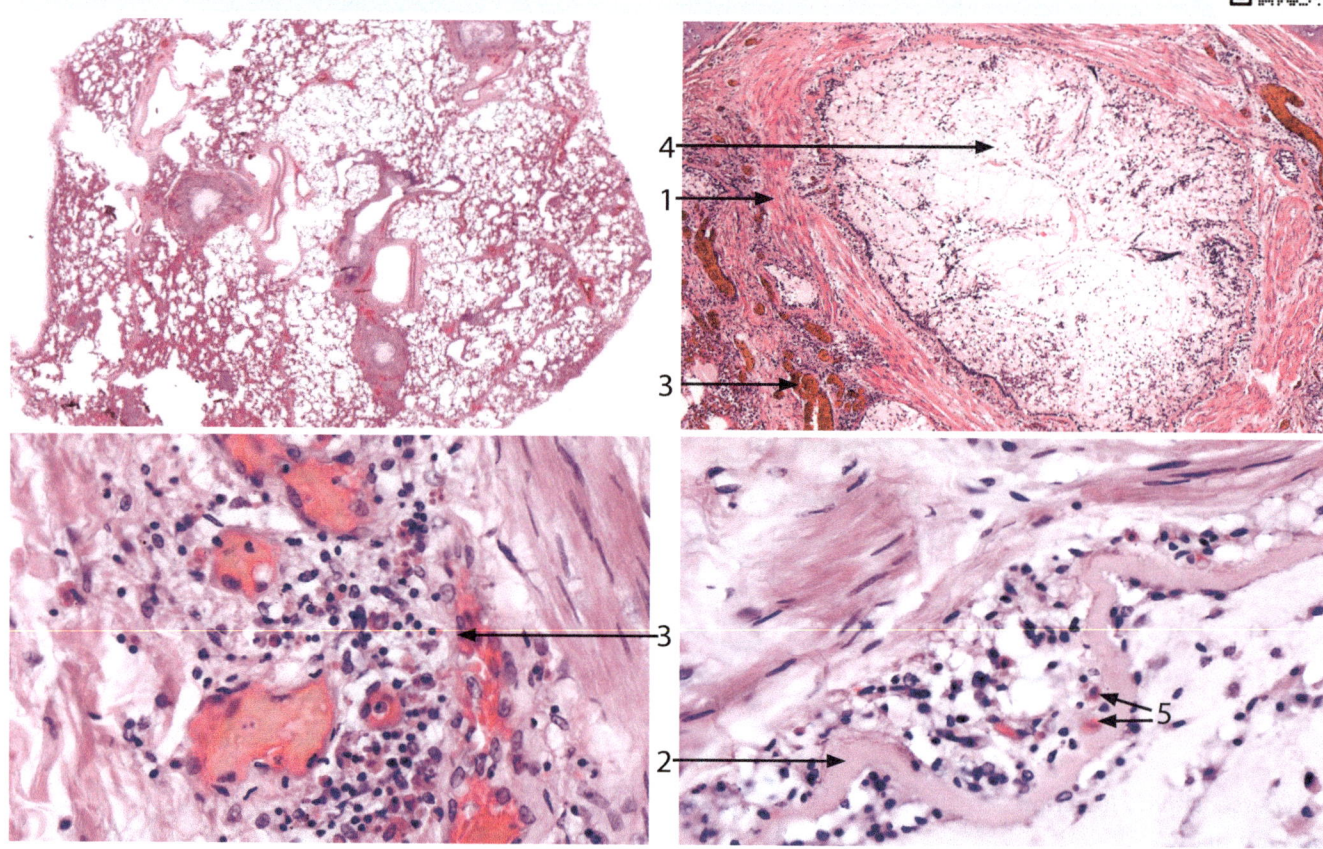

Macroscopy: Overinflated, distended lungs in severe and fatal asthma (status asthmaticus), occlusion of the airways by thick and tough mucus plugs

Microscopy: Tissue/organ: Lungs
  - Thickening of bronchi and bronchioles due to hypertrophy and/or hyperplasia of the bronchial wall smooth muscle[1]
  - Increase in bronchial glands size, and number of goblet cells (goblet cell metaplasia) of the epithelium, sub-basement membrane fibrosis/thickening[2], increased vascularity[3] (see left lower picture)
  - In acute exacerbation, intrabronchial mucus plugs[4], edema, and bronchoconstriction lead to lumen obstruction
  - Variable number of eosinophils in mucosa and submucosa[5]
  - In cytology bronchoalveolar lavage (BAL) specimens find:
  - Spiral-shaped mucus plugs detached from subepithelial mucous glands of the bronchi (Curschmann spirals), variable number of eosinophils, Charcot-Leyden crystals (crystalline needle-like precipitates originating from submerged eosinophils)

Definition: **Asthma:** A chronic respiratory disease caused episodically by an immunological response associated with reversible bronchial obstruction via chronic inflammation and increased mucus production, and increased sensitivity of the airways to a variety of stimuli

Types of Asthma:
  - Atopic asthma: Classic example of IgE-mediated (type I) immediate hypersensitivity reaction
  - Drug-induced asthma: E.g. uncommon aspirin-sensitive asthma, associated with recurrent rhinitis and nasal polyps
  - Occupational asthma: May be triggered by fume inhalation, e.g. plastics, wood, toluene, include type I hypersensitivity reaction

Immunopathology

Entity:	7.1 Bronchial Asthma
Stain:	Hematoxylin - Eosin

Etiology/Pathogenesis:
Allergic extrinsic/atopic bronchial asthma:
- IgE-mediated (type 1) hypersensitivity reaction, high prevalence in childhood, industrialized nations
- Triggers can be divided into seasonal (pollen, mold) or non-seasonal (dust mites, animals, fumes)

Non-allergic intrinsic/non-atopic bronchial asthma: Infections (esp. viral), inhalative noxae (fumes), cold air, reflux, stress/exercise-induced asthma, aspirin, NSAIDs

Clinical Info/Symptoms:
Chronic cough, dyspnea, expiratory wheezing, humming, chest tightness, symptoms can be worsened when exposed to certain triggers such as allergen, stress or exercise

Diagnostics:
Anamnesis, physical exam, lung function tests (f.e. spirometry)
- Spirometry: Measurement of FEV1 (Forced expiratory volume in one second)
  FVC (Forced vital capacity)
  Reduced FEV1/FVC ratio (normal range for adults > 0.75, children >0.9)
- Peak flow meter: Measurement of peak expiratory flow (PEF)
- Bronchial provocation tests: methacholine, mannitol
- Bronchodilator responsiveness: Symptoms can be reversed when inhaling corticosteroids
- Allergy tests
- Severity assessment accordingly to required treatment level to gain symptom control and reduce asthma exacerbations, classified in mild, moderate and severe asthma

Therapy:
- Treatment based on severity, different levels of therapy

Medications:
- SABAs = Short-acting beta-agonists (bronchodilator): salbutamol, fenoterol, terbutalin
- LABAs = Long-acting beta-agonists (bronchodilator): salmeterol, formoterol
- ICS = Inhaled corticosteroids: budesonide, fluticasone
- LAMAs = Long-acting muscarinic antagonists: Tiotropiumbromid, ipratropium bromide
- LTRA = Leukotriene receptor antagonist: Montelukast
- Anti-IL-5-Ab: Mepolizumab, Reslizumab, Anti-IgE-Ab: Omalizumab
- Milder symptoms (less than twice/month): initially controlled with ICS
- Symptoms > twice/month: ICS plus SABA
- For more severe symptoms: Combinations of ICS and LABA

Radiology:

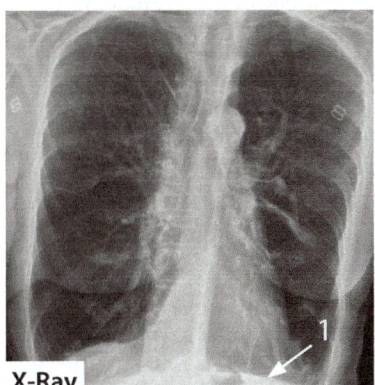
X-Ray

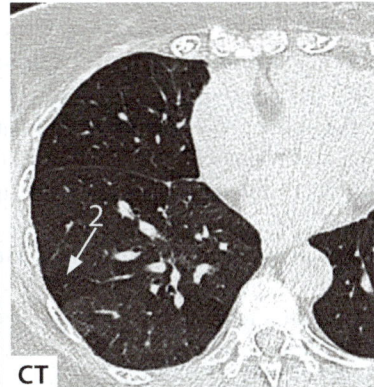
CT

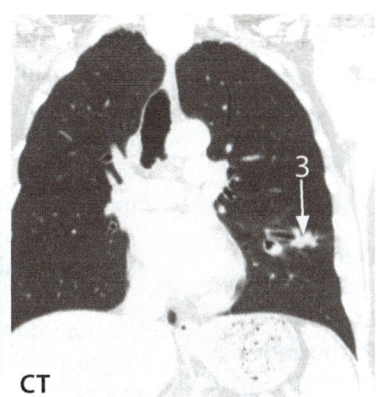
CT

General: Majority of patients without significant radiologic abnormalities. Primary purpose of imaging: Evaluation for complications, in particular, allergic bronchopulmonary aspergillosis (ABPA)

Chest X-Ray: Signs of hyperinflation with flattening of diaphragmatic contours (marked displacement below level of heart (frontal projection)[1], abnormal depth of retrosternal clear space (lateral projection)

CT: Air trapping[2] presents as accentuated areas of lucency intermixed with normal lung (which is slightly increased in density during the expiratory phase. Mucoid impaction with density filling in branch airway[3] and bronchiectasis with wall thickening may be seen among the more characteristic findings in ABPA.

7 Immunopathology

Entity: 7.2 Rheumatic Myocarditis
Stain: Hematoxylin - Eosin

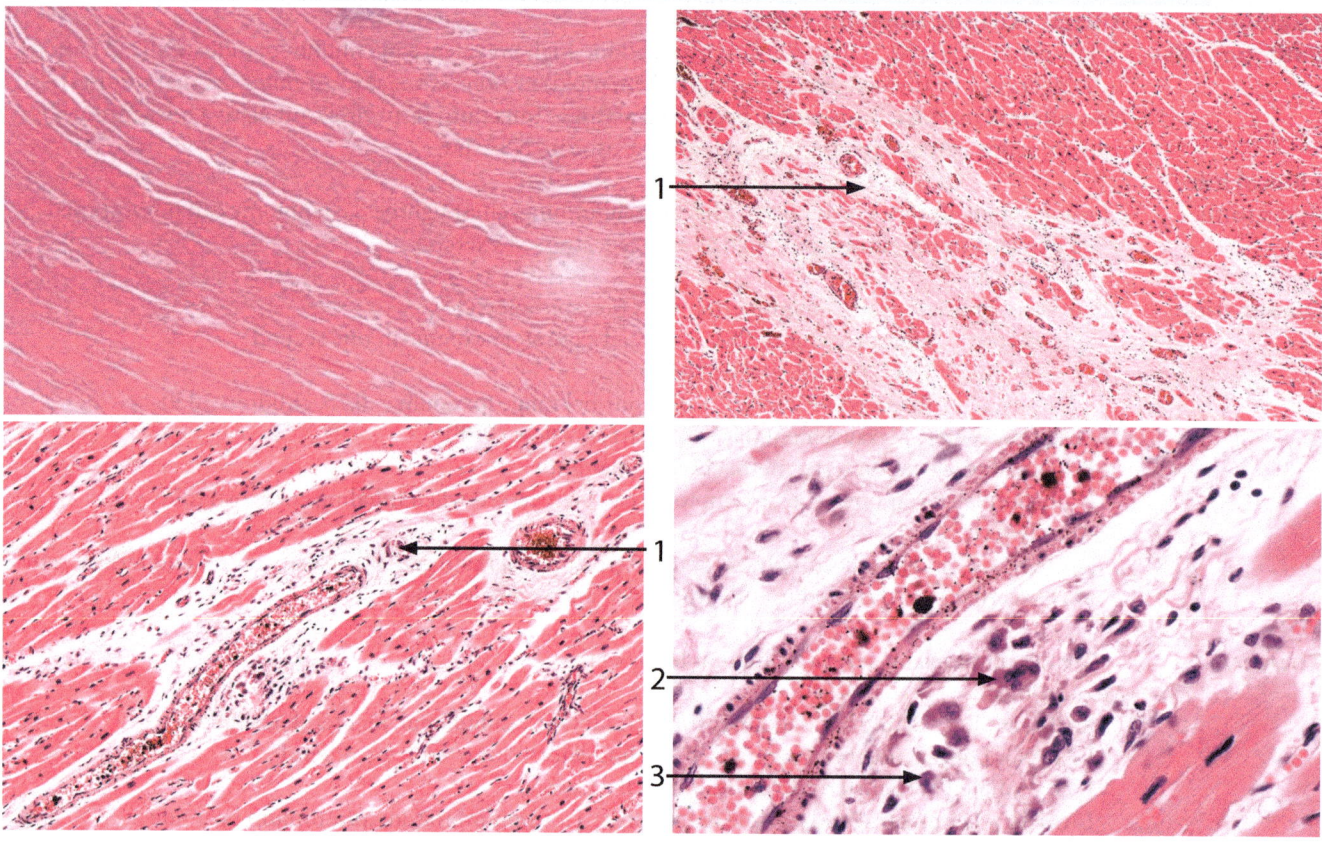

Macroscopy: Chronic myocarditis: defect-healed/defective tissue repair with dilatation of the usually hypertrophic heart chambers, small disseminated gray-white scars

Microscopy:
- Tissue/organ: Myocardium
- Distinct myocardial vascular-associated loose accumulations of inflammatory cells (Aschoff nodules)[1]
- Aschoff nodules with plump-looking activated macrophages (Aschoff giant cells)[2]
- Aschoff giant cells: Can be mono- or multinucleated
- Anitschkow cells[3]:
- Macrophages with bar-shaped condensed chromatin (owl eyes or caterpillar nucleus)
- Scattered lymphocytes (T-lymphocytes) and isolated plasma cells
- Final stage (not shown): Interstitial scarring, minimal inflammatory infiltrate

Definition: Poststreptococcal (rheumatic fever) immune-mediated myocarditis

Etiology/Pathogenesis:
Most commonly associated with:
- Streptococcal pharyngitis (strep throat)
- Infection with group A β-hemolytic streptococci → molecular mimicry → auto-antibodies react against bacterial antigens → cross-reaction with myocardial antigens (Hypersensitivity reaction type II - antibody-mediated) → immune-mediated inflammation of the myocardium and endocardium (including heart valves)
- Other immune-mediated reactions: postviral, systemic lupus erythematosus (SLE), drug hypersensitivity (e.g. methyldopa, sulfonamides), transplant rejection

Immunopathology

Entity:	**7.2 Rheumatic Myocarditis**
Stain:	*Hematoxylin - Eosin*

Clinical Info/Symptoms:
Fever, decreased performance,
SPECK (S = subcutaneous nodes, P = polyarthritis, E = erythema annulare, C = chorea, K = carditis)

Cardiac complications: Heart failure, arrhythmia, valve damage (mostly mitral valve regurgitation)

Diagnostics:
- Jones Criteria (SPECCA (S = Subcutaneous nodules, P = Polyarthritis, E = Erythema annulare, C = Chorea, CA = CArditis)
- Antistreptolysin-O-Titer, Anti-Desoxyribonukleotidase B, anti-DNase B
- Electrocardiogram (ECG)
- Echocardiography (ECHO)

Therapy:
- Antibiotic therapy with penicillin V
- NSAIDs
- Glucocorticoids
- Surgical reconstruction/repair/replacement in the course of cardiac valve destruction

Radiology:

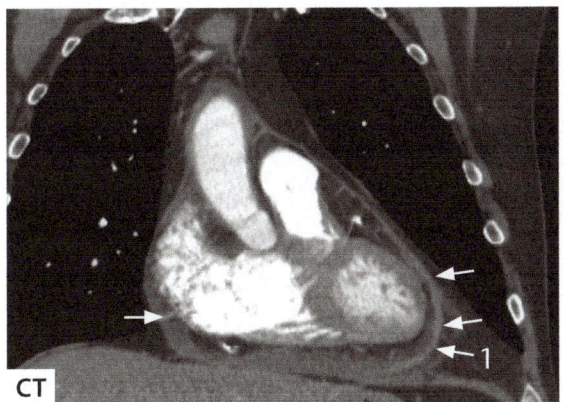
CT

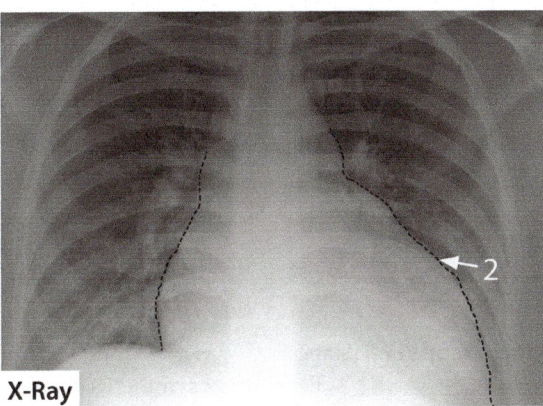
X-Ray

General:
- Radiologic findings depend on the stage of infection and location of involvement.
- In acute presentations, perimyocarditis may be indicated by presence of a pericardial effusion.
- Chronic damage can progress to a dilated cardiomyopathy

CT:
- Coronal cross-section shows abnormal pericardial thickening and enhancement due to exudative material[1]

Chest X-Ray:
- Enlarged silhouette of heart[2] (dominated by the left atrium and ventricle) with increased vascular markings from pulmonary edema

Immunopathology

Entity: 7.3 Lymphocytic Thyroiditis (Hashimoto's Thyroiditis)
Stain: Hematoxylin - Eosin

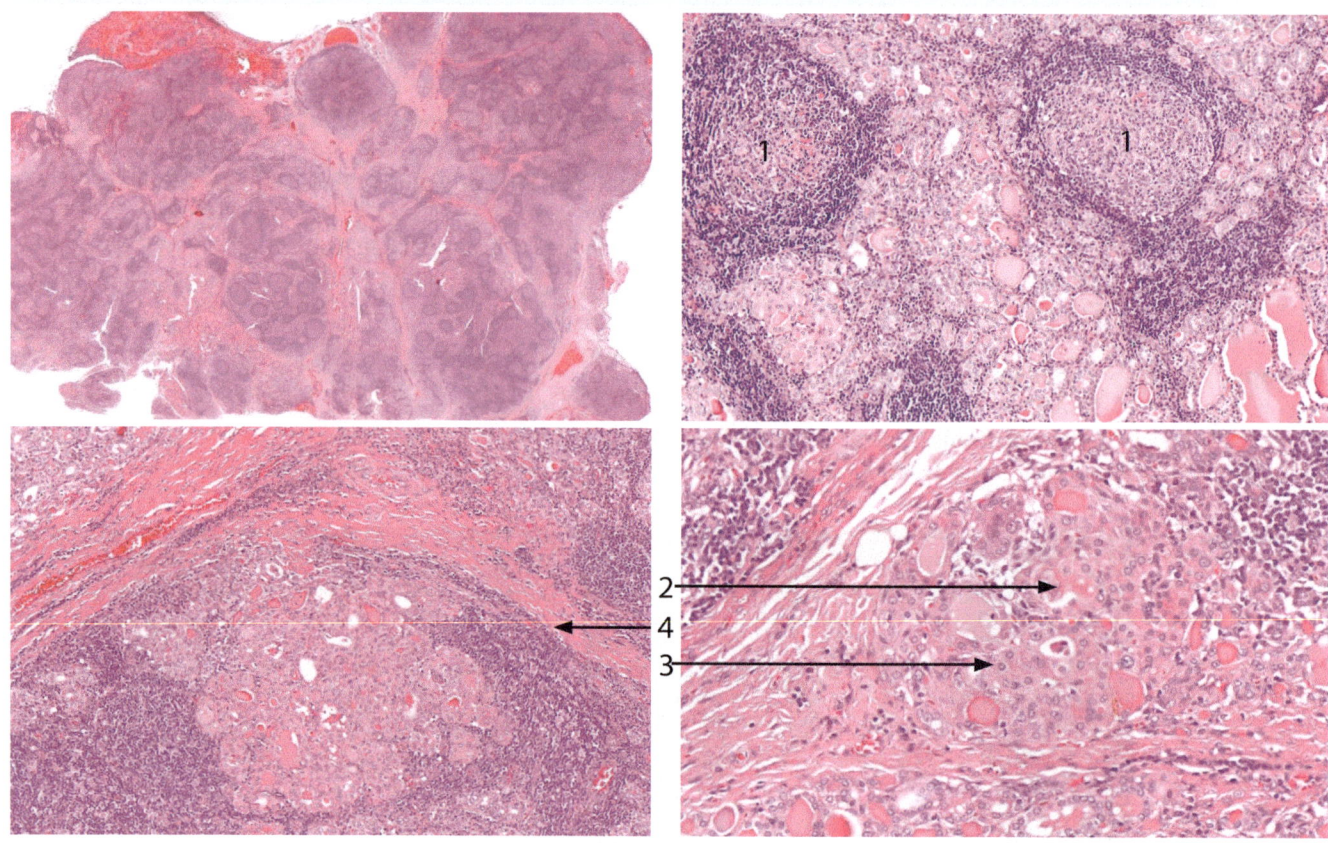

Macroscopy:	Stages: – Early stage: symmetrical enlargement (goiter, weight typically 40 g or more), cut surface beige or yellowish, firm (lymphoid tissue) – Later stage (elderly patients): atrophic, small thyroid, hard cut surface – Fibrous-atrophic variant: very small thyroid gland (1-6 g), firm cut surface, histologically extensive destruction of thyroid parenchyma with fibrosis
Microscopy:	– Tissue/organ: Thyroid gland – Extended nodular lymphoplasmacellular infiltrates with formation of secondary follicles[1] – Inflammatory permeation and destruction of thyroid follicles (colloid evident in lumen)[2] – Oxyphilic/oncocytic change can be seen in follicular cells (oncocytic metaplasia)[3] – Oxyphilic cells have reduced/no synthesis function of thyroglobulin – In the late stages, often fibrosis[4]/atrophy of thyroid gland
Definition:	Common organ-specific, antibody-mediated, inflammatory disease with formation of autoantibodies against thyroid antigens that alter thyroid function
Etiology/Pathogenesis:	– One of two major forms of autoimmune thyroiditis (along with Graves' disease) – Hashimoto's: most common form of thyroiditis, prevalence of 5-10% (f:m = 9:1), women between 30-50 years are often affected – Frequent association with other autoimmune diseases and certain HLA-markers (HLA-DR3, DR4, DR5), may be familial

Immunopathology

Entity:	7.3 Lymphocytic Thyroiditis (Hashimoto's Thyroiditis)
Stain:	Hematoxylin - Eosin

Clinical Info/Symptoms: Often asymptomatic in early stages, transient hashitoxicosis can occur, and later stages may evolve to hypothyroidism

Diagnostics: TPO antibodies (90%), Tg antibodies (50%), TSH, fT3, fT4, sonography

Therapy: L-Thyroxin Substitution

Radiology:

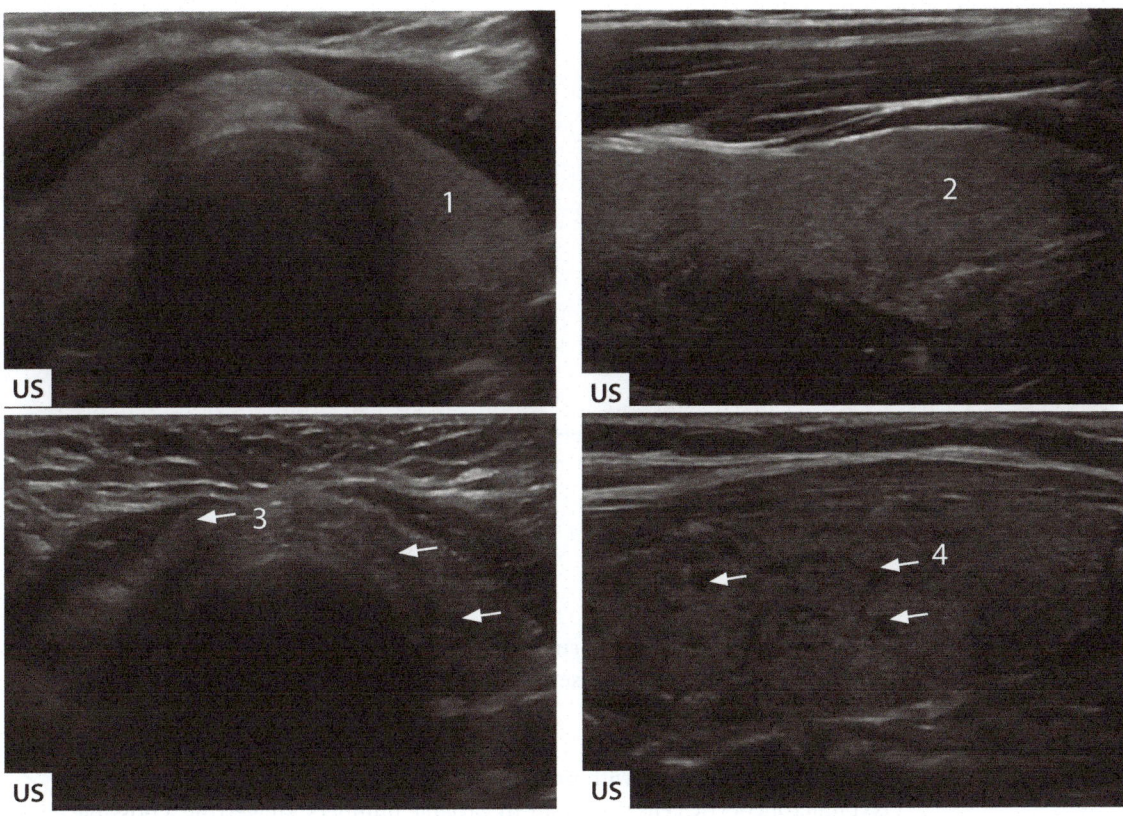

General:
- Features can vary widely depending on the severity and phase of disease
- Main utility of radiologic imaging (ultrasound) is for screening or surveillance of a discrete nodule
- Nuclear medicine studies (e.g. radioactive iodine and 18F FDG-PET) are not useful in this disease

Ultrasound:
- Normal thyroid: Homogeneous and smoothly marginated gland as seen in transverse[1] and sagittal[2] sections
- Hashimoto's thyroiditis: Can show diffuse heterogeneity[3,4]

7 Immunopathology

Entity: 7.4 Graves' Disease
Stain: Hematoxylin - Eosin

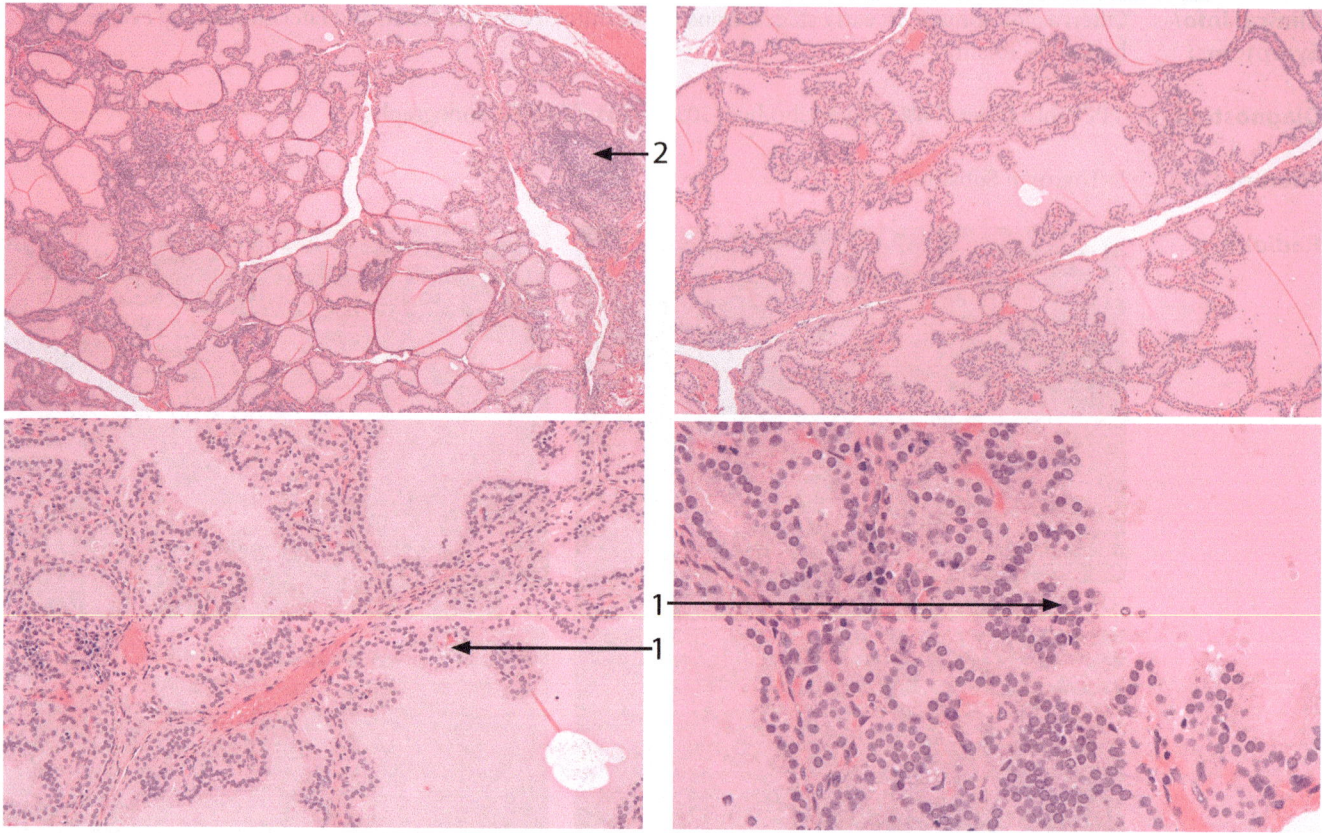

Macroscopy:	– Thyroid hyperplasia: the outer surface is hyperemic and swollen
	– Cut surface presents with diffuse enlargement with hyperemic ("juicy") appearance
Microscopy:	
	– Tissue/organ: Thyroid gland
	– Follicles are hyperplastic, with prominent papillary infoldings[1]
	– Oxyphilic/oncocytic cells can occur in variable numbers, suggesting a possible evolution toward Hashimoto thyroiditis
	– Aggregates of lymphoid tissue with germinal center formation[2] are found in the stroma
Definition:	– Most common cause of hyperthyroidism, resulting from overstimulation by autoantibodies against TSH receptor (TRAb)
Etiology/ Pathogenesis:	– One major form of autoimmune thyroid disease (the other being Hashimoto's thyroiditis)
	– Thyroid-stimulating immunoglobulins activate TSH receptors → overstimulation → overproduction of thyroid hormones → hyperthyroidism
Clinical Info/ Symptoms:	– Weight loss, muscle weakness, heat intolerance, irritability, fatigue, goiter, mostly increase in appetite
	– Children: most common cause of hyperthyroidism
	– Elderly patients: atrial fibrillation
	– Graves ophthalmopathy: autoimmune disorder of the periorbital tissue, exophthalmos occur in about 60% of patients with ophthalmopathy
	– Late clinical manifestation: localized dermopathy – pretibial myxedema and thyroid acropachy (swelling of extremities and clubbing fingers and toes caused by periosteal new bone formation)

Immunopathology

Entity:	7.4 Graves' Disease
Stain:	Hematoxylin - Eosin

Diagnostics:
- TSH levels decreased, T3/T4 levels increased, TRAb (TSH/Thyrotropin receptor antibody)
- Imgaing studies: Ultrasound, Scintigraphy with markedly increased uptake in radiotracers

Therapy:
- Beta-blockers (e.g. propranolol) for adrenergic symptom control (palpitations, tremor, anxiety)
- Antithyroid drugs: methimazole, propylthiouracil for pregnant patients during first trimester
- Radioactive iodine therapy
- Surgical resection

Radiology:

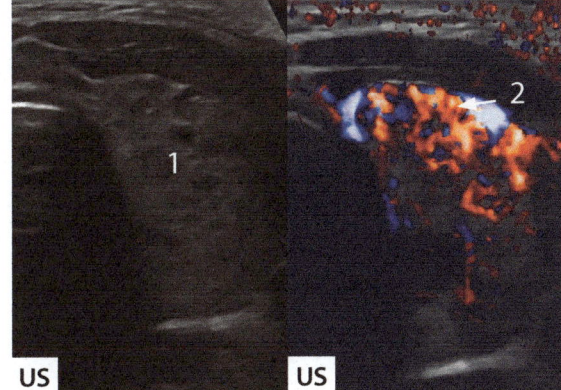
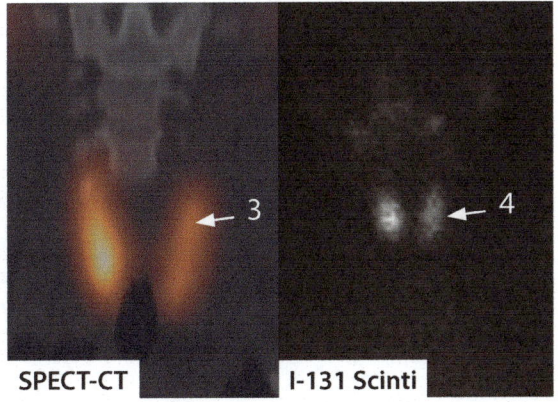

US | US | SPECT-CT | I-131 Scinti

Ultrasound:
- Heterogeneous and enlarged gland[1] with abnormally increased vascularity demonstrated by exuberant color Doppler signal[2] (see 7.3 for normal sonographic comparison)

Nuclear medicine:
- Evaluation by Tc-99m pertechnetate fused with SPECT-CT[3] and I-131 scintigraphy[4]:
Markedly increased uptake in radiotracers, allows for quantification of disease activity to calibrate dosages of radioactive iodine ablation therapy

	Mechanism	Symptoms	Laboratory Values	Therapy
Graves' Disease Hyperthyroidism: B and T mediated autoimmunity to the TSH receptor (TRAb) Excess stimulation and thyroid hormone production Type II Hypersensitivity	↑Thyroid function and growth	Goiter, weight loss, tachycardia, warm, moist skin, fine tremor	TSH↓ T4↑ TRAb↑ Anti-TPO and Anti-TG may be elevated	Beta blocker, Methimazole, Propylthiouracil (pregnancy), Radioiodine ablation, Surgical removal of thyroid gland
	Immune complex deposition	Pretibial myxedema		
	Cytokine release, inflammation	Graves' Ophthalmopathy		
Hashimoto's Thyroiditis Hypothyroidism: Autoimmune-mediated destruction of thyroid gland by B and T lymphocytes Development of Ab to thyroglobulin (Tg) and thyroid peroxidase (TPO)	Slowing of metabolism	Fatigue, bradycardia, cold intolerance, weight gain, constipation, cognitive dysfunction, can result in myxedema coma	TSH↑ T4↓ Anti-Tg Ab↑ Anti-TPO Ab↑	Levothyroxine
	Accumulation of matrix substance	Dry skin, hoarseness, edema (periorbital), puffy facies		

7 Immunopathology

Entity: 7.5 Temporal/Giant Cell Arteritis
Stain: Hematoxylin - Eosin

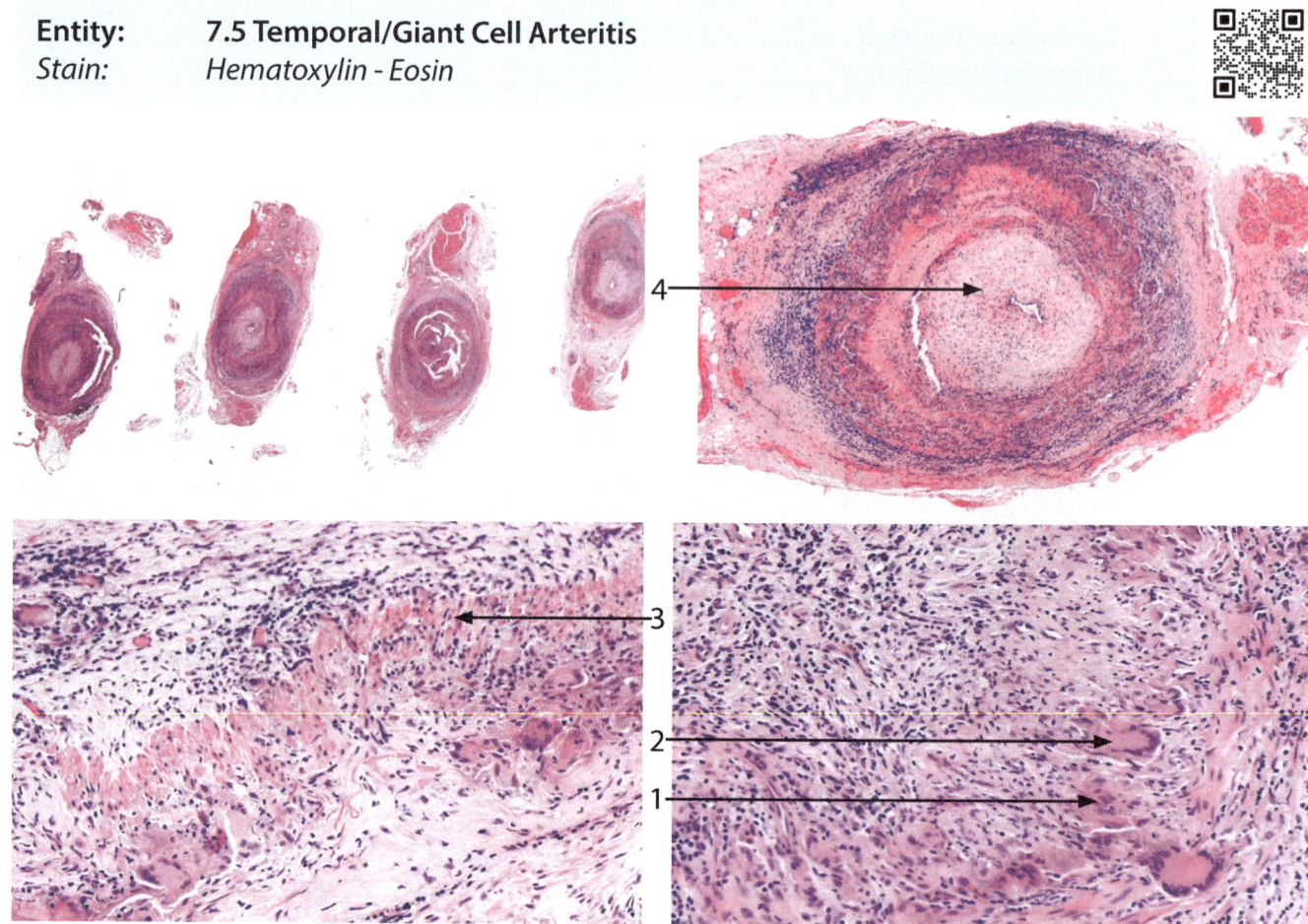

Macroscopy: Possibly abnormally tortuous, visible and firm temporal arteries

Microscopy: Tissue/organ: Artery, muscular type
- Partial fragmentation of the vascular wall of a medium-sized artery (artery: intima, media, adventitia) due to an inflammatory infiltrate that contains multinucleated giant cells[1], epithelioid cells, histiocytes, and lymphocytes mainly found at the intima/media border
- Multinucleated giant cells: Partly Langhans type[2] (contains nuclei arranged in a semicircle fashion), partly foreign-body type (disordered nuclei)
- Fragmentation[3], degeneration and dissolution of the internal elastic layer of the artery
- Intimal thickening and reduction of luminal diameter[4] (with possible thrombosis)
- Characteristic granuloma formation

Definition: **Vasculitis:** Inflammation of the blood vessels
Temporal giant cell arteritis (also called Horton's Disease): A chronic inflammatory disorder which may be caused by a T-cell mediated immune reaction against (uncertain) vessel wall antigens

Etiology/Pathogenesis:
- Mainly affects larger blood arterial vessels (e.g. temporal arteries, carotid arteries, aorta)
- The hypothesis of a cellular immune response is supported by the characteristic granulomatous inflammatory morphology and the prompt response to cortisone therapy.
- Vasculitis of large and medium-sized arteries, which most often involves the branches of the external carotid artery
- Blindness is possible if ophthalmic artery is affected
- Predominantly older women (75%) affected (most common form of vasculitis among older individuals in the United States)
- Risk increases with age

Immunopathology

Entity:	7.5 Temporal/Giant Cell Arteritis
Stain:	Hematoxylin - Eosin

Two pathomechanisms of primary vasculitis:
- Immune-mediated inflammation and invasion of the vascular wall by infectious agents; non-infectious vasculitis can also be triggered indirectly by pathogens (deposition of immune complexes in the vessel wall or cross-reactive immune reaction)
- Giant cell arteritis: presumably T-cell-mediated immune response against vascular antigens, evidence of anti-endothelial and anti-smooth muscle antibodies in 60% of patients, cellular immune etiology is supported by presence of characteristic granulomas

Clinical Info/Symptoms: Headache, tender hard superficial temporal artery, jaw claudication (discomfort/pain while chewing food), visual disturbances (double vision, vision loss)

Diagnostics: Duplex sonography, ESR with fall depression> 50mm / h, CRP, creatine kinase, no disease-specific fschen autoantibodies, sonography, biopsy (confirmation of diagnosis)

Diagnosis according to American College of Rheumatology criteria (3 criteria must be met)
- Age> 50 years
- New or changed headache
- Pressure pain port or hardened temporal artery
- ESR> 50 mm/h
- Biopsy: vasculitis with mononuclear or giant cell infiltration

Therapy: High dose of prednisolone even if suspected (acute), methotrexate or tocilizumab (chronic) Complication: Blindness in 20% of cases with involvement of the central retinal artery, (therefore it should be intervention with high-dose prednisolone for simultaneous changes in the visual field)

Radiology:

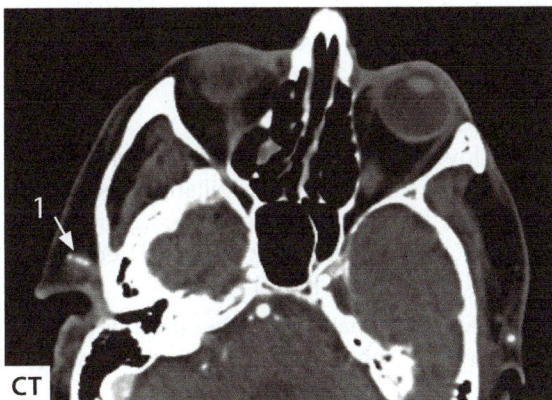
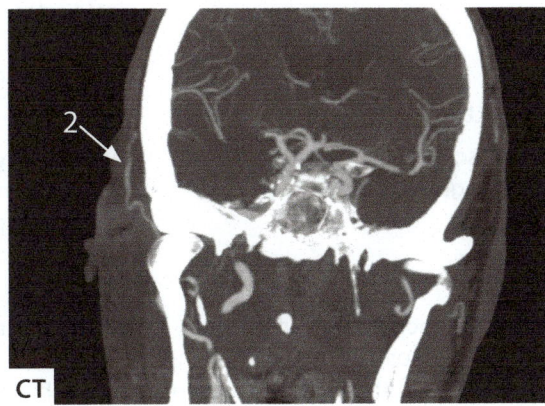

CT:
- Giant cell arteritis has a propensity for involving the superficial temporal artery.
- Inflammation is indicated by soft tissue density surrounding the vessels in their extraparotid courses over the zygoma[1] (normally, these areas should only have hypodense subcutaneous fat
- Abnormal irregular dilation of affected vessel is better depicted on a maximum-intensity projection reformat in the coronal plane[2] (same patient), focusing on the tortuous artery on the right

7 Immunopathology

Vasculitis, or inflammation of the blood vessel wall, can occur as part of another disease process (secondary vasculitis), or can occur as the primary etiology of a disease (primary vasculitis). The classification of primary vasculitides is frequently revised, but there are several classic primary vasculitides with stable definitions, and those will be addressed here. The most commonly encountered primary vasculitis is giant cell/temporal arteritis, and is presented as case 7.5. Of note, diagnosis is not made by histopathologic findings alone; patient demographics, clinical findings, and sometimes laboratory findings are needed to arrive at the correct diagnosis.

The primary vasculitides are generally classified by the size of the vessels involved. The three classic small vessel vasculitides do not show antibody deposition in the vessels, but patients' serum often contain Anti-Neutrophil Cytoplasmic Antibodies (ANCA), which cross-react with neutrophils' contents. Testing for these previously involved immunofluorescence microscopy studies, but typical laboratory serum testing for anti-PL3 and anti-MPO have now replaced visualizing ANCA.

Overview Vasculitis Types

Disease	Demographics	Clinical	Histology	Antibodies
LARGE VESSEL				
Temporal/giant cell arteritis	>50 yo	Headache, jaw pain, risk of blindness!	Branches of carotid (e.g. temporal artery); granulomatous inflammation	
Takayasu arteritis	<50 yo	Pulseless disease (weak upper extremity pulses)	Aorta and large branches, starts as inflammation of vasa vasorum, then into tunica media, tunica intima	
MEDIUM VESSEL				
Polyarteritis nodosa (PAN)	Adult	Wide variety of symptoms across organ systems, often spares lung, if kidney is involved the glomeruli are spared	Medium sized arteries; acute phase with polys and fibrinoid necrosis, segmental pattern (not entire circumference of vessel); eventual fibrosis	
Kawasaki disease	Children	Fever, rash, enlarged cervical nodes, erythema of oral mucosa, conjunctiva, palms and soles	Acute necrotizing vasculitis of the entire wall, tends to cause thrombi, can involve coronaries, risk of myocardial infarction!	
SMALL VESSEL				
Microscopic polyangiitis	Adults	Varied, many organs involved, including lung and kidney at capillary level	Arterioles, capillaries, venules; pulmonary capillaritis, necrotizing glomerulonephritis; neutrophil infiltration and fibrinoid necrosis, NO granulomas	Anti-MPO (p-ANCA)
Eosinophilic granulomatosis with polyangiitis	Adults with asthma/allergic rhinitis and peripheral blood eosinophilia	Varied, can involve many organs, including skin rash, GI bleed, glomerular sclerosis	Small vessels; neutrophils and fibrinoid necrosis eosinophils in vessel wall surrounding tissue	Anti-MPO (p-ANCA)
Granulomatosis with polyangiitis	Adults	Upper and/or lower respiratory tract symptoms, and glomerulonephritis	Triad often seen: -Respiratory tract (upper and/or lower) small vessel granulomatous vasculitis -Necrotizing granulomas in respiratory tract tissue -Glomerulonephritis	Anti-PR3 (c-ANCA)

While the small-vessel vasculitides in the table are "pauci-immune," with no antibodies detected within the vessel wall, small-vessel vasculitis can also be due to direct deposition of antibody complexes with resulting wall damage and inflammation. Increased circulating antibody complexes may be due to an autoimmune disease such as lupus and rheumatoid disease, or to a viral disease such as chronic viral hepatitis; these can produce a wide variety of symptoms. Henoch-Schonlein purpura, due to deposition of IgA complexes, favors the skin, joints, and kidneys, most often in children, and most often follows an upper respiratory tract infection.

Immunopathology

Entity:	7.6 Vascular Rejection Of Kidney Transplant
Stain:	Hematoxylin - Eosin

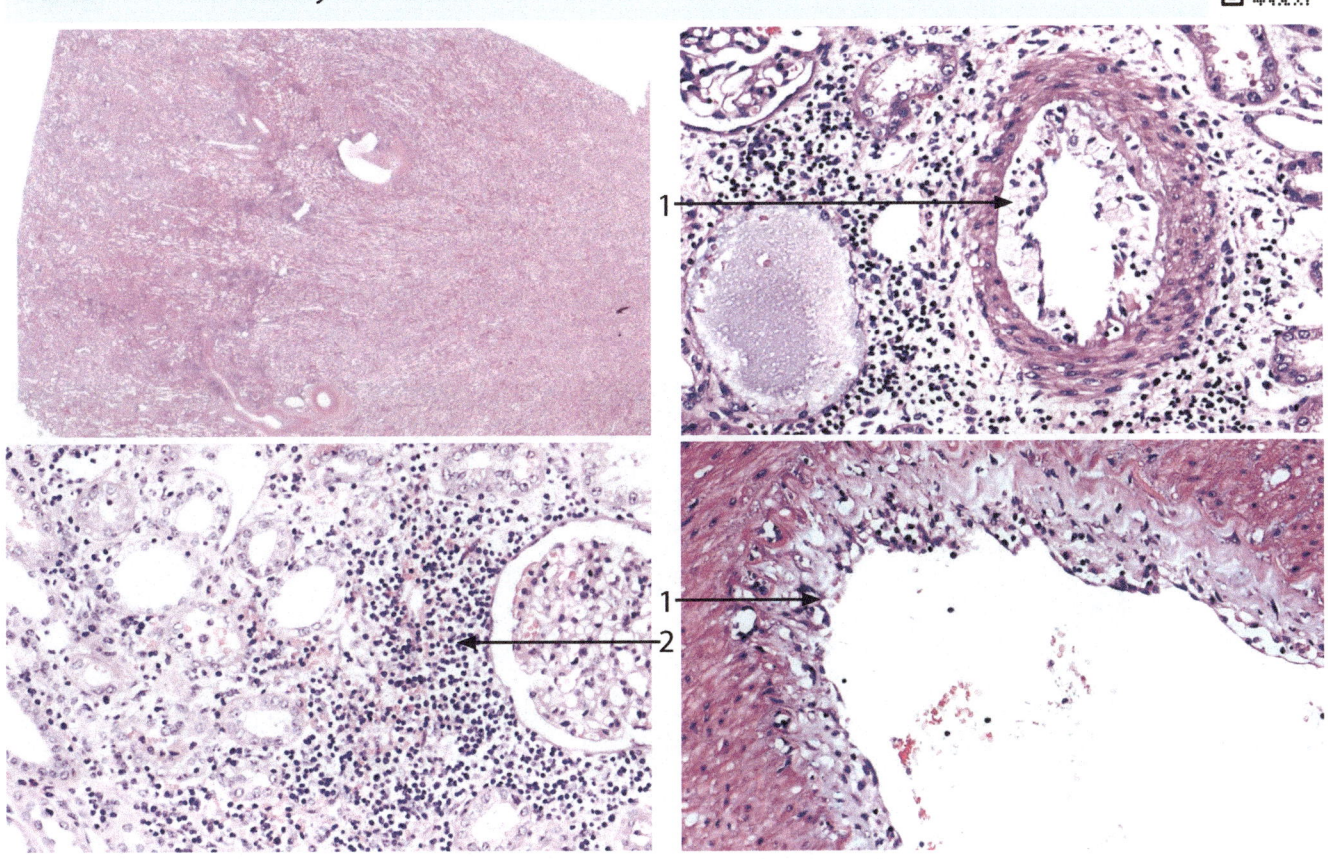

Macroscopy:	Kidney explant: in acute rejection, partly mottled, yellowish/reddish discolored kidney transplant, in vascular rejection often hemorrhagic geographic necrosis
Microscopy:	Tissue/organ: Kidney - Signs of vascular rejection in the renal parenchyma: - Inflammation of the blood vessels (endothelialitis) associated with - Swelling of the endothelium of small and medium-sized arteries, - Subendothelial foam cells[1] - Thickening (fibrosis) of the intima - Tubulointerstitial rejection (cellular rejection) with interstitial, mainly lymphocytic infiltrate[2] and inflammatory infiltrates in the tubules
Definition:	- **Organ rejection:** Immunological response leading to pathological changes in allograft; different rejection types (hyperacute, acute, chronic) - **Humoral rejection:** antibody-mediated (Type II hypersensitivity reaction); associated with hyperacute rejection (within minutes up to 48 hours post transplant) - **Cellular rejection:** T-lymphocytes (Type IV hypersensitivity reaction); associated with acute rejection (week to up to 6 months post transplant)
Etiology/ Pathogenesis:	- Chronic rejection characterized by both humoral and cellular immune responses - **Vascular rejection:** Rejection-induced intimal thickening by deposits of collagen I and III; varying degrees of intimal inflammation from absent to evident; T cell-mediated rejection or antibody-mediated rejection may underlie - **Tubulointerstitial rejection:** Lymphocytic inflammation of the parenchyma with tubulitis - **Glomerular rejection** (equivalent to arterial or vascular rejection): Glomerulonephritis may be T cell/antibody mediated

Immunopathology

Entity: 7.6 Vascular Rejection Of Kidney Transplant
Stain: Hematoxylin - Eosin

Clinical Info/Symptoms: Kidney transplantation: most common organ transplantation performed, as living and deceased donation performed, immunosuppressive therapy necessary to prevent a rejection reaction Rejection events: hyperacute (<hours), acute (days - weeks) or chronic (weeks - years)

Pain over the transplant (acute), continuous loss of organ functio

Diagnostics: Duplex sonography, hematology, urine sediment, biopsy

Therapy: Triple drug therapy with cyclosporine / tacrolimus, prednisolone, mycophenolate mofetil

Radiology:

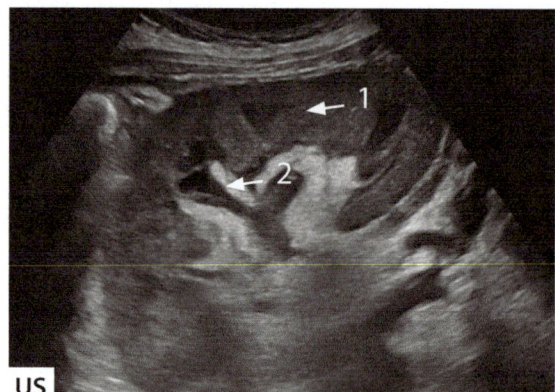
US

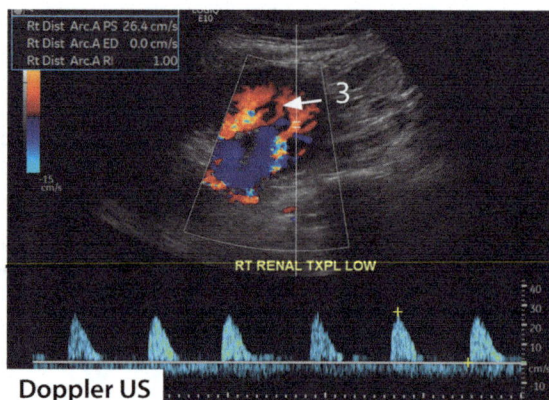
Doppler US

General:
Ultrasound routinely used for evaluation of renal transplant dysfunction; while numerous findings and hemodynamic parameters can be analyzed, no single abnormality is necessarily diagnostic
Ultrasound alos useful for pre-procedural planning to rule out relative contraindications (occluded vessel, severe hydronephrosis, or enveloping fluid collection)
Image-guided biopsies are performed for suspected rejection

Ultrasound (grayscale):
Increased echogenicity[1] of graft parenchyma and urothelial thickening[2] along the collecting system

Ultrasound (duplex Doppler)[3]:
Abnormal hemodynamic parameters such diminished diastolic flow and elevated intrarenal resistive indices (RI) greater than 0.7-0.8

Pathologic Regeneration
Shaolei Lu, Annette Zimpfer, Stephanie Barak, Jao Ou

8.1 Leukoplakia

8.2 Carcinoma in-situ and Squamous Cell Carcinoma of the Esophagus

8.3 Barrett's Esophagus

8.4 Barrett's Esophagus - Cancer (Adenocarcinoma)

8.5 Chronic Gastritis with Intestinal Metaplasia and Dysplasia

8.6 Cervical Intraepithelial Neoplasia, Grade 2-3

8 Pathologic Regeneration

Many tissues of the body are able to regenerate to replace cells that are lost or otherwise damaged. Epithelial tissues routinely regenerate, since they line surfaces of the body that are exposed to the external environment (e.g. skin, oral mucosa, lower gynecological tract) or harsh environments (e.g. gastric mucosa exposed to HCl). Regeneration of tissues requires cell division, and each time a cell divides, there is a risk of erroneous DNA replication. While there are robust, complex pathways within the cell that detect and repair DNA replication errors, excessive regeneration increases the likelihood of a DNA error being missed and passed on to daughter cells. This error may allow for other errors to go unchecked, and over time, the accumulation of these DNA errors may result in a malignancy.

Excessive cell replication and tissue regeneration is often seen when the tissue is exposed to unusually harsh environmental factors, or when a tissue is subject to a chronic and/or recurrent inflammatory response. In this chapter, we will review some examples of tissue regeneration that lead to a disease state. Additionally, we will review the course of human papilloma virus (HPV) infection; HPV is an environmentally-acquired, sexually-transmitted virus. Some HPV strains are considered high-risk; these take advantage of the regenerative properties of the stratified squamous epithelium of the uterine cervix, using the renewal of the epithelium to propagate and spread to other hosts

Concepts of Pathological Regeneration

Dysplasia:	A disorder of differentiation in tissues or organs **Congenital:** Abnormal development (e.g. cystic kidney dysplasia) **Acquired:** (Epithelial) anomaly of growth and maturation (e.g. cervical dysplasia, squamous epithelial dysplasia, described as as intraepithelial neoplasia)
Atypia:	Umbrella term for abnormal cellular features (see table below)
Metaplasia:	Conversion of a differentiated tissue into another differentiation pattern
Cervical Intraepithelial Neoplasia (CIN):	Abnormal growth with potential (facultative) precancerous transformation of cervical cells, synonymous with cervical dysplasia
Carcinoma in-situ (CIS):	Pre-invasive carcinoma, obligatory precancerous condition

Histological/Cytological Signs of Dysplasia (Architectural Disorder)	Features of Cytological Atypia
Irregular epithelial layer	Abnormal variation in cell size and shape
Loss of alignment of the basal cells	Increased nuclear to cytoplasmic ratio
Teardrop-shaped rete ridges	Atypical mitosis
Increase in the number of mitoses	Hyperchromasia of the nuclei
Premature keratinization in single cells (dyskeratosis)	Enlargement and polymorphism (anisonucleosis) of the nucleus
Keratin pearls within the rete ridges	Increased basophilia

Dysplasia (Based on the Example of Stratified Squamous Epithelium)

Mild dysplasia	Cellular atypia in the basal third of the squamous epithelium
Moderate dysplasia	Cellular atypia in the basal and middle third of the squamous epithelium, maturation of the upper third of the epithelium is intact
Severe dysplasia/ Carcinoma in-situ	Cellular atypia in the entire height of the squamous epithelium, but no evidence an invasion (i.e. breaking the basement membrane)
Invasive Carcinoma	Breakthrough of the basement membrane → carcinoma

Pathologic Regeneration

Entity:	8.1 Leukoplakia
Stain:	Hematoxylin - Eosin

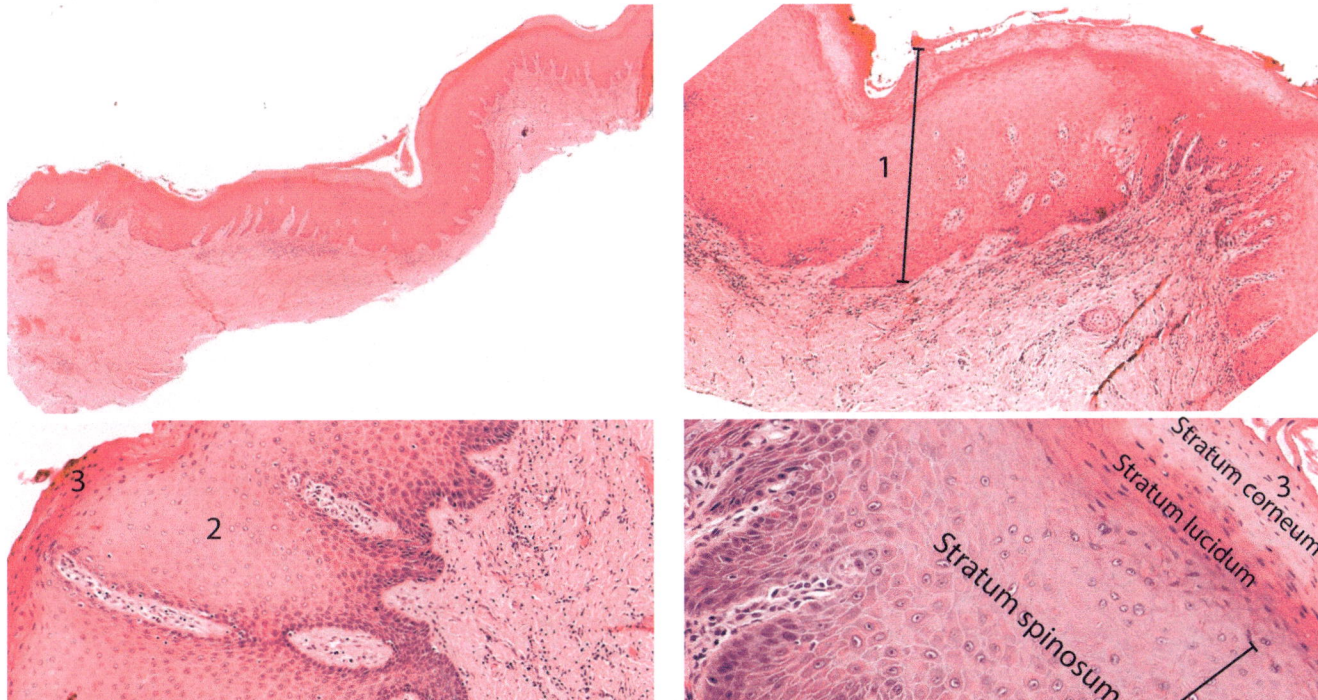

Macroscopy:	White, plaque-like changes on the surface of the mucous membrane that cannot be wiped away
Microscopy:	Tissue/organ: Non-keratinized squamous epithelium – Squamous epithelial hyperplasia (thickened epithelium)[1] – Acanthosis[2]: Thickening of the stratum spinosum layer – Hyperkeratosis: Keratinization of non-keratinizing squamous epithelium – Parakeratosis[3]: Nuclei are retained within the stratum corneum – No atypia or dysplasia present
Definition:	**Leukoplakia:** sharply defined, non-wipeable white area, typically in oral cavity (including tongue, lips) or in the genital area
Etiology/ Pathogenesis:	Risk factors: tobacco, alcohol, mechanical factors, vitamin deficiency, chronic infections, commonly associated with HIV; A precancerous lesion with possibility of regression or development into detectable dysplasia
Clinical Info:	Two clinical patterns for oral leukoplakia: – Homogeneous leukoplakia (uniform, flat appearance) – Non-homogeneous leukoplakia (irregular surface with eroded areas)
Symptoms:	Whitish plaque, cannot be wiped off
Diagnostics:	Clinical examination, brush biopsy, excisional biopsy (confirmation of diagnosis)
Therapy:	Excision in toto, laser, cryotherapy
Radiology	No specific radiologic manifestations of leukoplakia, more often an incidental finding that prompts assessment by direct visualization (i.e. endoscopy), or assessment for a mass lesion under the plaque

8 Pathologic Regeneration

Entity: 8.2 Carcinoma in-situ and Squamous Cell Carcinoma of the Esophagus
Stain: Hematoxylin - Eosin

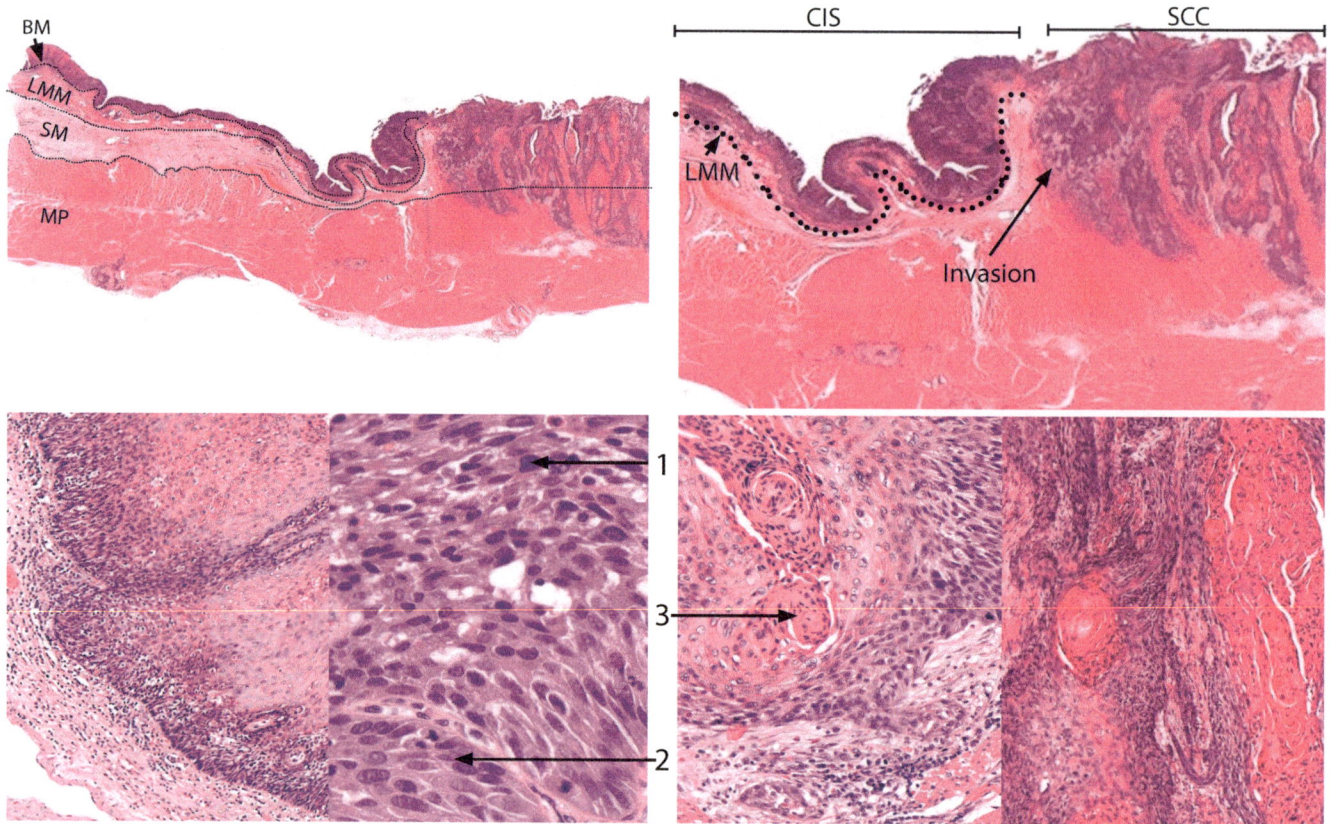

Macroscopy: Macroscopic appearance of esophageal squamous cell carcinoma varies depending on depth of invasion:
- Superficial carcinomas: Plaque-like, whitish thickening of the mucosa
- Deeply invasive/advanced carcinomas: Shows extension into/beyond the muscularis propria
- Polypoid/exophytic or ulcerating/endophytic masses

Microscopy: Tissue/organ: Esophagus

Squamous dysplasia and CIS:
- Severe cytologic atypia with increased nuclear:cytoplasmic ratio, nuclear and cellular pleomorphism[1]
- Loss of polarity; loss of maturation/cell stratification [2]
- Increased mitotic rate in basal layer, and mitoses seen in upper third

Transition to invasive squamous cell carcinoma:
- Basement membrane (BM) penetrated by tumor cell aggregates and/or single tumor cells, with focal keratinization (keratin pearls, typical of well-differentiated squamous cell carcinomas)[3]
- Ulcerating and endophytic carcinoma: tumor invading through muscularis mucosae (MM) into the submucosa (SM) and into the muscularis propria (MP)
- Tumor cells with glassy eosinophilic cytoplasm, sharp cell borders with intercellular bridges (squamous differentiation)
- Desmoplastic stromal reaction[5] with mixed inflammatory infiltrate

Definition: Esophageal malignancy, arising from squamous epithelium; characterized by a progression through multiple grades of dysplasia to invasive carcinoma

Etiology/ Pathogenesis: Smoking, ethanol etc. → dysplasia-carcinoma sequence (dysplasia → carcinoma in situ → carcinoma)
Other risk factors: Consumption of food that contains polycyclic aromatic hydrocarbons, hot foods, betel quid, radiation, achalasia, Fanconi anemia

Pathologic Regeneration

Entity:	8.2 Carcinoma in-situ and Squamous Cell Carcinoma of the Esophagus
Stain:	*Hematoxylin - Eosin*

Clinical Info/Symptoms: Range from asymptomatic to dysphagia, hematemesis, retrosternal pain, weight loss

Diagnostics: Esophagogastroduodenoscopy, endosonography, CT

Therapy: Endoscopic resection (≤ T1N0M0), neoadjuvant (radio) chemotherapy (≥T3), esophageal resection/esophagectomy + lymphadenectomy depending on the location

Radiology:

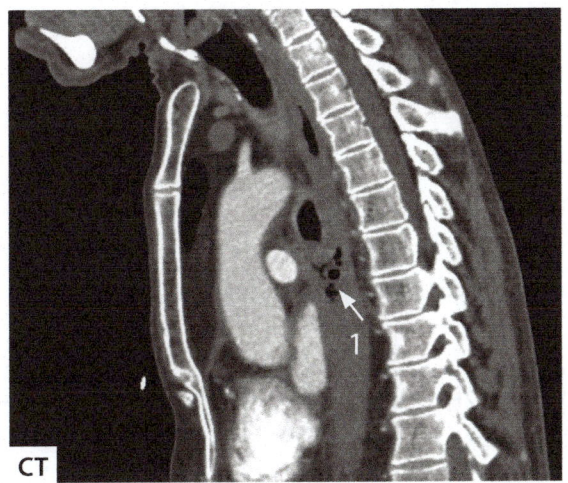

General:
- Majority of SCCs present radiologically as advanced lesions because the esophagus lacks a serosal barrier to prevent spread of tumor into the mediastinum and throughout chest and neck.
- The tracheobronchial tree is a particularly common site of invasion.

CT[1]:
- Note presence of bubbly air with no recognizable fat plane between the esophagus and trachea

8 Pathologic Regeneration

Entity: 8.3 Barrett's Esophagus
Stain: Hematoxylin - Eosin

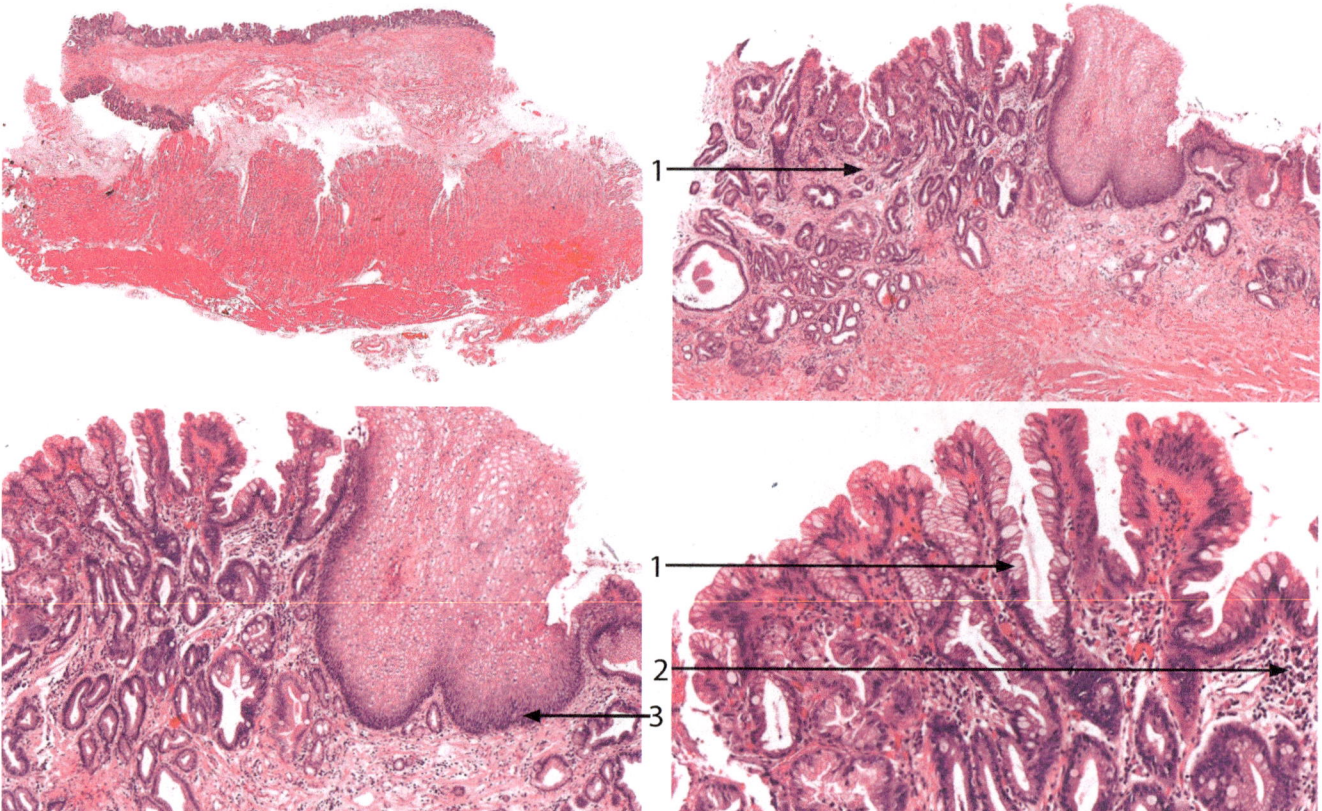

Macroscopy:	Reddish, salmon-colored, tongue-shaped mucosa with irregular borders surrounded by normal (white) squamous epithelium above the gastroesophageal junction (GEJ)
Microscopy:	Tissue/organ: Esophagus and gastroesophageal junction

Intestinal metaplasia: Squamous epithelium replaced by columnar epithelium with goblet cells[1]
Plasma cells and isolated granulocytes[2] in the stroma

Gastroesophageal junction:
    Adjacent gastric mucosa (with mucous glands and specialized gastric glands) without intestinal metaplasia, but with mild chronic inflammation[2] in the stroma
    Acanthotic esophageal squamous mucosa with thickening of the basal cell layer[3]
    (basal cell hyperplasia) as a sign of reflux

Definition: Barrett's esophagus: Diagnosis requires both a clinically evident lesion and biopsy showing intestinal metaplasia

Etiology/Pathogenesis:

Gastroesophageal reflux disease (GERD): Inflammation of the esophagus caused by the backflow of the gastric acid
    Barrett's esophagus detectable in approx. 10% of patients with GERD
    3-5% of cases long segment Barrett's, 10-15% short segment Barrett's
    Note: Barrett's esophagus is a precancerous disease

Chronic acid exposure → squamous epithelium in the lower esophagus transforms into a more resistant columnar epithelium with goblet cells (intestinal metaplasia)
Barrett's esophagus rarely progresses to adenocarcinoma

Pathologic Regeneration

Entity:	**8.3 Barrett's Esophagus**
Stain:	*Hematoxylin - Eosin*

Clinical Info/Symptoms: Heartburn postprandially or when lying down, acid regurgitation, dysphagia, dry cough

Diagnostics: Esophagogastroduodenoscopy with biopsy, 24h pH-metry, classification according to Los Angeles classification

Therapy: Small protein-rich meals, abdominal pressure reduction, proton pump inhibitors, fundoplication, hiatoplasty

Radiology:

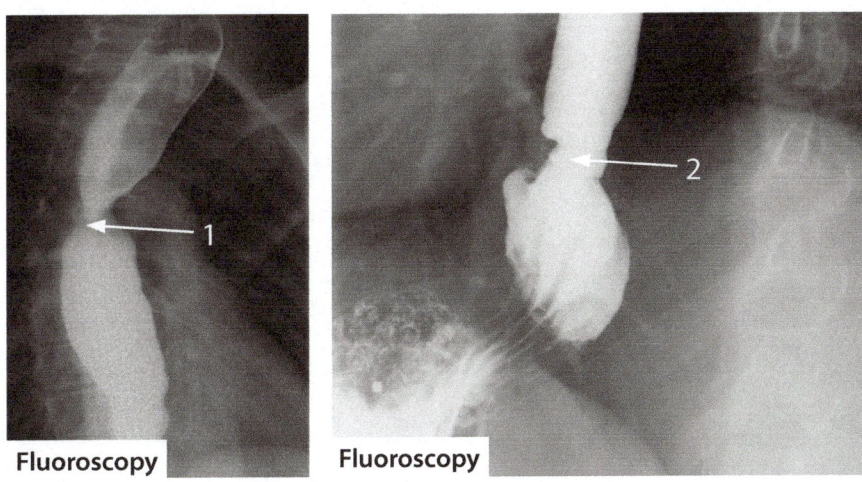

Fluoroscopy   Fluoroscopy

General:
- Barrett's esophagus is not commonly diagnosed by radiologic imaging; endoscopy is preferred method of visualization

Fluoroscopy (Imaging performed with the patient swallowing one or multiple boluses of contrast):
- A stricture in the mid-thoracic esophagus[1] has a fairly strong correlation with Barrett's esophagus
- Large and deep solitary ulcer[2] (depression along the gastroesophageal junction contour) also characteristic of Barrett's esophagus

8 Pathologic Regeneration

Entity: 8.4 Barrett's Esophagus - Cancer (Adenocarcinoma)
Stain: Hematoxylin - Eosin

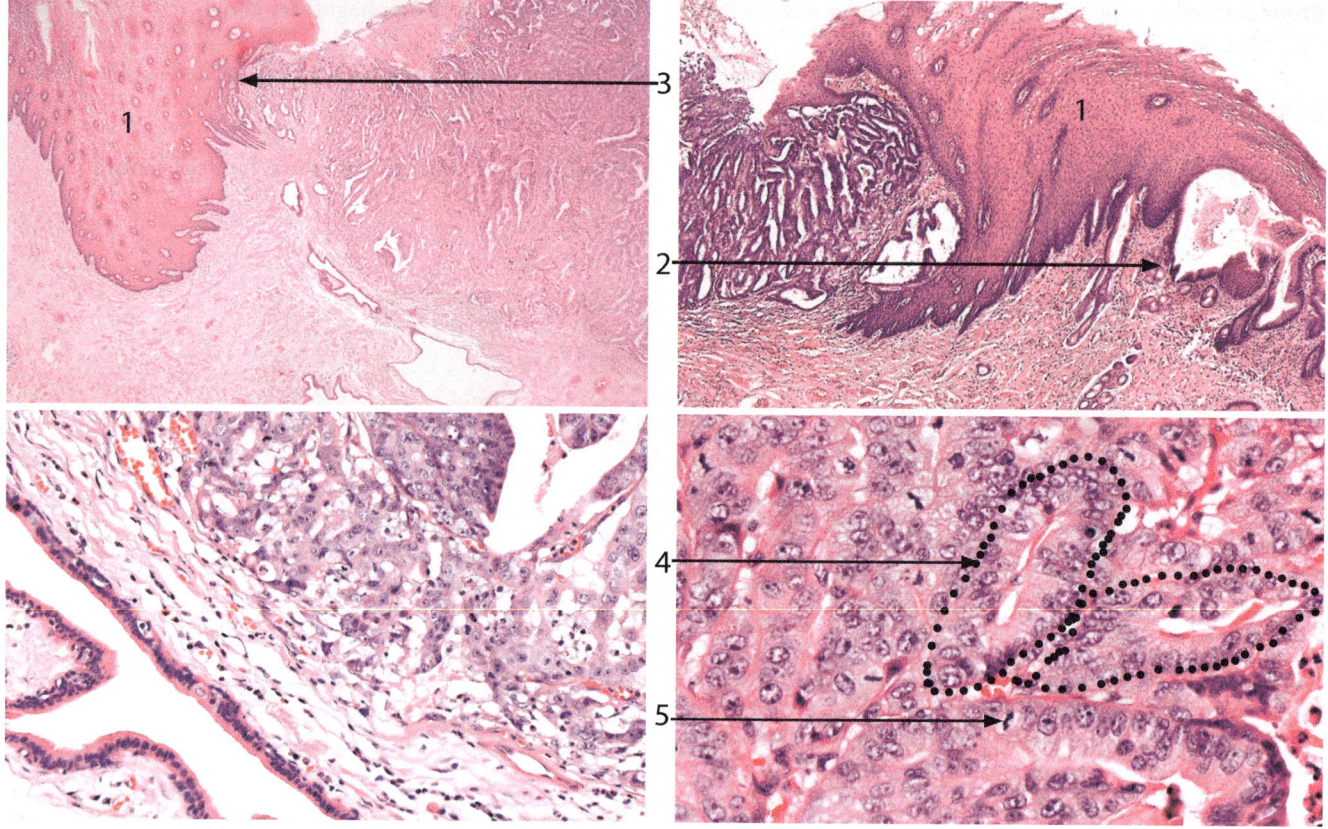

Macroscopy: Multiple or raised lesions, sometimes ulcerated or ulceropolypous, rarely growing purely exophytically, space-occupying, partially stenosing tumors in the distal third of the esophagus to the gastric junction (see macroscopy with squamous cell carcinoma of the esophagus in 8.2)

Microscopy:

Tissue/organ: Esophagus (gastroesophageal junction)
- Multilayered esophageal squamous epithelium[1] with signs of chronic reflux disease
- Gastric cardiac mucosa[2]
- Abrupt transition into a superficially ulcerated and stroma-invading adenocarcinoma[3], characterized by glandular formation[4]
- Merging of neoplastic gland lumens, gland complexity
- Significant nuclear atypia, with coarse, lumpy nuclear chromatin, may show prominent nucleoli and increased mitotic figures[5]

Definition: Carcinoma of glandular differentiation arising in the setting of Barrett's esophagus

Etiology/Pathogenesis: For the majority of adenocarcinomas of the lower esophagus or gastroesophageal junction:
  Initial insult is often chronic reflux disease, with eventual formation of Barrett's esophagus, followed by Barrett's esophagus with dysplasia
  Mechanism of reflux with chronic inflammation → metaplasia-dysplasia-carcinoma sequence

Clinical Info/Symptoms: Dysphagia, progressive weight loss, hematemesis, chest pain, vomiting

Diagnostics: Often an incidental finding during endoscopic biopsy for GERD, or in surveillance of known Barrett's esophagus

Therapy: Surgical resection/esophagectomy with lymphadenectomy, chemotherapy, chemoradiotherapy

Pathologic Regeneration

Entity:	8.4 Barrett's Esophagus - Cancer (Adenocarcinoma)
Stain:	Hematoxylin - Eosin

Radiology:

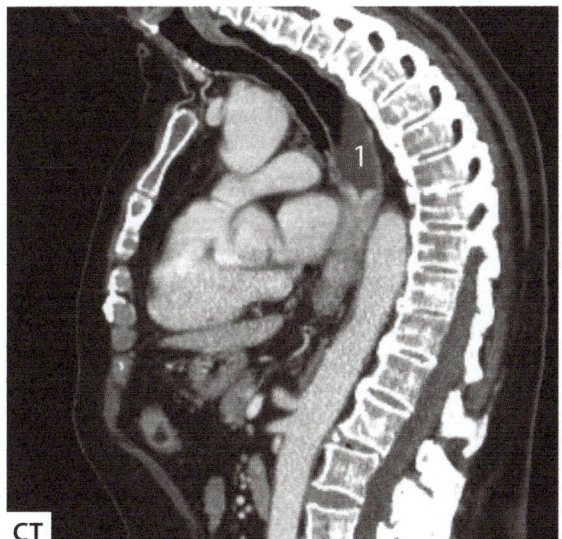 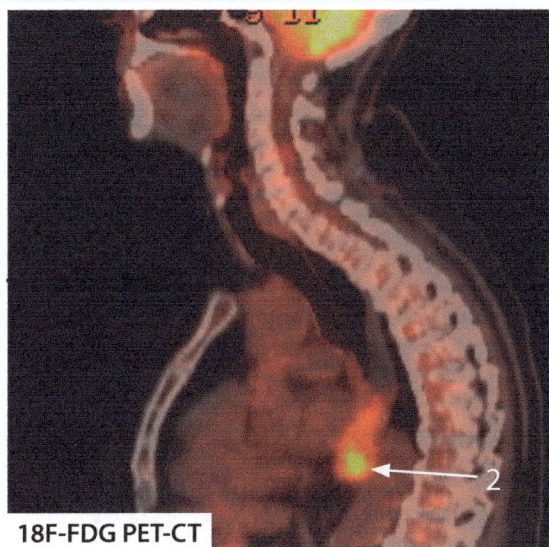

CT[1]:
- An obstructive stricture of the mid thoracic esophagus can become obstructive due to an underlying mass lesion; the esophagus wall is thickened with a "shelf-like" cutoff resulting in proximal dilation with an air-fluid level.

Nuclear medicine[2]:
- 18F-FDG PET-CT was used to determine abnormal focal hypermetabolic activity. indicating the presence of underlying malignancy

8 Pathologic Regeneration

Entity: 8.5 Chronic Gastritis with Intestinal Metaplasia and Dysplasia
Stain: Hematoxylin - Eosin

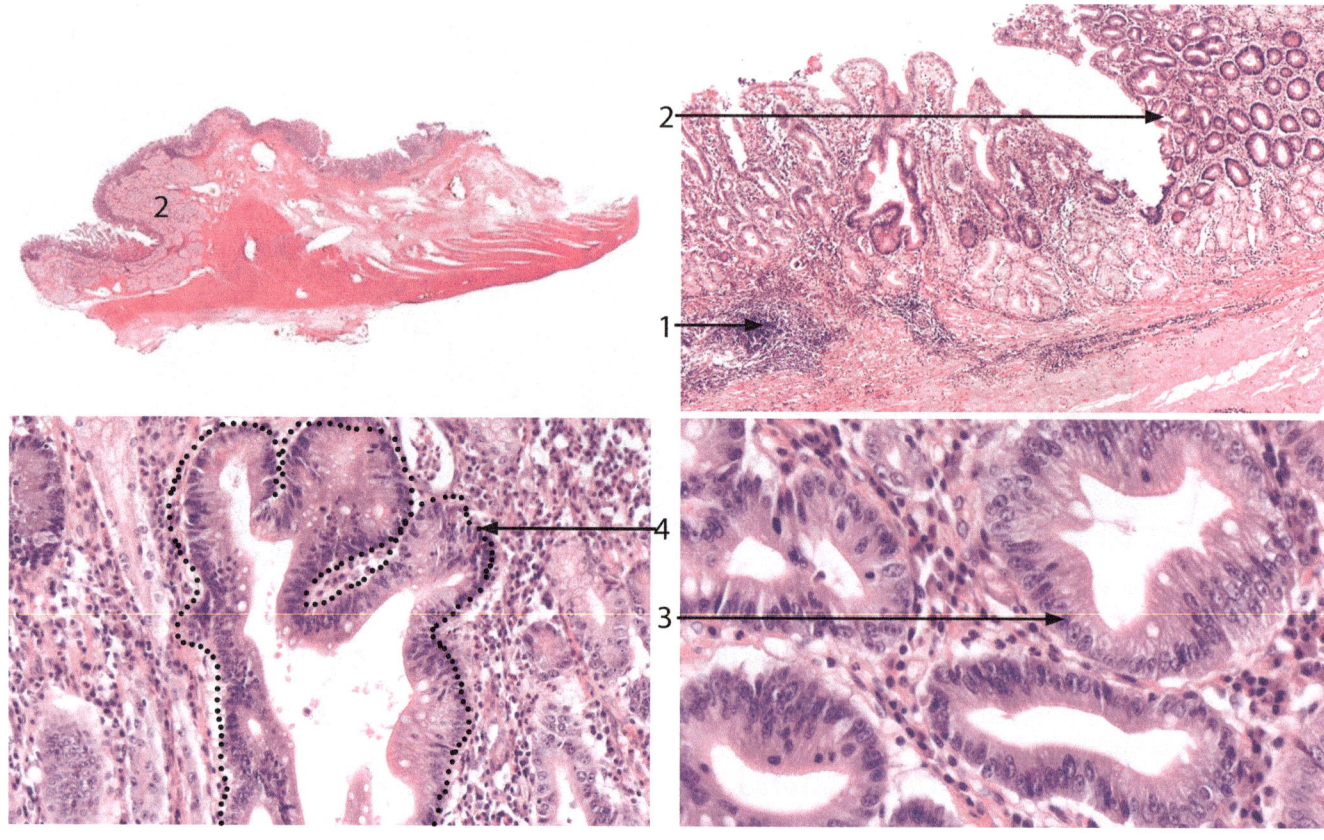

Macroscopy: Redness, erosions, scars, multiple elevations

Microscopy:
- Tissue/organ: Stomach
- Chronic lymphoplasmacytic inflammatory cell infiltrate[1] in the lamina propria with lymphoid follicle formation
- Intestinal metaplasia with replacement of the mucus-producing foveolar cells by brush border-bearing enterocytes, Paneth cells, and goblet cells of the small intestine[2]
- Dysplastic glands with neoplastic, sometimes stratified hyperchromatic epithelium, predominantly basally located nuclei[3], abnormal branching gland architecture[4] and back-to-back atypical glands

Definition: The sequence of steps in the evolution of gastric adenocarcinoma includes chronic gastritis, intestinal metaplasia, and dysplasia.

Etiology/Pathogenesis:

Gastritis:
- Inflammation of the mucosa of the stomach with an acute or chronic course, when prolonged irritation occurs.
- Even after replacement of the gastric epithelium by intestinal epithelium (intestinal metaplasia), gastritis is still a reversible change that often regresses once triggering agent is removed
- Complications: Dysplasia as a precancerous disease with risk of malignancy; MALT lymphoma (type B gastritis)

- Type A gastritis (autoimmune): anti-parietal cell antibodies, anti-intrinsic factor antibodies
- Type B gastritis (bacterial): Helicobacter pylori (very common)
- Type C gastritis (chemical): NSAIDs, bile reflux after partial gastric resection, alcohol, smoking

Pathologic Regeneration

Entity:	8.5 Chronic Gastritis with Intestinal Metaplasia and Dysplasia
Stain:	*Hematoxylin - Eosin*

Clinical Info/Symptoms: Upper abdominal pain, bloating, tarry stools, and coffee grounds vomiting with ulcer

Diagnostics: Esophagogastroduodenoscopy with biopsy demonstrating organisms (gold standard), also rapid urease test of tissue, 13-C breath test, detection of HP antigen in the stool

Therapy: Vitamin B-12 substitution (type A), antibiotic eradication therapy (type B, see gastric ulcer), Reduce noxa + proton pump inhibitor therapy (Type-C)

Radiology:

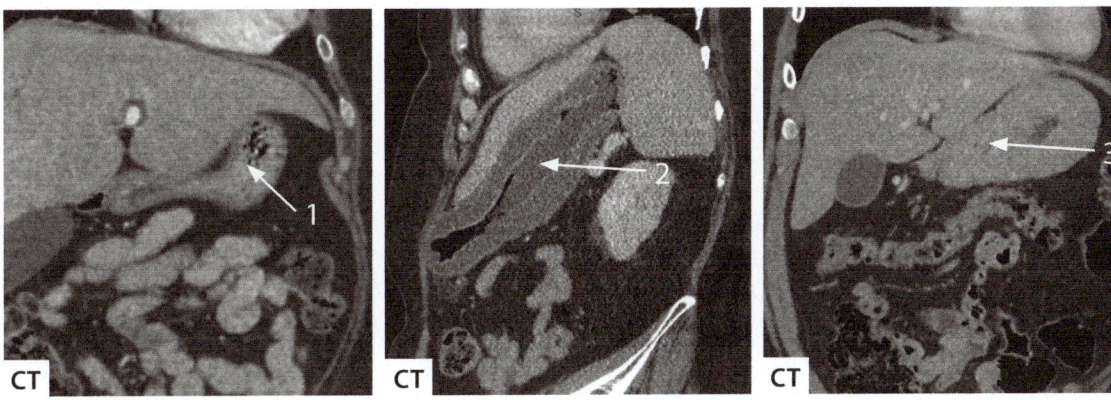

General:
- Radiologic findings are highly nonspecific on any modality, but can be generally recognized as an abnormal wall thickening.
- Since imaging cannot reliably determine the etiology, endoscopic evaluation with biopsies is necessary to directly assess any ulcers or masses.

CT:
- Normal appearance of a stomach wall by routine contrast-enhanced CT[1].
- The same patient reported acute pain several months later, showing new profound submucosal edema of the wall[2].
- In a chronic setting (years later), there is marked diffuse wall hypertrophy with generalized effacement of any recognizable rugal folds[3].

8 Pathologic Regeneration

Entity: 8.6 Cervical Intraepithelial Neoplasia, Grade 2-3
Stain: Hematoxylin - Eosin

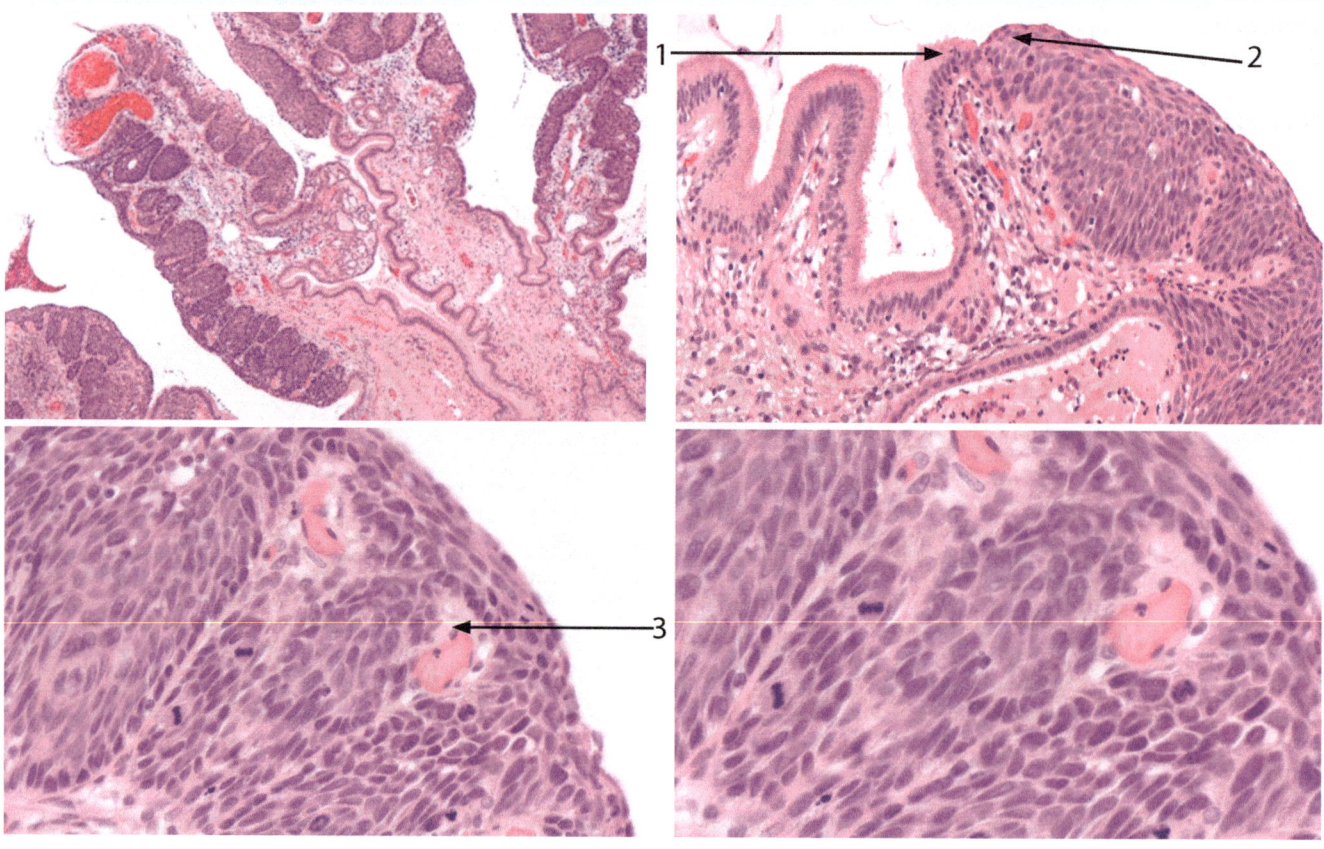

Macroscopy: Colposcopy: visual assessment of cervical mucosa
Acetic acid test (dilute 3-5% acetic acid solution):
  Vinegar-white epithelium: Minimal change with normal squamous epithelium and glandular epithelium, but protein-rich tissue turns white (dysplastic epithelium has a higher protein content)
  Dotting and mosaic: Using an acetic acid test, vascular patterns can be made visible
  Normal: Regular dotting and mosaic
  Abnormal: Irregular vascular pattern (irregular punctate and mosaics)

Lugol's iodine test:
  Physiological glycogen-containing cells of the squamous epithelium turn black/brown
  Atypical epithelium, which is glycogen deficient, turns yellow-whitish in color

Microscopy: Tissue/organ: Cervical transformation zone[1]

Microscopic stages of cervical intraepithelial neoplasia:
CIN1:
  Proliferation of atypical cells in the lower third of squamous epithelium
  Mild changes in polarity and basoapical epithelial layering
  Cell nuclei slightly enlarged, unequal in size, koilocytes
CIN2[2]:
  Proliferation of atypical cells in the lower 2/3 of the squamous epithelium
CIN3[3]:
  Atypical cells present throughout full thickness of epithelium
  Complete loss of epithelial stratification, severe cell atypia, mitotic figures in upper layers of epithelium
  Epithelial layer can show cellular features that overlap with carcinoma, with no baso-apical differentiation or polarity, mostly cells oriented vertically to the surface, but basement membrane is still intact

Pathologic Regeneration

Entity:	**8.6 Cervical Intraepithelial Neoplasia, Grade 2-3**
Stain:	*Hematoxylin - Eosin*

Transformation zone:
- Transition of endocervical glandular epithelium to non-keratinized squamous epithelium
- Physiological squamous cell maturing, reserve cell metaplasia, in addition to mature multilayered squamous and glandular epithelium

Definition:

Abbreviations (Bethesda Classification):
- **LSIL** - low grade squamous intraepithelial lesion
- **HSIL** - high grade squamous intraepithelial lesion, which includes CIN2-3

Neoplasia (new growth): Consisting of a clonal cell proliferation originated from one transformed cell due to certain (oncogenic) mutations and acquired the ability to divide independently of physiological stimuli (immortal cells)

Etiology/Pathogenesis:

Human papillomavirus (HPV) plays a key role in pathogenesis, especially high-risk HPV subtypes 16 and 18 (relative risk factor: 10)
- The basal cells of damaged or abraded mucosa can be infected by HPV virus.
- Proliferating HPV infection: Virus replicates and is discharged via the surface epithelium; morphological changes in mature squamous epithelium: CIN1 lesion with koilocytes (containing the virus particles)
- Transforming HPV infection: Viral DNA is integrated into host DNA, and transforms the cell morphologically → CIN/CIS (or endocervical adenocarcinoma in situ)

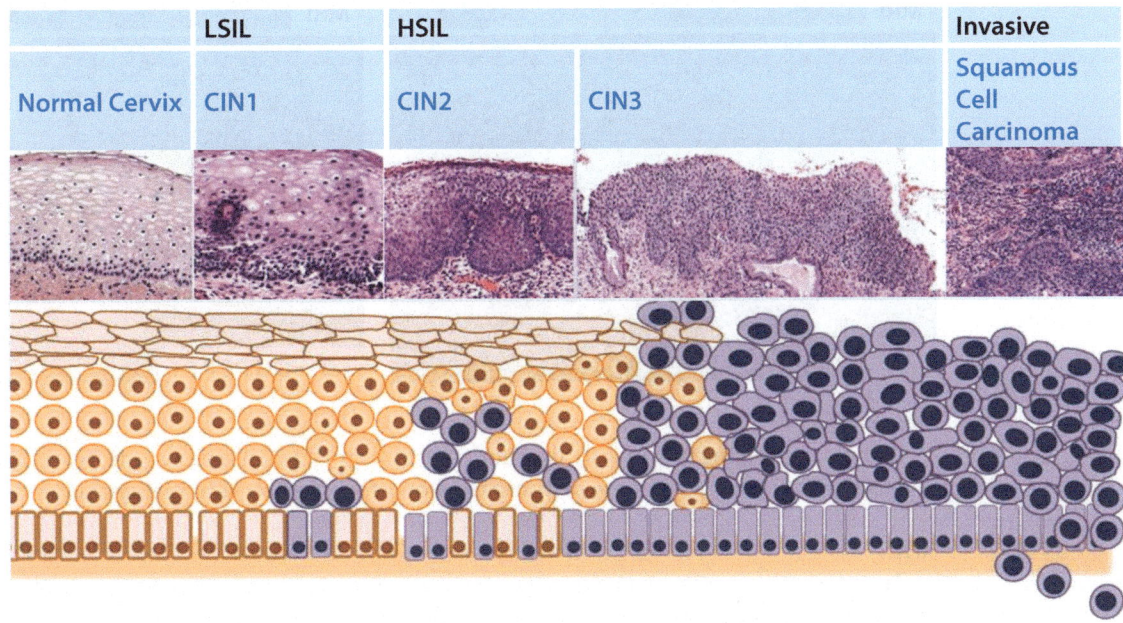

Note:
- The cervix has three surfaces, the ectocervical region with non-keratinized stratified squamous epithelium which is continuous to the vagina, the transformation zone with the transition from squamous to glandular epithelium and the endocervix (glandular, endocervical cells). Neoplasia predominantly occurs in the transformation zone, where squamous or glandular cells can be affected.

Neoplasia affecting the ectocervix/squamous mucosa:
- LSIL or HSIL or squamous cell carcinoma

Neoplasia affecting the endocervix/glandular tissue:
- Adenocarcinoma in situ or invasive adenocarcinoma of the cervix

8 Pathologic Regeneration

Entity: 8.6 Cervical Intraepithelial Neoplasia, Grade 2-3
Stain: Hematoxylin - Eosin

Clinical Info: Cervical carcinoma: malignant neoplasia of the cervix uteri, which usually has in situ lesion, so-called cervical intraepithelial neoplasia (CIN).
- Prevention: HPV vaccination recommended for all, ages 9-14, and screening for early detection at preliminary stages

Symptoms: Asymptomatic, postcoital bleeding, metrorrhagia, foul-smelling vaginal discharge (with co-infections), pain

Diagnostics: Pap-smear screening, HPV-DNA testing, colposcopy with biopsy, cone biopsy

Therapy: Depending on the pathology and stage and if fertility sparing or not: follow-up, loop electrosurgical excision procedure (LEEP), cone biopsy, laser ablation, radical hysterectomy, radiotherapy

Radiology:

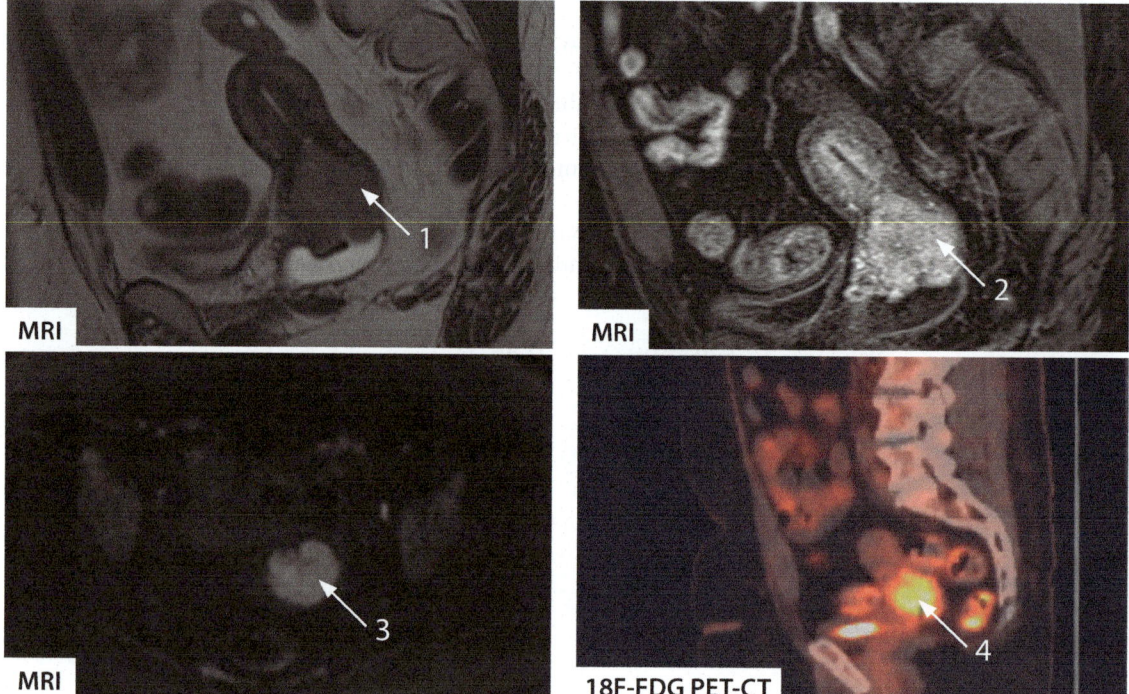

General:
- Radiologic imaging is primarily used for clinical staging, when invasive (degree of local extension or metastatic disease) in the case of a suspected or established cervical malignancy

MRI:
- Typical characteristics of an abnormal mass of the cervix includes T2 intermediate signal intensity compared to the uterine myometrium[1], relative hyperenhancement[2], and restricted diffusion[3].
- Key interpretation points include assessing the relationship of tumor to vagina, parametrium, pelvic sidewalls, and bladder or bowel

Nuclear medicine:
- 18F-FDG PET-CT shows corresponding abnormal hypermetabolic activity in the primary malignancy[4]
- Any similarly intense radiotracer accumulation detected in lymph nodes or distant organs provides significantly improved sensitivity and specificity for overall staging.

Pathologic Regeneration

Entity:	8.6 Cervical Intraepithelial Neoplasia, Grade 2-3
Stain:	Hematoxylin - Eosin

Extra: Pap test:
- Cytological examination method for evaluating cells from the cervical os and endocervix (gynecological check-up)
- Staining with Papanicolaou (Pap) staining (hematoxylin, orange, polychrome solution)
- Pap staining may be used for scrapings of other mucosa (e.g. anal canal, oral cavity); stain also used in cytologic examination of other body fluids (urine, pleural fluid, ascites, CSF)

Papanicolaou Staining Patterns

Structure	Coloring
Cell nuclei	Blue
Bacteria	Blue
Cytoplasm	Blue/green
Cytoplasm with keratin content	Red/orange
Collagen	Green

Pap Test - Cells

Cells		Morphology
Superficial Cells		Large cell body, small, pyknotic and highly condensed nuclei; fine chromatin
Large intermediate cells		Large cell body, nucleus slightly larger than superficial cell nucleus; fine nuclear chromatin
Small intermediate cells/Parabasal cells		Atrophic (post-menopausal) cell picture showing small intermediate cells and parabasal cells; smaller cell body; nucleus relatively larger than large intermediate cells; fine nuclear chromatin
Basal cells		Atrophic (post-menopausal) cell picture showing basal cells; smallest cell body with very little cytoplasm and large nucleus; fine nuclear chromatin, may show horizontal nuclear grooves
Endocervical cells		Glandular epithelium with eccentric nucleus and vacuolated cytoplasm, fine chromatin

8 Pathologic Regeneration

Entity: 8.6 Cervical Intraepithelial Neoplasia, Grade 2-3
Stain: Hematoxylin - Eosin

Bethesda System for Reporting Cervical Cytology	
Category	**Description**
Unsatisfactory for evaluation	This category is most commonly due to low cellularity of squamous cells, technical artifacts, or obscured cellular features (secondary to blood, inflammation, foreign material).
Normal (Negative for intraepithelial lesion or malignancy = NILM) 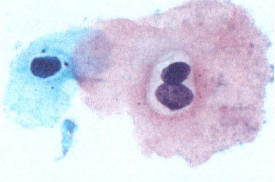	In addition to normal cervical cells, this category includes non-neoplastic findings such as organisms (e.g. Candida, Trichomonas, bacteria), atrophy, hormonal/treatment alterations, benign endometrial cells (reportable for women > 45 years old), metaplastic changes, and inflammation.
Atypical squamous cells of undetermined significance (ASC-US)	Atypical squamous cells show mild nuclear enlargement and focal nuclear changes (irregularity, hyperchromasia, multinucleation) that are suggestive, but insufficient for LSIL.
Atypical squamous cells cannot exclude HSIL (ASC-H)	Atypical cells in this category show features (small, hyperchromatic cells with increased nuclear:cytoplasmic (N:C) ratio) that are suggestive but insufficient for HSIL.
Low grade squamous intraepithelial lesion (LSIL) 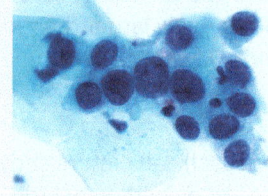	Classic LSIL cells (koilocytes) show enlarged, "raisinoid," hyperchromatic nuclei, at times with a characteristic perinuclear cytoplasmic halo (clearing). Multinucleation can also be present.
High grade intraepithelial lesion (HSIL)	HSIL cells are frequently smaller than LSIL cells, with markedly increased N:C ratio, irregular nuclear membranes, and coarse chromatin. These cells can be found singly or in syncytial aggregates.
Squamous Cell Carcinoma (SCC)	Marked atypia can be seen in squamous cell carcinoma, including tadpole-shaped cells, at times with keratinization (orange-tinged) and frequent background tumor diathesis (necrotic cellular debris).
Atypical glandular cells (AGC)	While Pap smears are not designed for the screening of glandular abnormalities, enlarged nuclei may be seen in atypical endometrial cells, while hyperchromasia, increased N:C ratio, and nuclear pseudostratification and overlapping can be identified in atypical endocervical cells.
Adenocarcinoma (AC)	Cervical adenocarcinoma in situ (AIS) shows features similar to atypical endocervical cells, but more overt and organized in irregular rosettes or "feathering" aggregates. The presence of tumor diathesis (necrotic debris) in addition to features of AIS raise concern for cervical adenocarcinoma. In rare cases, endometrial adenocarcinoma may also be identified in a Pap smear.

Epithelial Tumors

Shaolei Lu, Robert Barno, Jao Ou

9.1 **Papilloma (Oral)**

9.2 **Non-invasive Papillary Urothelial Carcinoma, low- and high-grade**

9.3 **Tubulovillous Adenoma of the Rectum with low-grade Dysplasia**

9.4 **Basal Cell Carcinoma (Nodular Type)**

9.5 **Prostate Cancer**

9 Epithelial Tumors

Epithelial tumors are the common tumors in the human body. The word "tumor" means "a swelling" and is generally used to describe a neoplastic mass.

Some neoplastic tumors are self-limited, and while they may cause issues by occupying space, they will not invade other tissues, and are unable to invade vascular spaces and metastasize; these are benign tumors. Our example is the oral papilloma. Malignant tumors are able to invade adjacent tissues, and may invade vessels and spread to lymph nodes or other organs as metastases. With epithelial tumors, the defining behavior of an invasive malignancy is the ability of the tumor cells to cross the epithelial basement membrane, gaining access to and invading through the adjacent tissue. An epithelial malignancy that has not yet crossed the basement membrane is referred to as an in-situ lesion; we will review a case of a non-invasive papillary urothelial carcinoma.

Some lesions may be classified as "pre-malignant," meaning that they have not yet crossed that basement membrane, but if left untreated long enough, would eventually invade. Adenomatous polyps of the colon are an example of this type of lesion. When they are sampled, they are not malignant, but they do indicate that the colonic epithelium has accumulated some genetic errors already, indicating the patient is at high risk of accumulating an additional DNA error, and making a polyp that will progress to a carcinoma and invade.

Properties of Solid Tumors

Properties	Benign Tumors	Malignant Tumors
Growth	Displacing, pushing	Infiltrative, locally destructive
Growth rate	Slow	Fast
Lymphovascular invasion	No	Yes
Perineural invasion	No	Yes
Metastasis	No	Yes

General Morphological Criteria for Benign and Malignant Tumors

Criteria	Benign Tumors	Malignant Tumors
Capsule	yes (typically present)	no
Mitoses	rare	frequent
Atypical mitosis (e.g. tripolar)	no	yes
Necrosis	rare	may be frequent
Resemblance to origin tissue	very similar	somewhat similar (well differentiated) to unrecognizable (poorly differentiated)
Atypia/dysplasia (see below, 'Features of atypia')	minimal	conspicuous, marked
Lymphatic invasion	no	possible
Blood vessel invasion	no	possible
Perineural sheath invasion	no	possible
Metastasis	no	possible

Features of Atypia

Abnormal variation in nucleus size (anisoneucleosis/anisokaryosis)

Increased nuclear-to-cytoplasmic (N:C) ratio

Hyperchromatic nuclei

Abnormal variation in the shape of the nucleus (nuclear pleomorphism)

Abnormal variation in cell size

Abnormal variation in cell shape (cellular pleomorphism)

Epithelial Tumors

Malignant Solid Tumors are Usually Classified by TNM Classification According to the Tumor Type

Code	Definition
Tumor	Primary tumor stage: classification typically T1-4; may reflect tumor size, invasion depth, or other characteristics, depending on the organ involved; Tis = carcinoma in situ
Node	Nodal status: presence of lymph node metastases. Nodal scoring varies depending on the organ, usually N0, N1, N2; some organs also score an N3. N0 means that none of the regional nodes are affected. N1, 2, or 3 represent increasing numbers of the involved nodes. Nx indicates that nodes were not evaluated. The modifier (sn) may be used to indicate that sentinel nodes were sampled.
Metastases	Distant metastases: Classification: 0 or 1 M0: no distant metastases. M1: distant metastases present (if using M1 in pathologic staging, histologic confirmation of the metastasis is required to use this code). Location of the metastasis may also be given in brackets (e.g. PUL = lungs, OSS = bones, HEP = liver)

Grading (G) Grading makes a statement about the degree of differentiation of the tumor (i.e. its similarity to the original tissue, from well-differentiated G1 (similar to the original tissue) to G3 (very little similarity to the original tissue)

Grading Code	Definition
G1	well-differentiated
G2	moderately differentiated
G3	poorly differentiated
G4	undifferentiated

ATTENTION: For some tumor entities there is only a two-stage grading system: low grade = well differentiated; high grade = poorly differentiated

Additional Codes
Lymphovascular invasion (LVI) coding (this staging code is still evolving, per AJCC 8th ed, 2017)

Lymphovascular invasion (LVI)	Definition
0	LVI no present/not identified
1	LVI present/identified, not otherwise specified (NOS)
2	Lymphatic and small vessel invasion only (L)
3	Venous (large vessel) invasion only (V)
4	Both lymphatic and small vessel AND venous (large vessel) invasion
9	Presence of LVI unknown/indeterminate

Resection status (R)

R0	Tumor removed entirely, no residual tumor
R1	Microscopic residual tumor
R2	Macroscopic residual tumor (at primary site or in nodes)
Rx	Resection status cannot be determined with certainty (e.g. tumor removed in a piecemeal fashion)

9 Epithelial Tumors

Resection status (R)

R0	Tumor removed entirely, no residual tumor
R1	Microscopic residual tumor
R2	Macroscopic residual tumor (at primary site or in nodes)
Rx	Resection status cannot be determined with certainty (e.g. tumor removed in a piecemeal fashion)

Prefixes of the TNM Classification

c	Clinical stage classification
p	Pathologic stage classification
yc	Clinical stage, classified after neoadjuvant therapy
yp	Pathologic stage, classified after neoadjuvant therapy
a	Stage classified after autopsy finding
r	Tumor is recurrent, after a disease-free interval

Example (according to TNM classification, AJCC 8th edition 2017):

Colon cancer with the stage:
G2, pT2, pN1a (1/15), V3, pM1 (HEP), R0 means:

Moderately differentiated, invasion into the muscularis propria, nodal metastasis present (in one of 15 sampled nodes), large vessel invasion only, histologically confirmed liver metastasis, all tumor completely removed

Selected Examples of Epithelial Tumors

Tissue	Benign	Malignant
Squamous epithelium	Squamous cell papilloma	Squamous cell carcinoma
Urothelium	Urothelial papilloma	Papillary urothelial carcinoma
Glandular epithelium	Adenoma	Adenocarcinoma

Epithelial Tumors

Entity:	9.1 Papilloma (Oral)
Stain:	Hematoxylin - Eosin

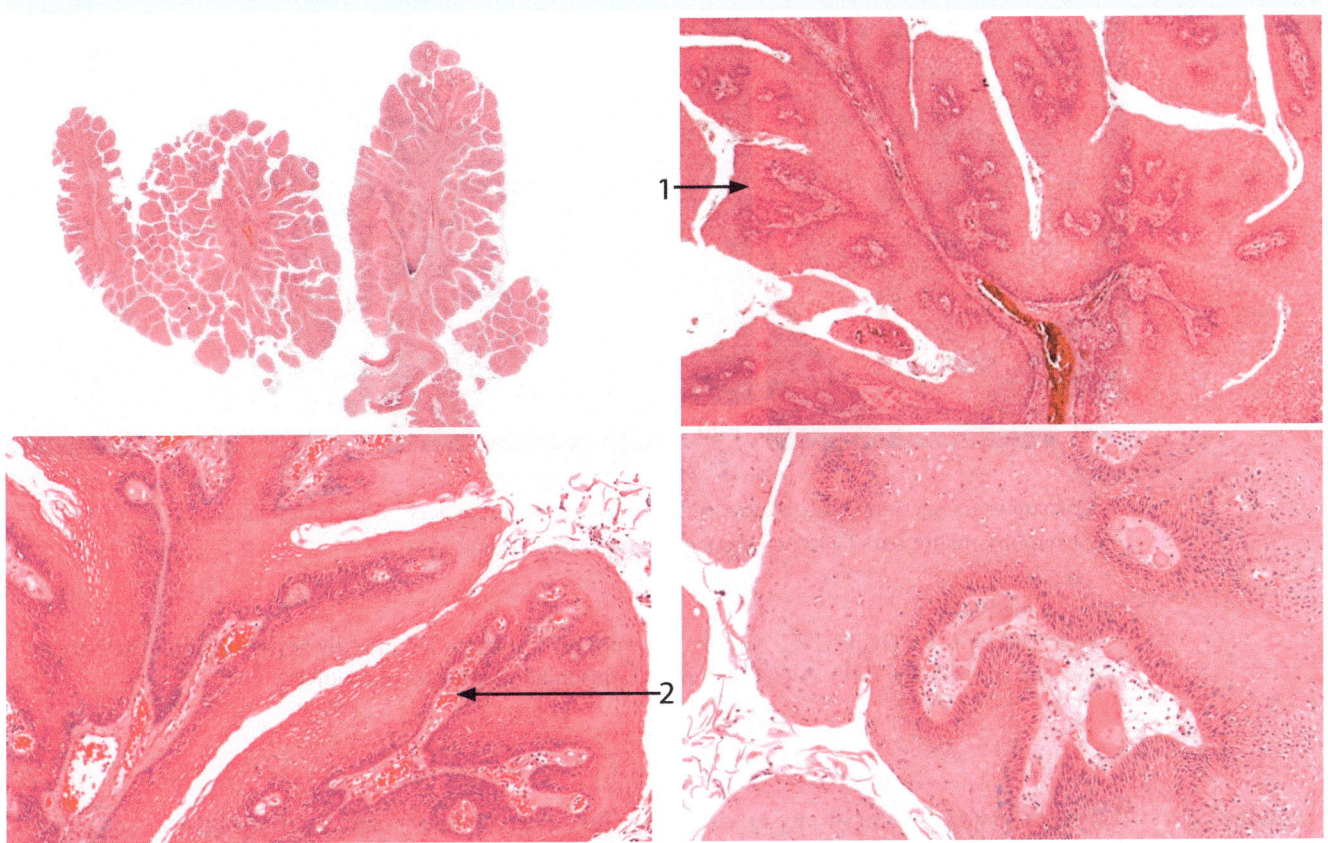

Macroscopy:	Pedunculated or broad-based tumor on the base with a fine shaggy surface and cauliflower-like/exophytic structure
Microscopy:	Tissue/organ: Oral mucosa (shown above) – Somewhat hyperplastic/thickened, non-keratinizing squamous epithelium[1] – No cellular atypia, appropriate maturation from basal layer to surface – Intact basement membrane, supported by branched core of well-vascularized connective tissue[2] – May rarely find koilocytes (epithelial cells with large, hyperchromatic raisinoid nucleus, surrounded by a light halo); indicative of HPV replication
Definition:	**Papilloma:** Benign tumor of the keratinizing and/or non-keratinizing squamous epithelium, with an exophytic growth pattern
Etiology/Pathogenesis:	Low-risk HPV infections (including HPV serotypes: 2, 6, 11, 57) causative in the development – In the area of the larynx, singular squamous epithelial papillomas and multiple papillomas (= juvenile laryngeal papillomatosis) are common in children – Rarely multiple squamous cell papillomas in adults – Recurrences are common
Clinical Info/Symptoms:	Mass with nasal/pharyngeal obstruction
Diagnostics:	Clinical detection, with biopsy or excision to confirm diagnosis and alleviate symptoms
Therapy:	Total excision, laser ablation, cryotherapy

9 Epithelial Tumors

Entity:	9.1 Papilloma (Oral)
Stain:	Hematoxylin - Eosin

Radiology:

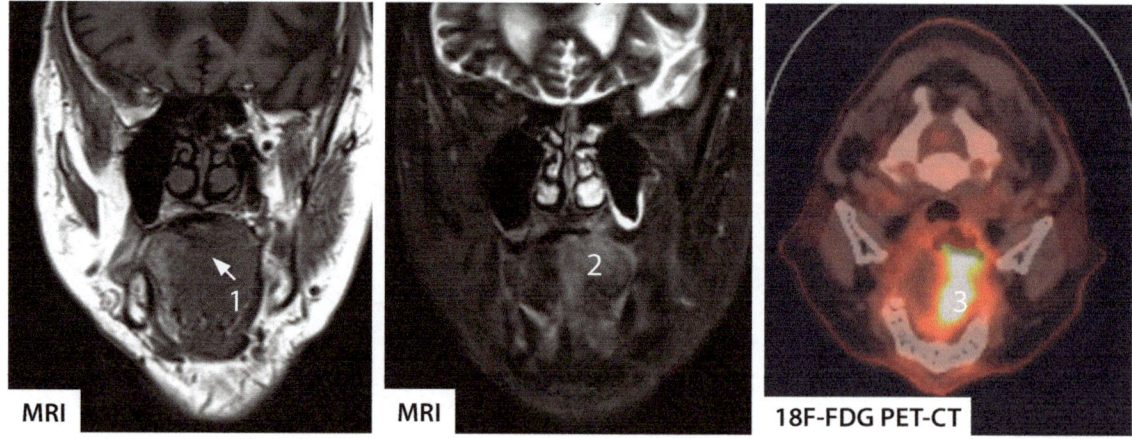

MRI — MRI — 18F-FDG PET-CT

MRI:
- Coronal cross-section: Amorphous mass involving the left aspect of the tongue shows T1 hypointensity[1] and T2 hyperintensity[2], indicating edema.

Nuclear medicine[3]:
- Followup by 18F-FDG PET-CT shows corresponding abnormal markedly hypermetabolic activity of the tumor, while the right side of the lingual musculature appears uninvolved

Entity:	9.2 Non-invasive Papillary Urothelial Carcinoma, low- and high-grade
Stain:	Hematoxylin - Eosin

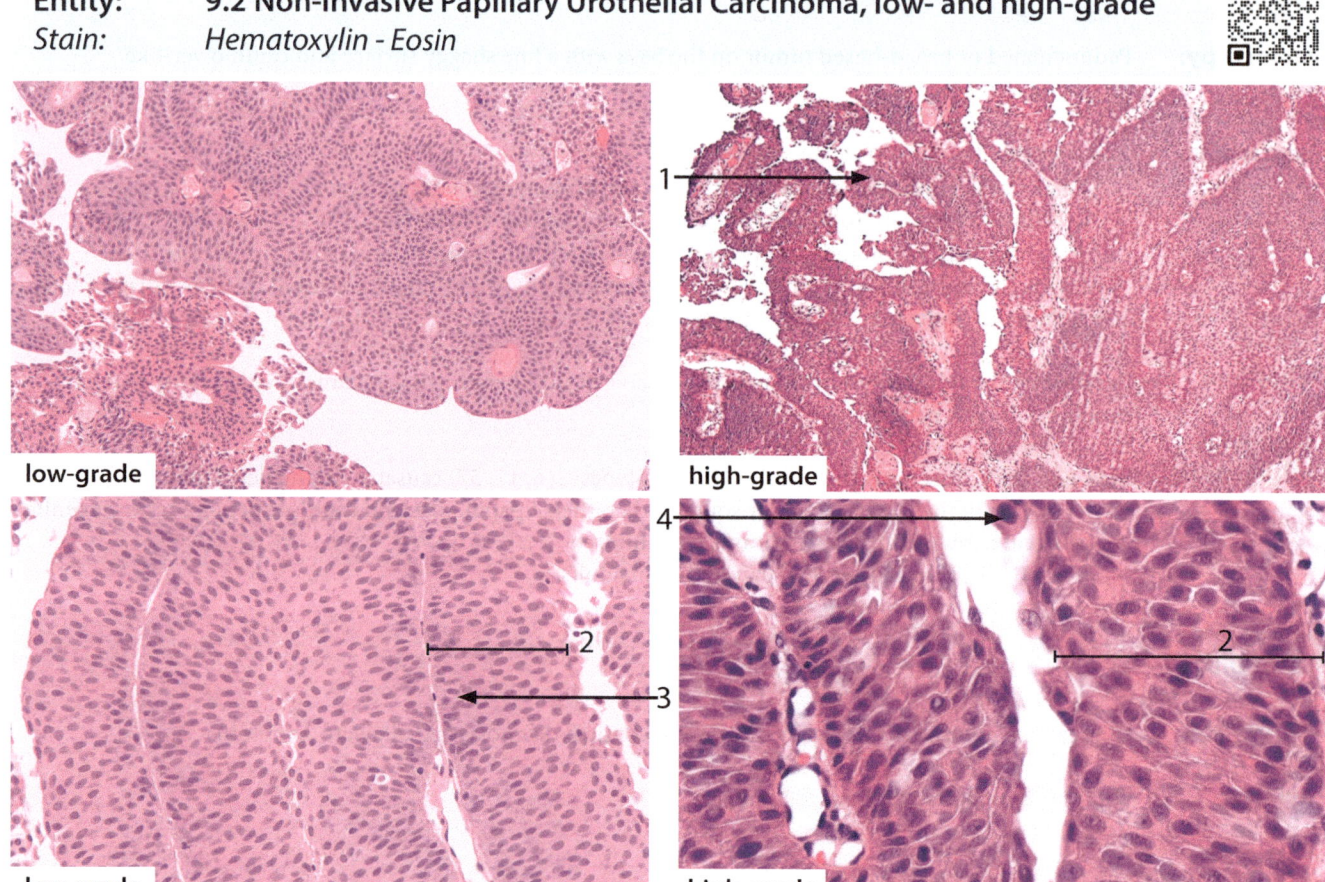

low-grade — high-grade

low-grade — high-grade

Epithelial Tumors

Entity:	9.2 Non-invasive Papillary Urothelial Carcinoma, low- and high-grade
Stain:	*Hematoxylin - Eosin*

Macroscopy: Cystoscopy: Fine, white papillary lesions in the urinary bladder

Microscopy: Tissue/organ: Urothelium (transurethral resection of the urinary bladder (TUR-B)
- Papillary architecture[1] with irregular, branched fibrovascular cores
- Atypical urothelium with > 8 cell layers[2]
- Low-grade: Orderly arranged cells[3], well-differentiated appearing, mild anisonucleosis/pleomorphism
- High-grade: Marked dysplasia[4], frequent mitotic figures

Dysplastic features can include:
- Nuclear pleomorphism
- Increased nuclear:cytoplasmic ratio
- Loss of epithelial polarity
- Focal mitoses in basal cells, may see mitoses in the upper third of epithelial layer
- Focal early invasion of submucosal connective tissue

Morphological spectrum of bladder tumors:
- Papillary tumors: Papilloma (benign), papillary urothelial neoplasia with low malignant potential (PUNLMP), non-invasive low-grade papillary carcinoma, non-invasive papillary urothelial carcinoma, invasive papillary urothelial carcinoma
- Flat urothelial lesion: Urothelial carcinoma in situ, invasive urothelial carcinoma

Definition: **Urothelial carcinoma:** Lesion originating from the urothelial cells that line the urinary tract, the renal pelvis, ureter, bladder or urethra can be affected.

Etiology/ Pathogenesis: Can arise in bladder, ureter, or renal pelvis
- Urothelial carcinoma risk factors include: Smoking, occupational exposure (aromatic amines/aniline dye industry), medication, Schistosomiasis, genetic (e.g. Lynch syndrome)

Strong association between certain genetic abnormalities and histological patterns:
- Gain-of-function mutations of fibroblast growth factor receptor 3 (FGFR3) associated with non-invasive low-grade papillary urothelial carcinoma
- Loss-of-function mutations in TP53 and retinoblastoma (RB) tumor suppressor genes are almost always seen in high-grade and muscle-invading tumors

Clinical Info/ Symptoms:
- Hematuria, pollakiuria, urgency symptoms, dysuria

Diagnostics:
- Urine test strips, urine cytology, sonography, urethrocystoscopy, ureterorenoscopy, biopsy or tissue removal for histology as part of a transurethral resection of the urinary bladder (TUR-B)

Therapy:
- Transurethral resection + intravesical chemo- (BCG instillation) / immunotherapy (<pT1) radical cystectomy (> pT1), chemotherapy

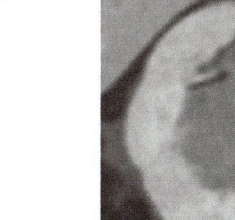
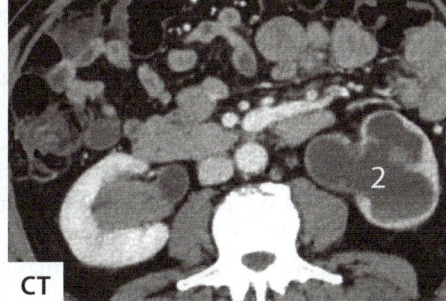

Radiology:

General: Urothelial masses are best demonstrated on cross-sectional imaging, with prescribed timing of contrast enhancement. Typical optimized acquisition to best discriminate urothelium: achieved around 90 to 100 seconds after intravenous injection

CT: On magnified inset from CT urogram[1], large enhancing soft tissue mass with lobulated margins fills the pelvicalyceal system of the right kidney. On the right image, similar but smaller nodules seen in left kidney result in conspicuous mechanical obstruction[2] of upper urinary tract

9 Epithelial Tumors

Entity: 9.3 Tubulovillous Adenoma of the Rectum with Low-grade Dysplasia
Stain: Hematoxylin - Eosin

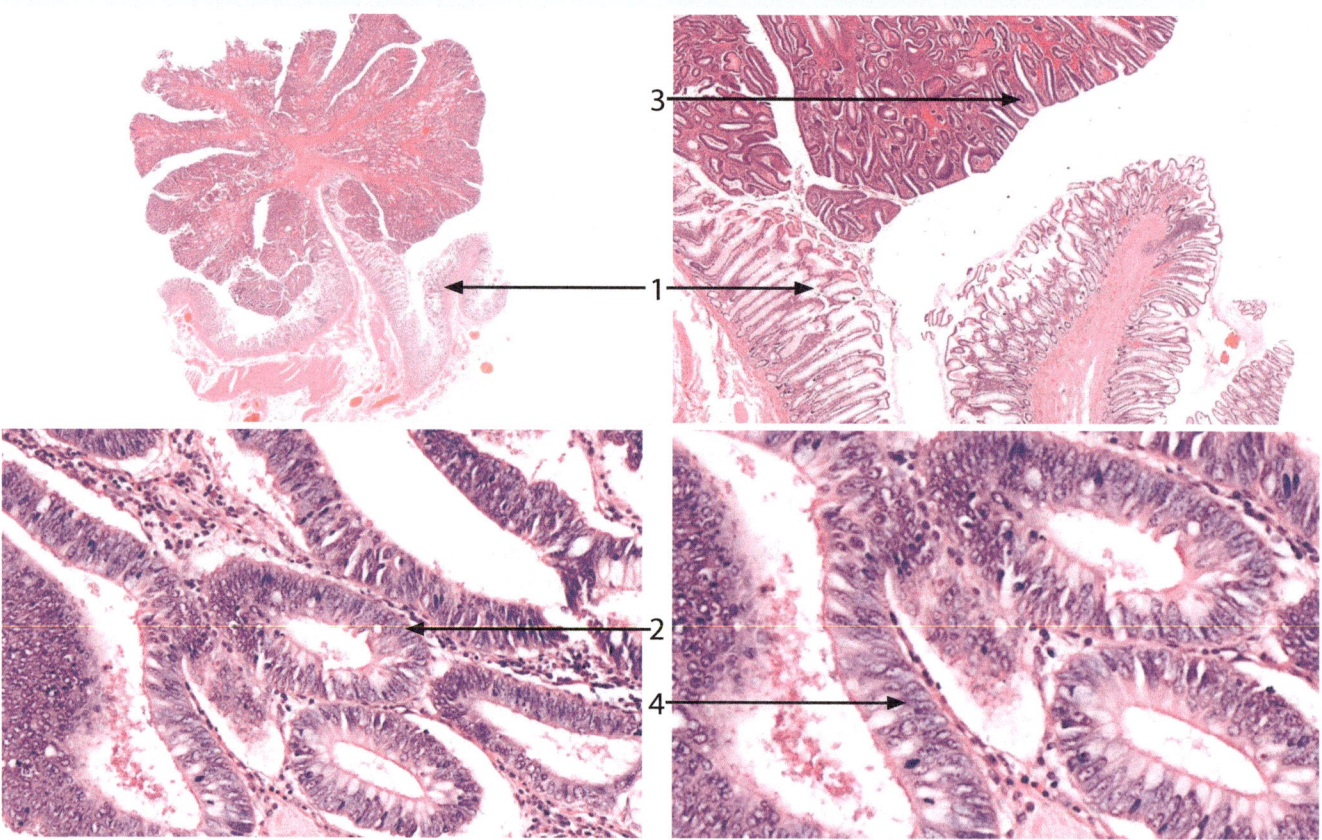

Macroscopy: Colonoscopy: Multiple, broad-based polyps (sessile or pedunculated mucosal protrusions), which bulge into the intestinal lumen

Microscopy: Tissue/organ: Rectal mucosa
- Colorectal type mucosa[1]
- Gland architecture: Tubulovillous (tubular[2] = tube-like; Villi[3] = finger-shaped protuberances)
- Abrupt transition from the normal crypt-arrangement of columnar epithelium into proliferating, dysplastic epithelium arranged on fibrovascular cores, with elongated, cigar-shaped, hyperchromatic nuclei with conspicuous nucleoli, mitoses; nuclear polarity is preserved (predominantly basally located nuclei)[4]
- No invasive growth (basement membrane intact, no involvement of the submucosa)
- Proliferating cells no longer limited to the base of crypts, may extend up to surface of mucosa

Definition: Neoplastic polyps of the gastrointestinal tract

Etiology/Pathogenesis: Depending on the histological type, characteristic genomic alterations can be associated with adenoma development: e.g. KRAS mutations in tubular adenomas

Colon or rectal carcinomas often arise from adenomatous precursors in a multi-stage process that can be called the "adenoma-carcinoma sequence".

Risk factors: Genetic predispositions, inflammatory bowel disease

Epithelial Tumors

Entity:	9.3 Tubulovillous Adenoma of the Rectum with Low-grade Dysplasia
Stain:	*Hematoxylin - Eosin*

Clinical Info/Symptoms: Asymptomatic (initially), weight loss, bloody/dark stools, constipation, mass effect

Diagnostics: Digital rectal examination, immunological blood-in-stool test (iFOBT), colonoscopy, sonography

Therapy: Mucosal stripping, en bloc colon resection with lymphadenectomy, deep anterior rectal resection + total mesorectal excision (rectum), chemotherapy

Radiology:

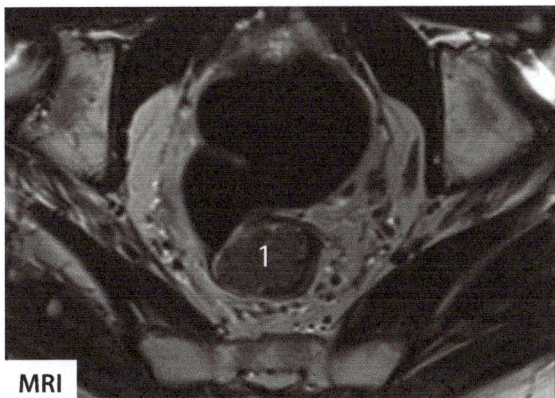 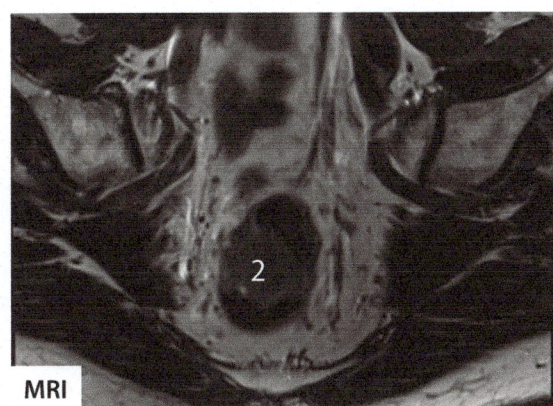

General:
- No specific radiologic characteristics for tubulovillous adenoma
- To determine if a tumor is locally advanced, MR imaging of the rectum is now essentially standard of care

MRI:
- Lobular soft tissue mass in the upper rectum with T2 intermediate signal protrudes into the lumen in the axial[1] and coronal[2] planes
- Example shows a relatively broad base of attachment that does not breach the wall into the surrounding mesorectal fat, allowing for the following provisional clinical staging: not locally advanced disease (i.e. T1/T2 under current AJCC TNM definitions)

9 Epithelial Tumors

Entity: 9.4 Basal Cell Carcinoma (Nodular Type)
Stain: Hematoxylin - Eosin

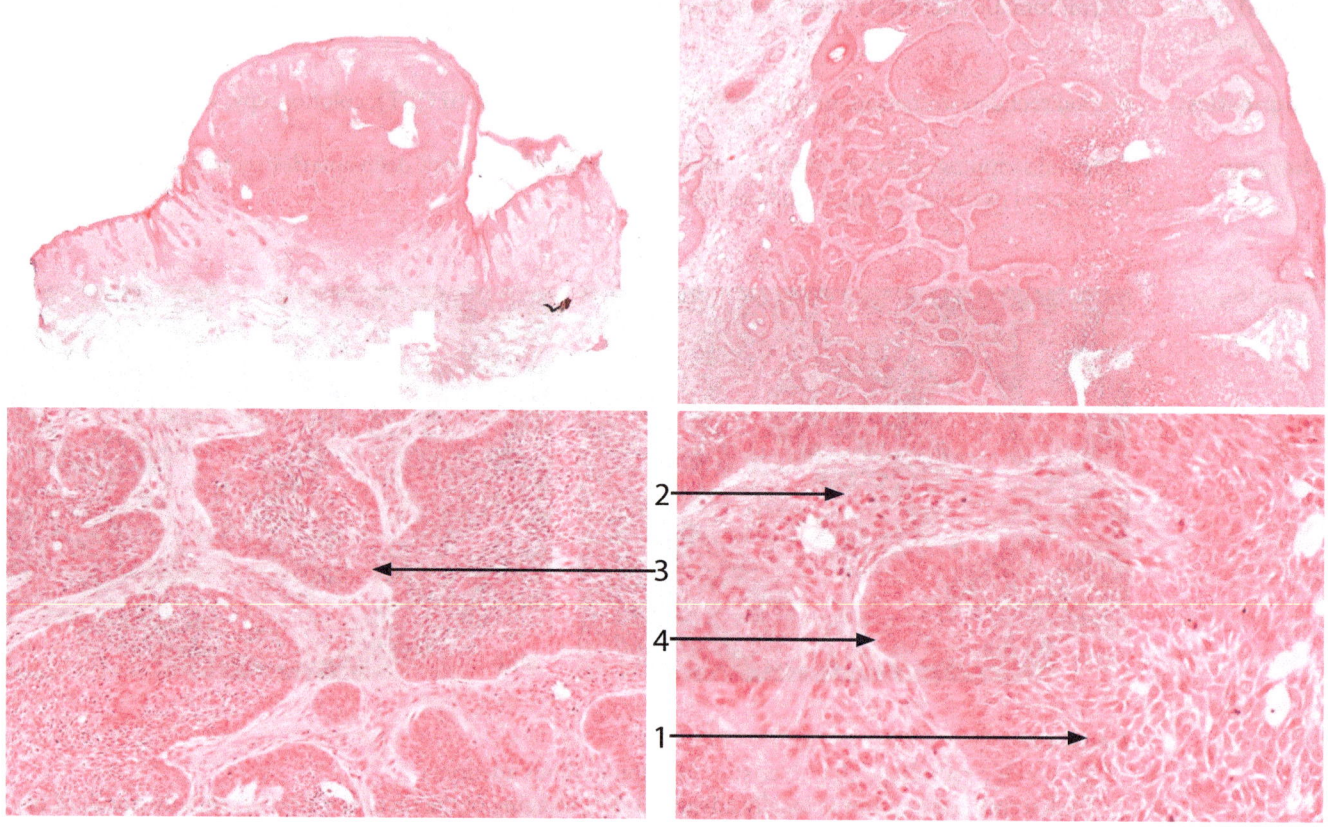

Macroscopy: Mother-of-pearl-colored skin lesion, possibly ulcerated with a pearl-like edge wall, often with telangiectasia, rarely pigmented

Microscopy: Tissue/organ: Skin
- Clusters of cells, basaloid-appearing, with nuclear hyperchromasia, anisonucleosis, mitoses, and increased nucleus-cytoplasm ratio[1]
- Invasion of the dermis, may show a desmoplastic stromal reaction[2]
- Islands and/or strands of oval basaloid tumor cells[3]
- Palisading basal nuclei[4] along the periphery of invasive cell nests
- Peritumoral retraction artifact between cell nests and stroma
- May show small bluish mucin-like areas between cells within nests
- May show a peritumoral inflammatory infiltrate

Growth pattern variants: Solid-nodular (often with surface ulceration), superficial/multicentric (skips along the surface of the skin), scirrhous or sclerodermic (morphea-like, infiltrative pattern)

Definition: Most common malignant epithelial skin tumor with an extremely low metastasis rate (<0.1% metastases, "semi-malignant"), but with locally aggressive and invasive growth pattern

Etiology/ Pathogenesis:

Location: Commonly in sun-exposed areas such as the face, cheeks and nose

Risk factors: UV exposure, sun sensitive skin, inorganic arsenic, associated with mutations that activate the Hedgehog pathway, immunosuppression and diseases with aberrations of the DNA repair genes, nevoid basal cell carcinoma syndrome (Gorlin-Goltz syndrome, multiple basal cell carcinomas in patients often <20 years of age)

Epithelial Tumors

Entity:	9.4 Basal Cell Carcinoma (Nodular Type)
Stain:	Hematoxylin - Eosin

Clinical Info/Symptoms: Skin nodules with central atrophy / ulceration and a pearl-like rim with / without telangiectasia; advanced cases may have locally extensive growth with destruction of adjacent tissues

Diagnostics: Clinical appearance, biopsy/excision (confirms diagnosis)

Therapy: Total excision; alternatively, radiation, laser, cryosurgery, imiquimod, or 5-fluorouracil

Radiology:

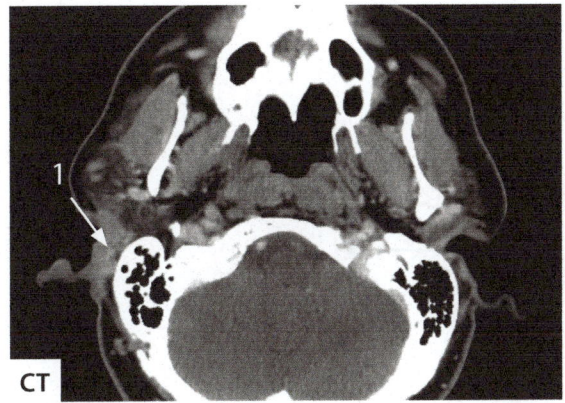
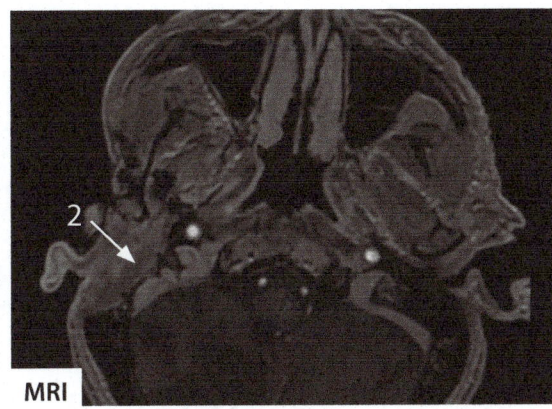

General:
- Can manifest as a soft tissue tumor involving skin surface, but can display locally aggressive behavior invading muscle or bone

CT:
- In this example, note asymmetry of the right periauricular region[1] that involves the skin but also penetrates to the scalp musculature.

MRI:
- Same patient on short term follow-up: further evidence of mass eroding into the calvarium and mastoid air cells[2]

9 Epithelial Tumors

Entity: 9.5 Prostate Cancer
Stain: Hematoxylin - Eosin

Triple stain

Macroscopy: Often multicentric, 95% start in the peripheral zone, may be palpable (firm) on rectal examination
Gross: homogeneous, spongy yellowish tissue

Microscopy:

Tissue/organ: Prostate
- Cellular atypia[1] (conspicuous nucleoli, nuclear hyperchromasia, irregular nuclear borders, loss of cell polarity)
- Absent underlying basal cell layer[2] (single row)
- Depending on grade, may show abnormal glandular architecture (cribriform growth, "back-to-back" glands); high-grade carcinoma may show sheets of cells or single cells
- Highly variable pattern of differentiation: spectrum ranges from circumscribed, well-differentiated glands, to fused small-caliber glands[4], to solid "sheet-like" growth (poorly differentiated)
- Initially local parenchymal spread, can subsequently extend to intraprostatic lymphatics and/or extend beyond prostatic capsule, with perineural invasion[4]

Immunohistochemistry (IHC):
- AMACR, NKX3.1, PSA, PSMA
- Triple stain (AMACR, p63, HMWCK) can be helpful to distinguish benign and neoplastic cells
- AMACR: red cytoplasmic staining for neoplastic cells[5]
- p63 and HWCK: highlights basal cells (brown), negative in prostate carcinoma

Definition: **Prostate carcinoma:** Malignant tumor (Adenocarcinoma) that usually arises from the epithelia of the peripheral zone

Etiology/Pathogenesis:
Most common malignant neoplasm in men (USA, Europe)
85% localized in the peripheral zone of the prostate
Increase in prevalence with increasing age, peak age of 70 years
Risk factors: Familial predisposition, hormonal factors, diet high in fat and fish

Epithelial Tumors

Entity:	9.5 Prostate Cancer
Stain:	Hematoxylin - Eosin

Diagnostics:

Calculation of the Gleason Score:

1. Assignment of a Gleason pattern (Gleason 1 - 5) to the different growth patterns
2. For prostate punch biopsies: the highest Gleason pattern in terms of area + the worst Gleason pattern (the most + the worst) = Gleason score (values between 2 - 10)
3. For prostatectomies: the highest Gleason pattern in terms of area + the second most common Gleason pattern = Gleason score (values between 2 - 10)
4. With uniform morphology, duplicate the pattern to have the score, e.g. Gleason 4 + 4 = 8

Gleason Classification Based on a Histological Pattern

Gleason Pattern	Histology
Gleason 1	Small uniform glands
Gleason 2	Enlarged areas of the stroma between the glands
Gleason 3	Marked inflation of cells at the glandular margins
Gleason 4	Irregular large number of neoplastic cells, isolated glands
Gleason 5	Absence of glands, cell layers from neoplastic cells

Gleason Score

Calculated Score	Differentiation Grade
2-4	Well-differentiated carcinoma
5-6	Moderately differentiated carcinoma
7	Moderately to poorly differentiated carcinoma
8-10	Poorly / undifferentiated carcinoma

ISUP/WHO Grade Group Classification System

ISUP/WHO Grade Groups	Calculated Gleason Score
I	1-6
II	3+4 = 7
III	4+3 = 7
IV	8
V	9-10

ATTENTION:
- Prostatic intraepithelial neoplasia (PIN) considered as precursor lesion
- Intraepithelial proliferation within the ducts or acini with cellular atypia (f.e. hyperchromasia)
- Subtypes: flat, tufted, cribriform, micropapillary
- IHC: Positive staining of basal cells[6] (HMWCK, p63), AMACR highlights acinar cells

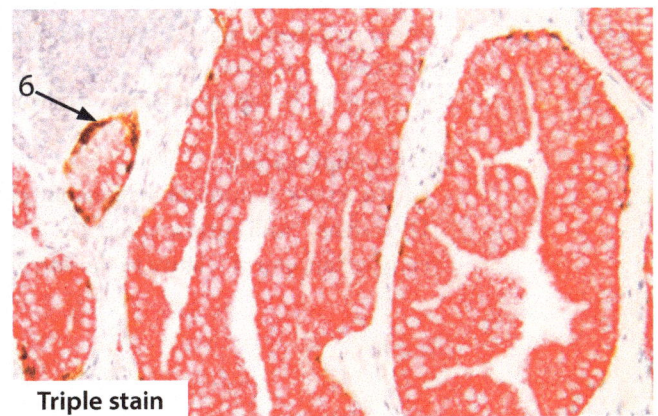

Triple stain

9 Epithelial Tumors

Entity:	9.5 Prostate Cancer
Stain:	Hematoxylin - Eosin

Clinical Info/Symptoms: Asymptomatic (initially), weight loss, urinary tract obstruction, hematuria, bone pain (with late stage metastases)

Diagnostics: Digital rectal examination (DRE), prostate-specific antigen (PSA), transrectal ultrasound scan (TRUS), MRI (PI-RADS classification), ultrasound-guided prostate punch biopsy (confirmation of diagnosis)

Therapy: Radical prostatectomy, brachytherapy, hormone therapy, active surveillance. Regular early diagnosis examinations should facilitate diagnosis at initial stages.

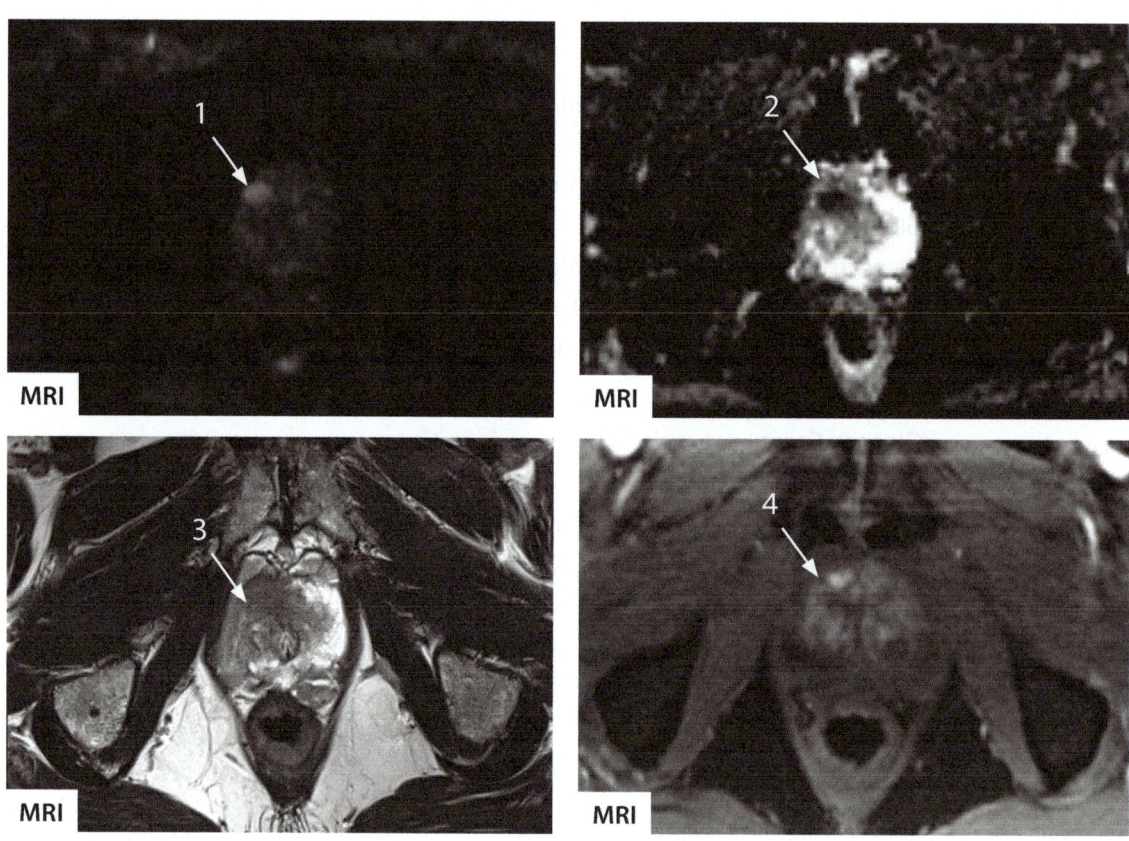

Radiology:

General:
- Multiparametric MR imaging is now a critical element in evaluating suspected or confirmed prostate cancer.
- PI-RADS (Prostate Imaging Reporting and Data System) system, version 2.1: Lesions are graded on degree of abnormality with some weighting based on location (e.g. peripheral versus transitional zone), and then assigned an overall score of 1 (very low) to 5 (very high) for likelihood to represent a clinically significant cancer.
- In addition to staging, imaging can be useful for directing targeted biopsies

MRI (example shown):
- Characteristic features of malignancy present on all key sequences: marked restricted diffusion (bright DWI signal[1] with corresponding ADC hypointensity[2]), ill-defined T2 hypointensity[3], and a core of early enhancement relative to the surrounding gland[4]

Non-Epithelial Tumors
Jesse Hart, Heejae Yang, Jao Ou

10.1 Lipoma

10.2 Cavernous Hemangioma (Liver)

10.3 Leiomyoma (Uterine)

10.4 Leiomyosarcoma

10.5 Melanocytic Nevus (Compound Type)

10 Non-Epithelial Tumors

While epithelial tumors are the most common in the body, non-epithelial tumors or neoplasms do occur, and can arise from various types of tissues. Soft tissue tumors, which are a group of non-epithelial tumors, can arise from muscle, fat, fibrous and vascular tissue. They can occur in any part of the body, however depending on the entity they do have preferred locations and different age prevalences. Soft tissue has a mesenchymal origin that comes from the mesoderm and ectoderm. Due to their origin (mesenchymal cells), it is important to keep in mind that the adult soft tissue does contain mesenchymal stem cells that have the ability to differentiate into various tissue types. Depending on different stimuli, such as genetics, environmental or infections, these tissues can develop into tumors or benign or malignant neoplasms, later ones are also often called sarcomas. According to the WHO classification soft tissue tumors can be classified into multiple groups. With a focus on clinical relevance for medical students, we have selected representative tumors to demonstrate the variety of entities that can be seen in this group.

Soft Tissue Tumors (selected from WHO)	Selected Examples
Adipocytic tumors	**Lipoma**, angiolipoma Atypical lipomatous tumor Dedifferentiated liposarcoma Myxoid liposarcoma Pleomorphic sarcoma
Fibroblastic and myofibroblastic tumors	Various types fibromas (elastofibroma, cellular angiofibroma) Fibroblastomas Lipofibromatosis Various types of fibrosarcoma (adult and infantile fibrosarcoma, myxofibrosarcoma)
So-called fibrohistiocytic tumors	Deep fibrous histiocytoma Plexiform fibrohistiocytic tumor Giant cell tumor of soft tissue
Vascular tumors	**Hemangiomas** Kaposi Sarcoma Angiosarcoma
Pericytic (perivascular) Tumors	Glomus tumor Myopericytoma Angioleiomyoma
Smooth muscle tumors	**Leiomyoma** **Leiomyosarcoma**
Skeletal muscle tumors	Rhabdomyoma Rhabdomyosarcoma (embryonal, alveolar, pleomorphic, spindle cell)
Gastrointestinal stromal tumor	Gastrointestinal stromal tumor
Chondro-osseus tumors	Soft tissue Chondroma Extraskeletal osteosarcoma
Peripheral nerve sheath tumors	Schwannoma Neurofibroma Perineurioma Malignant peripheral nerve sheath tumor
Tumors of uncertain differentiation	Intramuscular myxoma Synovial sarcoma Epithelioid sarcoma PEComa Undifferentiated sarcoma

Other non-epithelial tumors are also hematolymphoid tumors (such as lymphomas) or melanocytic tumors (**melanocytic nevus**, melanomas).

Embryology Review

Germ Layers and Their Derivates

Ectoderm
The outermost layer that gives rise to:
- Epidermis (including skin, hair, nails, adenohypophysis/anterior lobe, epidermis of the eye)
- Tooth enamel
- Neural ectoderm:
  → neural tube → brain, spinal cord (central nervous system)
  → neural crest → peripheral nerves (peripheral nervous system) and enteric nervous system, melanocytes, adrenal medulla, C-cells (parafollicular cells of the thyroid gland), neurohypophysis/posterior lobe, skull (craniofacial skeleton), facial cartilage and muscles

Mesoderm
Middle Layer, axial, paraaxial, intermediate, lateral plate mesoderm
- Axial skeleton
- Tendon
- Muscles
- Dermis
- Kidneys
- Adrenal Cortex
- Gonads
- Endothelium
- Red and white blood cells

Endoderm
Inner layer, forms into: Foregut, midgut, hindgut
- Viscera of organs
- Thyroid
- Parathyroids
- Thymus
- Liver
- Pancreas

Non-Epithelial Tumors

Entity:	10.1 Lipoma
Stain:	Hematoxylin - Eosin

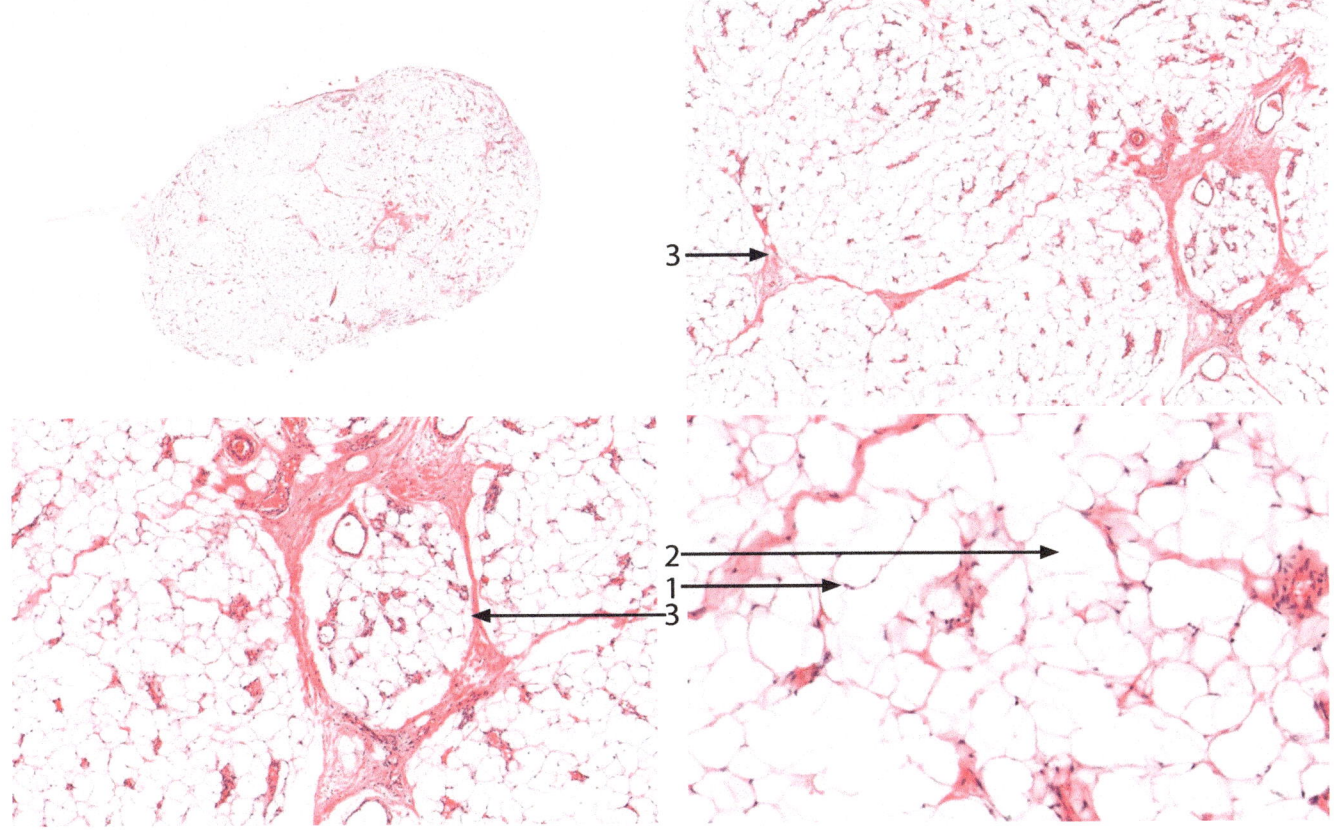

Macroscopy: Lobulation typical of adipose tissue (fat), grossly yellow and soft

Microscopy: Tissue/organ: May arise from mature adipose tissue anywhere in body
- Consists of mature adipocytes containing small nuclei[1] compressed to the edge of cell
- Clear cytoplasm with large solitary fat vacuole[2] (univacuolar)
- Cells are of similar size, homogeneous morphology
- Tissue encapsulated by delicate connective tissue septa[3], outlining circumscribed lobules

Definition: Lipoma: benign tumor arising from mature adipocytes

Etiology/Pathogenesis: Most common benign mesenchymal tumor, chromosomal aberrations in ~50% of solitary lipomas

Clinical Info/Symptoms: Painless, indolent, with slow growth, typically 2-3 cm in size, solitary or multiple, often superficial/subcutaneous, soft and mobile; deep intramuscular, intra-abdominal, and retroperitoneal lipomas are rare, must rule out low-grade malignancy (atypical lipomatous tumor/well-differentiated liposarcoma)

Diagnostics: Sonography (superficial lipomas), MRI or CT (deep lipomas), biopsy or excision (diagnostic)

Therapy: Excision in toto (symptomatic lipomas) or observation

Radiology:
General:
Incidental finding on imaging (mass with homogeneous macroscopic fat composition). If evaluation is requested for palpable abnormality, targeted ultrasound interrogation is modality of choice.
Ultrasound:
Ovoid mass[1] just beneath the skin surface
Lesion matches echogenicity and echotexture

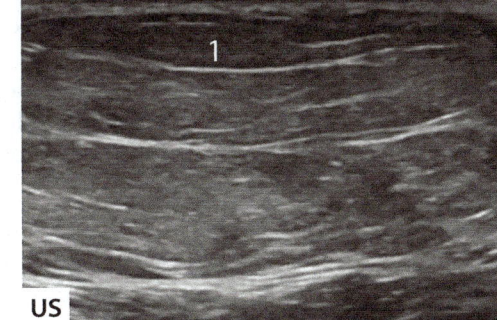

10 Non-Epithelial Tumors

Entity: 10.2 Cavernous Hemangioma (Liver)
Stain: Hematoxylin - Eosin

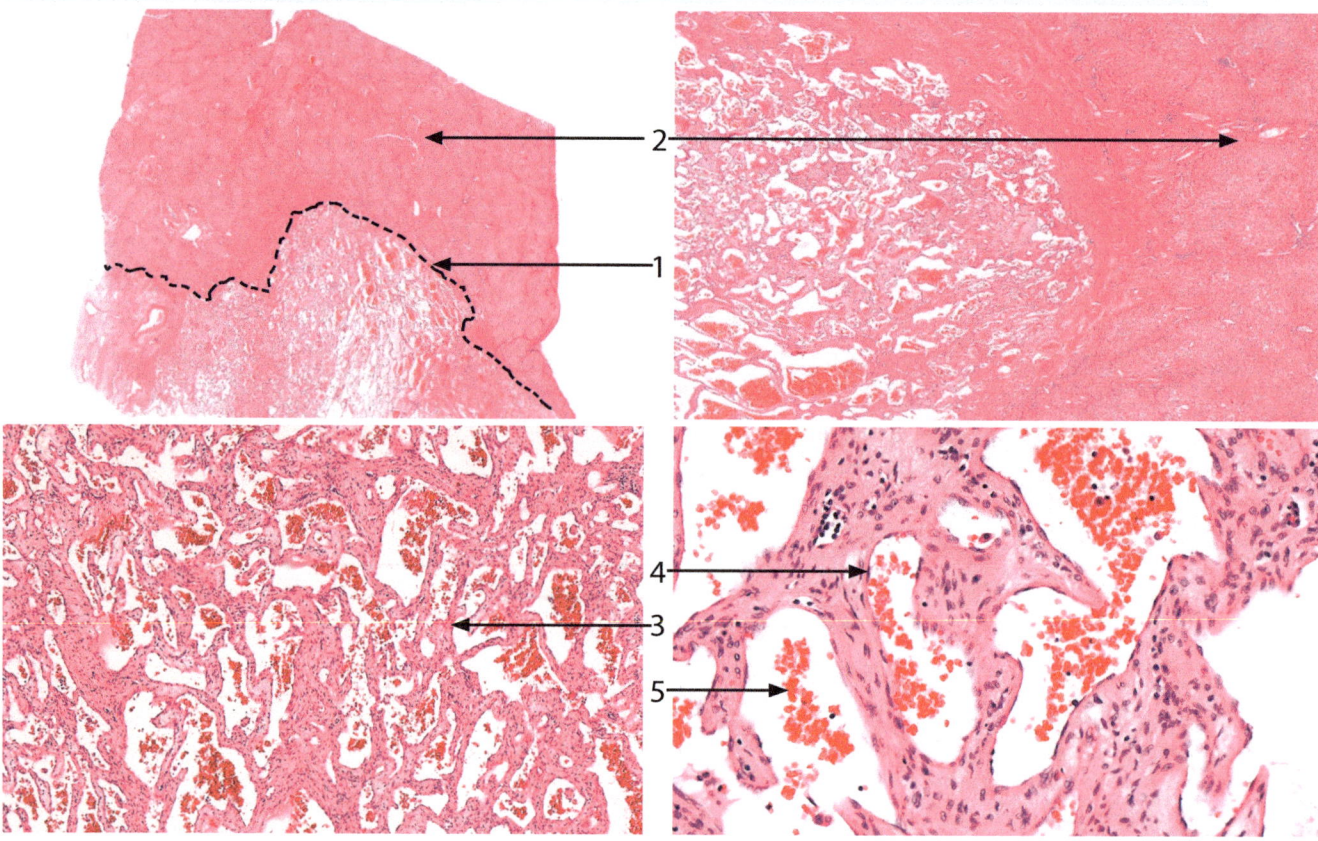

Macroscopy: Spongy structures (blood sponges) with a reddish color on the skin or in other organs (see Etiology), dark brown cut surface

Microscopy: Tissue/organ example: Liver, subserosal
- Hemangioma is sharply demarcated[1] from subserosal liver parenchyma[2]
- Composed of numerous vessels[3], lined by endothelium[4] and containing blood[5], with interspersed connective tissue stroma
- Endothelial cells show no atypia
- Various descriptive types; above is a "cavernous hemangioma" with wide vascular spaces

Definition: **Hemangioma:** Benign tumor of normal or abnormal blood vessels, different histological subtypes such as capillary (most common), cavernous, epithelioid, and lobular capillary (pyogenic granuloma)

Etiology/ Pathogenesis:
- May occur anywhere in the body, and seen in all age groups
- Often occurs in children, typically superficial head and neck; rarely parenchymal organs affected (liver, brain, spleen)
- Most common benign liver tumor in all age groups
- Pregnant patients at increased risk for growth and/or rupture during pregnancy

Syndromes involving hemangiomas:
- Von Hippel-Lindau syndrome: cavernous hemangiomas in the cerebellum, brain stem, retina, liver
- Kasabach-Merritt Syndrome: Giant Hemangiomas + Disseminated Intravascular Coagulopathy

153

Non-Epithelial Tumors

Entity:	10.2 Cavernous Hemangioma (Liver)
Stain:	Hematoxylin - Eosin

Clinical Info/Symptoms: Bright red, sharply demarcated raised vascular anomaly (superficial), mostly asymptomatic, with hemangiomas of the liver with increasing size sometimes epigastric discomfort and bleeding (with size> 5 cm, rupture and high risk of bleeding, bleeding shock)

Diagnostics: Clinic, sonography, MRI or CT (visceral and cerebral hemangiomas), excisional biopsy

Therapy: Propranolol (in childhood), cryotherapy, laser therapy or, rarely, surgical excision

Radiology:

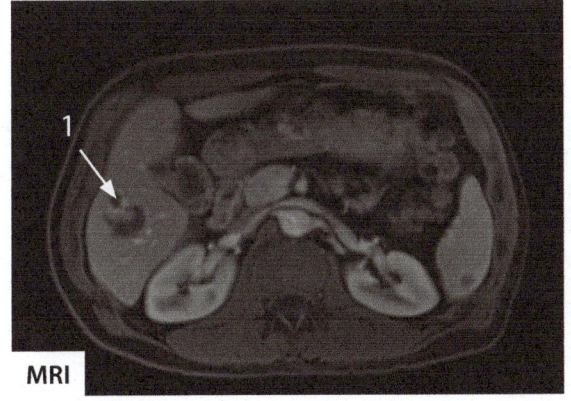
MRI

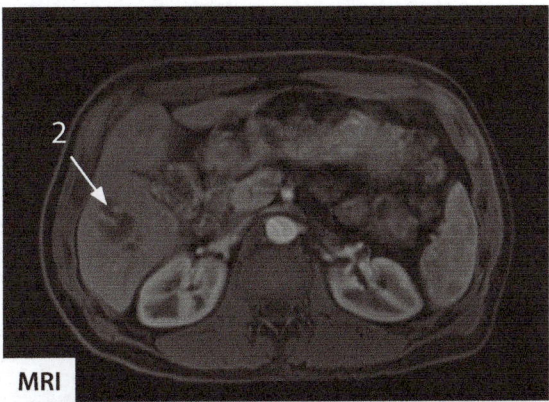
MRI

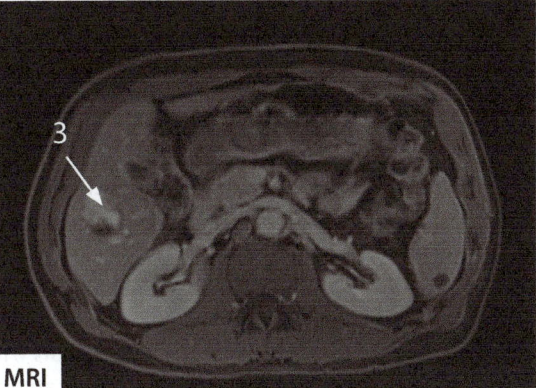
MRI

General:
- Liver masses are best evaluated by dynamic contrast-enhanced imaging (most often either CT or MR)
- Features demonstrated in a particular chronological order are linked to specific diagnostic patterns

MRI:
- Prescribed acquisitions that optimize assessment include a late arterial[1], portal venous[2], and delayed venous[3] phases
- Characteristic features of hemangioma:
Peripheral, nodular, and initially discontinuous enhancement of a lesion in the right hepatic lobe which progressively fills in the mass in a centripetal fashion

10 Non-Epithelial Tumors

Entity: 10.3 Leiomyoma (Uterine)
Stain: Hematoxylin - Eosin

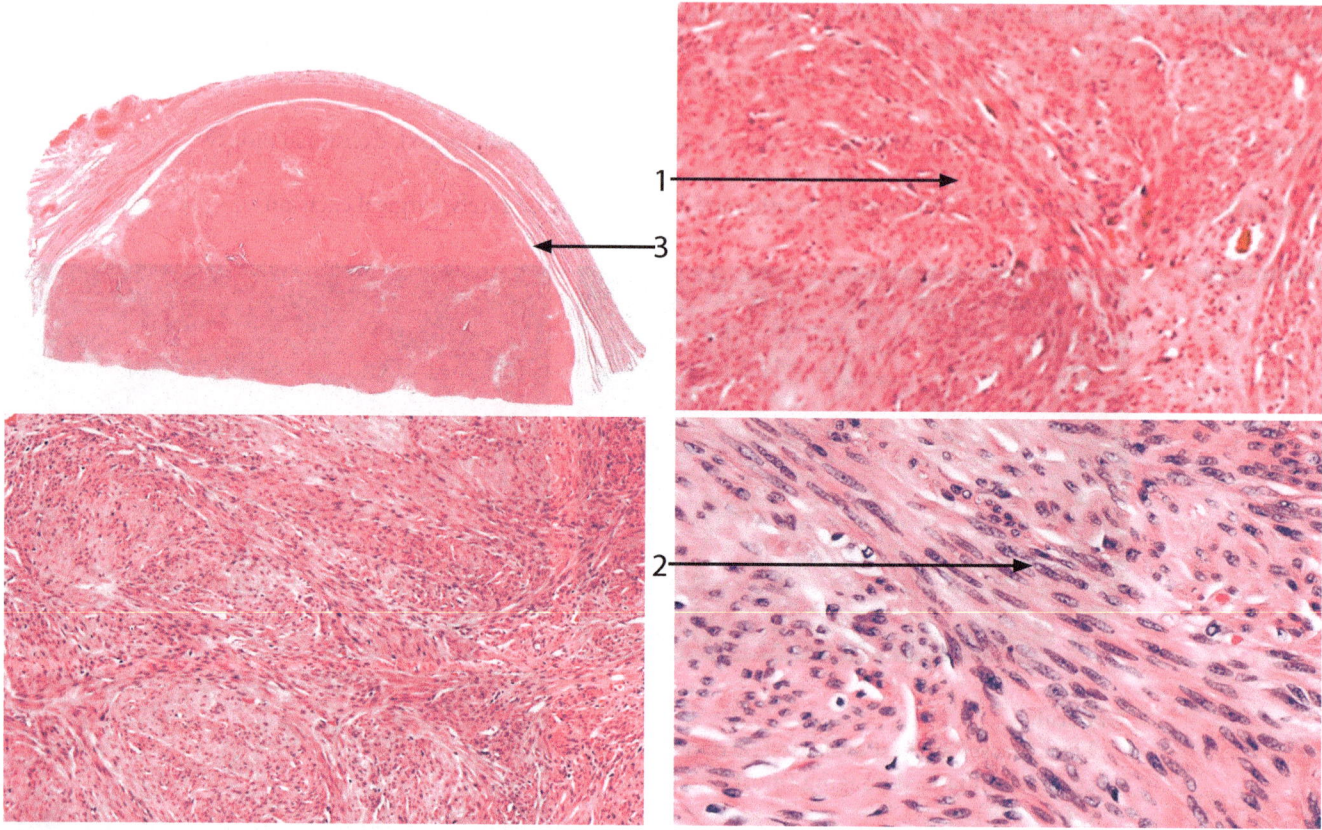

Macroscopy:	Sharply demarcated, well-circumscribed, rounded nodules (often several)
	Tan-gray-white whorled cut surfaces, may degenerate and show calcifications
Microscopy:	
	Tissue/organ: Uterine musculature (myometrium)
	– Fascicles (bundles) of smooth muscle cells[1], running in different directions
	– Bland smooth muscle cells with cigar-shaped nuclei[2] resemble normal smooth muscle cells, no or very rare mitoses, no cellular atypia
	– Spindle-like cells
	– Stroma containing collagen fibers
	– Focal hemorrhages or calcification possible, without necrosis
	– Well-circumscribed borders[3], occasional retraction artifact can be seen
	– Various subtypes: cellular, epithelioid, myxoid, fumarate hydratase-deficient
Definition:	**Uterine Leiomyoma:** Benign tumor of smooth muscle cells of the uterus, with estrogen and progesterone-dependent growth
Etiology/Pathogenesis:	MED12 mutation and HMGA2 overexpression are most common
	Rare: hereditary leiomyomatosis with renal cell carcinoma (HLRCC) due to autosomal dominant germline mutations in fumarate hydratase (FH) gene

Non-Epithelial Tumors

Entity:	10.3 Leiomyoma (Uterine)
Stain:	*Hematoxylin - Eosin*

Clinical Info: Classification by location (impacts treatment options):
- Location descriptors: Intramural, submucosal (may be pedunculated into cavity), subserosal (may be pedunculated, with risk of torsion)

Symptoms: Asymptomatic, or hypermenorrhea, dysmenorrhea, pelvic pain

Diagnostics: Bimanual palpation, sonography, hysteroscopy

Therapy: Observation, ulipristal acetate, myoma enucleation, myoma embolization, hysterectomy

Radiology:

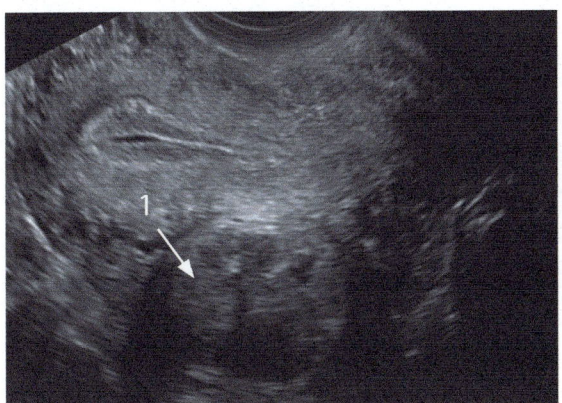 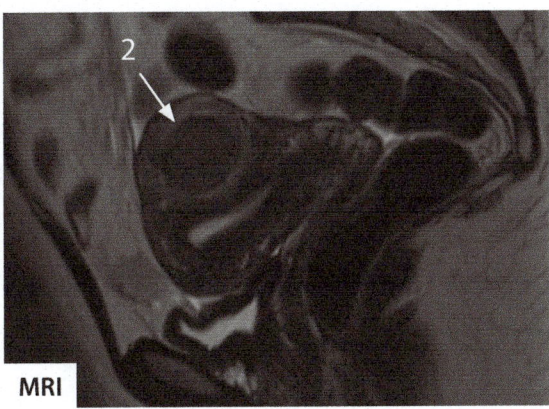

Ultrasound (transvaginal sonography)[1]:
- Subserosal mass arising from the posterior myometrium demonstrating heterogeneous shadowing (dark bands which partially obscure the rounded lesion).

MRI[2]:
- Corresponding imaging of the same patient, showing a rounded T2 intermediate-to-low signal mass.

10 Non-Epithelial Tumors

Entity: 10.4 Leiomyosarcoma
Stain: Hematoxylin - Eosin

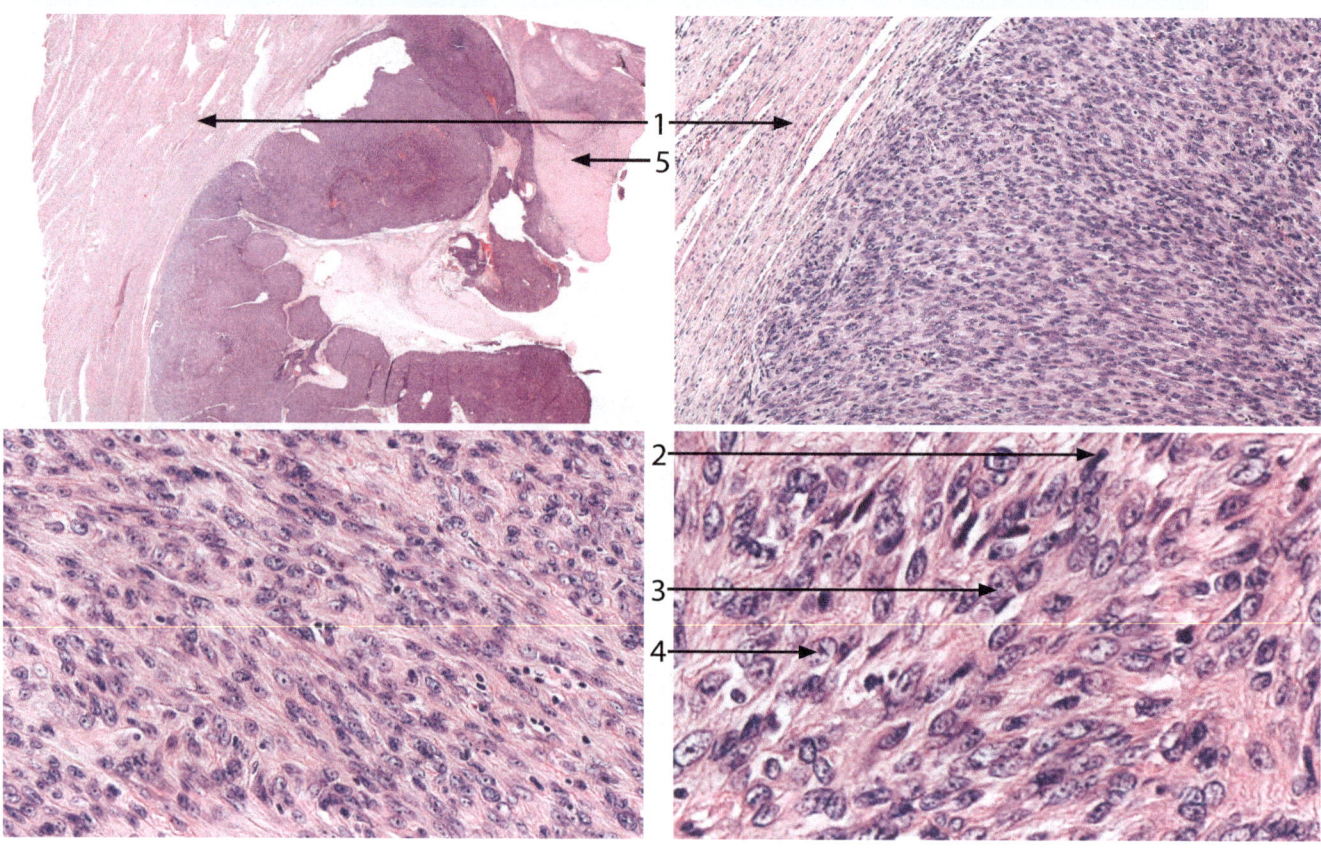

Macroscopy: Soft, tan-yellow, with infiltrative or poorly circumscribed borders, can show necrosis and hemorrhage

Microscopy: Tissue/organ: Commonly found in uterine musculature (myometrium)[1]
- Depending on degree of differentiation, may be organized in smooth muscle fascicles similar to leiomyomas
- Lesion with infiltrative borders
- Smooth muscle cells with cytologic atypia

Signs of malignancy:
- Increased and atypical mitoses[2]
- Atypical cells with cigar-shaped nuclei[3], high nuclear:cytoplasmic ratio, hyperchromasia, prominent nucleoli[4]
- Vascular invasion, regions of necrosis[5] may be present

Definition: **Leiomyosarcoma:** Malignant smooth muscle tumor

Etiology/Pathogenesis: **Morphologic subtypes:** Conventional (spindle), epithelioid, myxoid

- Multiple locations: Myometrium (most common), pelvic retroperitoneum, larger blood vessels (inferior vena cava, large veins of the lower extremity, etc.), gastrointestinal tract, lower extremities, any location containing smooth muscle
- Favored to arise de novo rather than arising via malignant transformation from a benign leiomyoma
- In contrast to leiomyomas, leiomyosarcomas have complex karyotypes with copy number alterations

Non-Epithelial Tumors

Entity:	10.4 Leiomyosarcoma
Stain:	Hematoxylin - Eosin

Clinical Info/ Symptoms: Clinical presentation depending on location: Weight loss, bleeding, mass effect

Diagnostics: Sonography, CT, MRI, biopsy / excisional biopsy (confirmation of diagnosis), TNM or FIGO Classification

Therapy: Excision in toto, poor response to radio- and chemotherapy

Radiology:

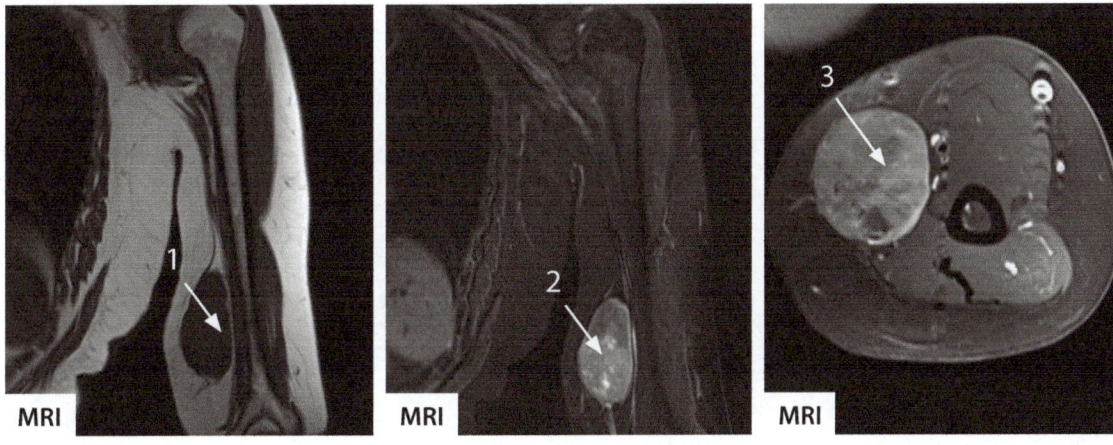

General:
- Highly variable in appearance, and therefore not necessarily distinguishable from other soft tissue tumors

MRI (left upper extremity):
- Lobular mass, T2 hypointense to surrounding fat[1]
- Mass then becomes relatively T2 hyperintense after selective fat-suppression[2] revealing subtle internal cystic changes
- Mass then enhances in a mildly heterogeneous fashion[3] with confirmation of internal necrosis (triangular dark area).

10 Non-Epithelial Tumors

Entity: 10.5 Melanocytic Nevus (Compound Type)
Stain: Hematoxylin - Eosin

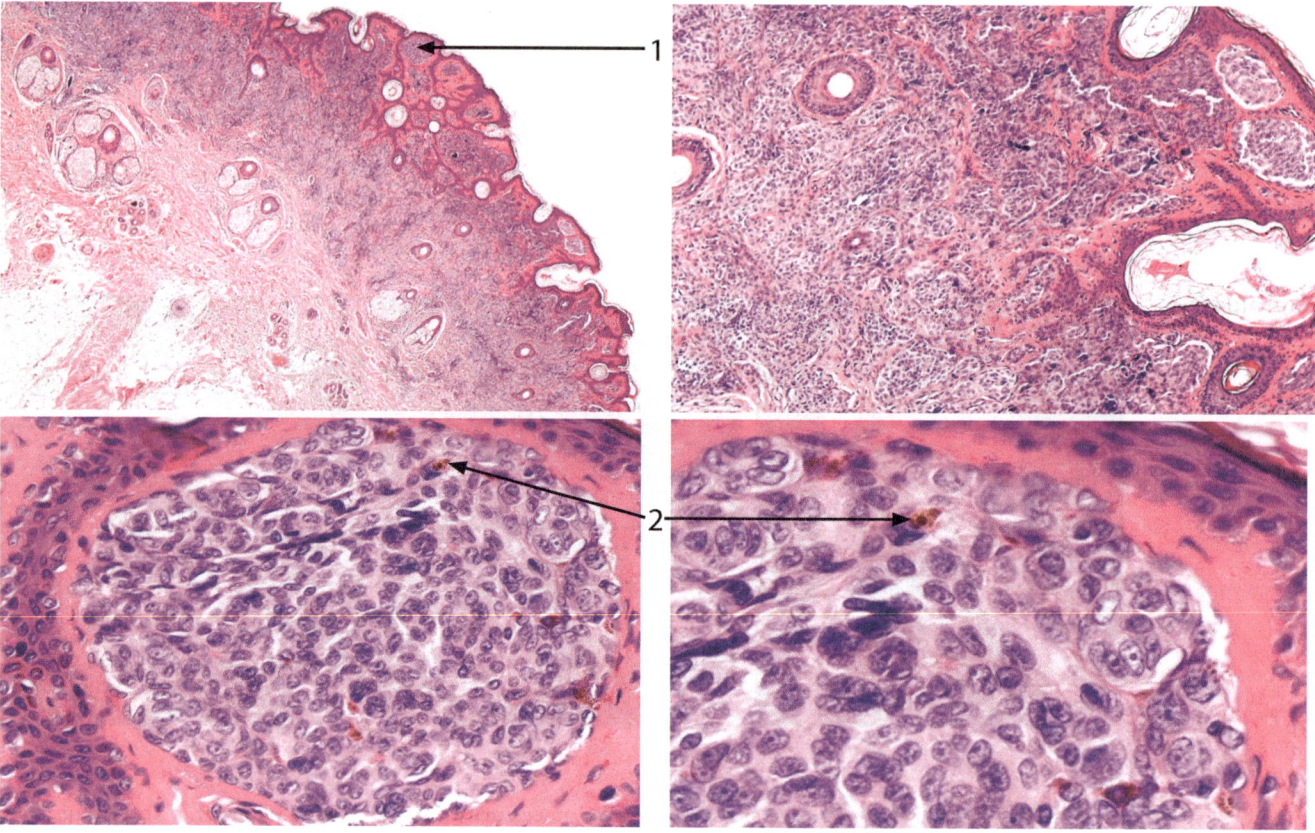

Macroscopy:	Brown/black macules or papules, usually <5 mm in diameter, uniform in appearance; example above is a compound type nevus
Microscopy:	**Classification:** Junctional nevi: Nests of melanocytes at the dermal-epidermal junction only Compound nevi: Nests of melanocytes at the junction, and nests or single cells in the dermis Dermal nevi: Nests or single melanocytes in the dermis only Congenital nevus: Compound or dermal nevus with prominent extension along adnexal structures Tissue/organ: Skin tissue Nest-like growth[1] with symmetrical distribution of the cell nests Relatively homogeneous/monomorphic cells, with abundant eosinophilic cytoplasm, relatively large nucleus, and prominent nucleolus In compound and dermal types, cells mature downward, i.e. cells mature (become smaller) deeper in the dermis Very low mitotic activity, no mitoses at deeper aspect, no atypical mitoses Melanin pigment[2] frequently identified but not required for diagnosis
Definition: Etiology/ Pathogenesis:	**Nevus:** Benign, congenital or acquired, circumscribed proliferation of melanocytes in skin or mucous membranes
Clinical Info/ Symptoms: Diagnostics:	Nevi are neoplasms, with acquired mutations in BRAF, NRAS, and other genes Sharply demarcated skin lesion, usually pigmented, typically asymptomatic though may be pedunculated and prone to irritation. Dermoscopy, biopsy/excisional biopsy (confirmation of diagnosis)
Therapy:	Important in practice: differentiation of benign melanocytic nevi from malignant melanoma Control, excision in toto (if malignancy is suspected or if the patient wishes)

Appendix

List of Abbreviations

References

© The Author(s), under exclusive license to Springer-Verlag GmbH, DE, part of Springer Nature 2024
J. Claus et al. (eds.), *General Pathology Student Guide*, https://doi.org/10.1007/978-3-662-67962-3_11

List of Abbreviations

Ab	Antibody
ABI	Ankle-Brachial-Index
ABPA	Allergic bronchopulmonary aspergillosis
AC	Adenocarcinoma
ACE	Angiotensin-converting enzyme
ADC	Apparent diffusion coefficient
AICD	Automated implantable defibrillator
AJCC	American Joint Committee on Cancer
ALT	Alanine transaminase
ANCs	Acute necrotic collections
APFCs	Acute peripancreatic fluid collections
aPTT	Activated Partial Thromboplastin Time
approx.	Approximately
ASA	Acetylsalicylic acid
ASC-H	Atypcal squamous cells, cannot exclude high-grade squamous intraepithelial lesion
ASCUS	Atypical squamous cells of undetermined significance
ASCVD	Atherosclerotic vascular disease
BAL	Bronchoalveolar lavage
BAX	Bcl-2 Associated X-protein
BCG	Bacille Calmette-Guerin
Bcl	B-cell lymphoma
BM	Basement membrane
BNP	Brain natriuretic peptide
BP	Blood pressure
BOO	Bladder outlet obstruction
BPE	Benign prostatic enlargement
BPO	Benign prostatic obstruction
BRAF	v-Raf murine sarcoma viral oncogene homolog B1
BUN	Blood Urea Nitrogen
CAD	Coronary artery disease
CBC	Complete blood count
CHD	Coronary heart disease
CIN	Cervical intraepithelial neoplasia
CK	Creatine kinase
CMV	Cytomegalovirus
CNS	Central nervous system
COPD	Chronic obstructive pulmonary disease
CPA	Chronic pulmonary aspergillosis
CRP	C-reactive protein
CSF	Cerebrospinal fluid
CT	Computer tomography
DAD	Diffuse alveolar disease
DNA	Deoxyribonucleic acid
DOAC	Direct oral anticoagulants
DIC	Disseminated intravascular coagulation
DRE	Digital rectal examination
DVT	Deep vein thrombosis
DWI	Diffusion-weighted imaging
ECG	Electrocardiogram/electrocardiography
ECHO	Echocardiography, an ultrasound of the heart
E. coli	Escherichia coli
e.g.	From latin exemplī grātiā meaning "for example"
ER	Estrogen Receptor
ERCP	Endoscopic retrograde cholangiopancreatography
esp	Especially
ESR	Erythrocyte sedimentation rate
ESWL	Extracorporeal shock wave lithotripsy

List of Abbreviations

etc.	Et cetera
EVAR	Endovascular aneurysm repair
FAS	Fas Cell Surface Death Receptor
FDG	Fluorodeoxyglucose, a radiotracer used for the positron emission tomography (PET)
FeNO	Fractional exhaled nitric oxide
FEV	Forced expiratory volume
FFP	Fresh frozen plasma
FGFR3	Fibroblast growth factor receptor 3
FH	Fumarate hydratase
FVC	Forced vital capacity
GERD	Gastroesophageal reflux disease
GFR	Glomerular filtration rate
GI	Gastrointestinal
GIT	Gastrointestinal tract
H. pylori	Helicobacter pylori
HbA1c	Glycated hemoglobin, used to monitor the average blood sugar over the past three months
HEP	Liver
HLRCC	Hereditary leiomyomatosis and renal cell cance
HMGA2	High Mobility Group AT-Hook 2
HP	Helicobacter pylori
HPV	Human papillomavirus
HSIL	High-grade squamous intraepithelial lesion
HSV	Herpes simplex virus
HU	Hounsfield Unit
HUS	Hemolytic uremic syndrome
H&E	Hematoxylin and Eosin
HGPRT	Hypoxanthine-guanine phosphoribosyltransferase
HLA	Human leukocyte antigens
ICP	Intracranial pressure
ICS	Inhaled corticosteroids
i.e.	From Latin "id est" and means "that is"
iFOBT	Immunological fecal occult blood test
IL	Interleukin
IV	Intravenous
INR	International normalised ratio
ISUP	International Society of Urological Pathology
KRAS	Ki-ras2 Kirsten rat sarcoma viral oncogene homolog
LABA	Long-acting beta-agonists
LAMA	Long-acting muscarinic antagonists
LDL	Low-density lipoprotein
LSIL	Low grade squamous intraepithelial lesion
LTRA	Leukotriene receptor antagonist
LTBI	Latent tuberculosis infection
LUTS	Lower urinary tract symptoms
LV	Left ventricle
LVI	Lymphovascular invasion
MALT	Mucosa-associated lymphoid tissue
MED12	Mediator of RNA polymerase II transcription subunit 12 homolog
MI	Myocardial infarction
min	Minute
MM	Muscularis mucosae
MP	Muscularis propria
MRI	Magnetic resonance imaging
MRSA	Methicillin-resistant Staphylococcus aureus
MSU	Monosodium urate
N:C ratio	Nuclear-to-cytoplasmic ratio
N. meningitidis	Neisseria meningitidis

List of Abbreviations

NIHSS	National Institute of Health Stroke Scale
NRAS	Neuroblastoma ras viral oncogene homolog
NSAIDs	Non-steroidal anti-inflammatory drugs
NYHA	New York Heart Association
OSS	Bones
PAD	Peripheral arterial occlusive diseas
Pap	Papanicolaou
PCN	Percutaneous nephrostomy
PCR	Polymerase chain reaction
PDE	Phosphodiesterase
PE	Pulmonary embolism
PEComa	Perivascular epithelioid cell neoplasms
PEF	Peak expiratory flow
PET	Positron emission tomography
PI-RADS	Prostate imaging–reporting and data system
PO	Per os (by mouth)
PUL	Lungs
PUNLMP	Papillary urothelial neoplasia with low malignant potential
PSA	Prostate-specific antigen
PTLA	Percutaneous transluminal angioplasty
PYR	Pyrrolidonyl Arylamidase
RB	Retinoblastoma
RV	Right ventricle
SABA	Short-acting beta-agonists
SCC	Squamous cell carcinoma
SFU	Society of Fetal Urology
SLE	Systemic lupus erythematosus
SM	Submucosa
S. pneumoniae	Streptococcus pneumoniae
SPECT	Single-photon emission computerized tomography
Spp.	Species
STEMI	ST-elevation myocardial infarction
T2DM	Type 2 Diabetes mellitus
Tc-99	Technetium-99
TEE	Transesophagea echocardiography
TTE	Transthoracic echocardiography
TMA	Thrombotic microangiopathy
TP53	Tumor protein P53
TRUS	Transrectal ultrasound scan
TSH	Thyroid stimulating hormone
TRAb	TSH/Thyrotropin receptor antibody
TURB	Transurethral resection of the bladder
TURP	Transurethral resection of the prostate
URS	Ureterorenoscopy
UV	Ultraviolet Radiation
WBC	White blood cell count
WHO	World Health Organization
WON	Walled-off necrosis

References

Chapter 1:

Forrest JA, Finlayson ND, Shearman DJ. Endoscopy in gastrointestinal bleeding. Lancet. 1974;2(7877):394-397. doi:10.1016/s0140-6736(74)91770-x

Gorter RR, Eker HH, Gorter-Stam MA, et al. Diagnosis and management of acute appendicitis. EAES consensus development conference 2015. Surg Endosc. 2016;30(11):4668-4690. doi:10.1007/s00464-016-5245-7

Lim WS, van der Eerden MM, Laing R, et al. Defining community acquired pneumonia severity on presentation to hospital: an international derivation and validation study. Thorax. 2003;58(5):377-382. doi:10.1136/thorax.58.5.377

Neogi T, Jansen TL, Dalbeth N, et al. 2015 Gout classification criteria: an American College of Rheumatology/European League Against Rheumatism collaborative initiative [published correction appears in Ann Rheum Dis. 2016 Feb;75(2):473]. Ann Rheum Dis. 2015;74(10):1789-1798. doi:10.1136/annrheumdis-2015-208237

Metlay JP, Waterer GW, Long AC, et al. Diagnosis and Treatment of Adults with Community-acquired Pneumonia. An Official Clinical Practice Guideline of the American Thoracic Society and Infectious Diseases Society of America. Am J Respir Crit Care Med. 2019;200(7):e45-e67. doi:10.1164/rccm.201908-1581ST

Chapter 2:

Ammirati E, Frigerio M, Adler ED, et al. Management of Acute Myocarditis and Chronic Inflammatory Cardiomyopathy: An Expert Consensus Document. Circ Heart Fail. 2020;13(11):e007405. doi:10.1161/CIRCHEARTFAILURE.120.007405

Ashraf N, Kubat RC, Poplin V, et al. Re-drawing the Maps for Endemic Mycoses. Mycopathologia. 2020;185(5):843-865. doi:10.1007/s11046-020-00431-2

Brandt ME, Warnock DW. Epidemiology, clinical manifestations, and therapy of infections caused by dematiaceous fungi. J Chemother. 2003;15 Suppl 2:36-47. doi:10.1179/joc.2003.15.Supplement-2.36

Cano MV, Hajjeh RA. The epidemiology of histoplasmosis: a review. Semin Respir Infect. 2001;16(2):109-118. doi:10.1053/srin.2001.24241

Chapman SW, Bradsher RW Jr, Campbell GD Jr, Pappas PG, Kauffman CA. Practice guidelines for the management of patients with blastomycosis. Infectious Diseases Society of America. Clin Infect Dis. 2000;30(4):679-683. doi:10.1086/313750

Galgiani JN, Ampel NM, Blair JE, et al. Executive Summary: 2016 Infectious Diseases Society of America (IDSA) Clinical Practice Guideline for the Treatment of Coccidioidomycosis. Clin Infect Dis. 2016;63(6):717-722. doi:10.1093/cid/ciw538

Hector RF, Laniado-Laborin R. Coccidioidomycosis--a fungal disease of the Americas. PLoS Med. 2005;2(1):e2. doi:10.1371/journal.pmed.0020002

Kang M, Chippa V, An J. Viral Myocarditis. In: StatPearls. Treasure Island (FL): StatPearls Publishing; November 20, 2023.

Lockhart SR, Toda M, Benedict K, Caceres DH, Litvintseva AP. Endemic and Other Dimorphic Mycoses in The Americas. J Fungi (Basel). 2021;7(2):151. Published 2021 Feb 20. doi:10.3390/jof7020151

Perfect JR, Dismukes WE, Dromer F, et al. Clinical practice guidelines for the management of cryptococcal disease: 2010 update by the infectious diseases society of america. Clin Infect Dis. 2010;50(3):291-322. doi:10.1086/649858

Petrikkos G, Skiada A, Lortholary O, Roilides E, Walsh TJ, Kontoyiannis DP. Epidemiology and clinical manifestations of mucormycosis. Clin Infect Dis. 2012;54 Suppl 1:S23-S34. doi:10.1093/cid/cir866

References

Queiroz-Telles F, Esterre P, Perez-Blanco M, Vitale RG, Salgado CG, Bonifaz A. Chromoblastomycosis: an overview of clinical manifestations, diagnosis and treatment. Med Mycol. 2009;47(1):3-15. doi:10.1080/13693780802538001

Rosenberg M, Patterson R, Mintzer R, Cooper BJ, Roberts M, Harris KE. Clinical and immunologic criteria for the diagnosis of allergic bronchopulmonary aspergillosis. Ann Intern Med. 1977;86(4):405-414. doi:10.7326/0003-4819-86-4-405

Saccente M, Woods GL. Clinical and laboratory update on blastomycosis. Clin Microbiol Rev. 2010;23(2):367-381. doi:10.1128/CMR.00056-09

Saha DC, Goldman DL, Shao X, et al. Serologic evidence for reactivation of cryptococcosis in solid-organ transplant recipients. Clin Vaccine Immunol. 2007;14(12):1550-1554. doi:10.1128/CVI.00242-07

Sedhai YR, Lamichhane A, Gupta V. Agranulocytosis. In: StatPearls. Treasure Island (FL): StatPearls Publishing; May 23, 2023.

Shah A, Panjabi C. Allergic Bronchopulmonary Aspergillosis: A Perplexing Clinical Entity. Allergy Asthma Immunol Res. 2016;8(4):282-297. doi:10.4168/aair.2016.8.4.282

Skalski JH, Kottom TJ, Limper AH. Pathobiology of Pneumocystis pneumonia: life cycle, cell wall and cell signal transduction. FEMS Yeast Res. 2015;15(6):fov046. doi:10.1093/femsyr/fov046

Sorrell TC, Ellis DH. Ecology of Cryptococcus neoformans. Rev Iberoam Micol. 1997;14(2):42-43.

Vincent JL, Moreno R, Takala J, et al. The SOFA (Sepsis-related Organ Failure Assessment) score to describe organ dysfunction/failure. On behalf of the Working Group on Sepsis-Related Problems of the European Society of Intensive Care Medicine. Intensive Care Med. 1996;22(7):707-710. doi:10.1007/BF01709751

Wang JL, Patterson R, Rosenberg M, Roberts M, Cooper BJ. Serum IgE and IgG antibody activity against Aspergillus fumigatus as a diagnostic aid in allergic bronchopulmonary aspergillosis. Am Rev Respir Dis. 1978;117(5):917-927. doi:10.1164/arrd.1978.117.5.917

Wheat LJ, Conces D, Allen SD, Blue-Hnidy D, Loyd J. Pulmonary histoplasmosis syndromes: recognition, diagnosis, and management. Semin Respir Crit Care Med. 2004;25(2):129-144. doi:10.1055/s-2004-824898

Wheat LJ, Freifeld AG, Kleiman MB, et al. Clinical practice guidelines for the management of patients with histoplasmosis: 2007 update by the Infectious Diseases Society of America. Clin Infect Dis. 2007;45(7):807-825. doi:10.1086/521259

Chapter 3:

Abrams P. LUTS, BPH, BPE, BPO: A Plea for the Logical Use of Correct Terms. Rev Urol. 1999;1(2):65.

Agustí A, Celli BR, Criner GJ, et al. Global Initiative for Chronic Obstructive Lung Disease 2023 Report: GOLD Executive Summary. Eur Respir J. 2023;61(4):2300239. Published 2023 Apr 1. doi:10.1183/13993003.00239-2023

Criteria Committee, New York Heart Association, Inc. Diseases of the Heart and Blood Vessels. Nomenclature and Criteria for diagnosis, 6th edition Boston, Little, Brown and Co. 1964, p 114.
©1994 American Heart Association, Inc.

Dahm P, Brasure M, MacDonald R, et al. Comparative Effectiveness of Newer Medications for Lower Urinary Tract Symptoms Attributed to Benign Prostatic Hyperplasia: A Systematic Review and Meta-analysis. Eur Urol. 2017;71(4):570-581. doi:10.1016/j.eururo.2016.09.032

Dolgin M, Association NYH, Fox AC, Gorlin R, Levin RI, New York Heart Association. Criteria Committee. Nomenclature and criteria for diagnosis of diseases of the heart and great vessels. 9th ed. Boston, MA: Lippincott Williams and Wilkins; March 1, 1994.

Fernbach SK, Maizels M, Conway JJ. Ultrasound grading of hydronephrosis: introduction to the system used by the Society for Fetal Urology. Pediatr Radiol. 1993;23(6):478-480. doi:10.1007/BF02012459

References

Jackson G, Montorsi P, Cheitlin MD. Cardiovascular safety of sildenafil citrate (Viagra): an updated perspective. Urology. 2006;68(3 Suppl):47-60. doi:10.1016/j.urology.2006.05.047

Lam CS, Solomon SD. The middle child in heart failure: heart failure with mid-range ejection fraction (40-50%). Eur J Heart Fail. 2014;16(10):1049-1055. doi:10.1002/ejhf.159

Levey AS, Coresh J, Balk E, et al. National Kidney Foundation practice guidelines for chronic kidney disease: evaluation, classification, and stratification [published correction appears in Ann Intern Med. 2003 Oct 7;139(7):605]. Ann Intern Med. 2003;139(2):137-147. doi:10.7326/0003-4819-139-2-200307150-00013

Perez C, Scrimshaw S & Munoz A. Technique of endemic goiter surveys. In Endemic Goiter, pp. 369±383. Geneva: WHO, 1960.

Peterson S, Sanga A, EkloÈf H, Bunga B, Taube A, GebreMedhin M. et al. Classification of thyroid size by palpation and ultrasonography in field surveys. Lancet 2000 355 106±110.

WHO, UNICEF & ICCIDD. Indicators for assessing iodine deficiency disorders and their control through salt iodization. WHO/NUT/94.6. Geneva: WHO 1994.

Chapter 4:

Brown F, Modi P, Tanner LS. Lofgren Syndrome. In: StatPearls. Treasure Island (FL): StatPearls Publishing; July 31, 2023.

FONTAINE R, KIM M, KIENY R. Die chirurgische Behandlung der peripheren Durchblutungsstörungen [Surgical treatment of peripheral circulation disorders]. Helv Chir Acta. 1954;21(5-6):499-533.

Gorman EW, Perkel D, Dennis D, Yates J, Heidel RE, Wortham D. Validation Of The HAS-BLED Tool In Atrial Fibrillation Patients Receiving Rivaroxaban. J Atr Fibrillation. 2016;9(2):1461. Published 2016 Aug 31. doi:10.4022/jafib.1461

Kirchhof P, Benussi S, Kotecha D, et al. 2016 ESC Guidelines for the management of atrial fibrillation developed in collaboration with EACTS. Eur J Cardiothorac Surg. 2016;50(5):e1-e88. doi:10.1093/ejcts/ezw313

Lane DA, Lip GY. Use of the CHA(2)DS(2)-VASc and HAS-BLED scores to aid decision making for thromboprophylaxis in nonvalvular atrial fibrillation. Circulation. 2012;126(7):860-865. doi:10.1161/CIRCULATIONAHA.111.060061

Mills JL Sr, Conte MS, Armstrong DG, et al. The Society for Vascular Surgery Lower Extremity Threatened Limb Classification System: risk stratification based on wound, ischemia, and foot infection (WIfI). J Vasc Surg. 2014;59(1):220-34.e342. doi:10.1016/j.jvs.2013.08.003

National Institute of Neurological Disorders and Stroke (U.S.). NIH Stroke Scale. [Bethesda, Md.?] :National Institute of Neurological Disorders and Stroke, Dept. of Health and Human Services, USA, 2011.

Pisters R, Lane DA, Nieuwlaat R, Vos CB de, Crijns HJGM, Lip GYH. A novel user-friendly score (HAS-BLED) to assess 1-year risk of major bleeding in patients with atrial fibrillation: the Euro Heart Survey. Chest. 2010;138(5):1093-1100.

Rutherford RB, Baker JD, Ernst C, et al. Recommended standards for reports dealing with lower extremity ischemia: revised version [published correction appears in J Vasc Surg 2001 Apr;33(4):805]. J Vasc Surg. 1997;26(3):517-538. doi:10.1016/s0741-5214(97)70045-4

Chapter 5:

CRAIG JM, GITLIN D. The nature of the hyaline thrombi in thrombotic thrombocytopenic purpura. Am J Pathol. 1957;33(2):251-265.

Desch KC, Motto DG. Thrombotic thrombocytopenic purpura in humans and mice. Arterioscler Thromb Vasc Biol. 2007;27(9):1901-1908. doi:10.1161/ATVBAHA.107.145797

Fredrik Skjørten, Peter B. Kierulf, Miklos Degré, FORMATION OF HYALINE MICROTFIROMBI IN THE MOUSE, Acta Pathologica Microbiologica Scandinavica Section A Pathology, 10.1111/j.1699-0463.1970.tb03311.x, 78A, 3, (351-361), (2009).

References

George JN, Nester CM. Syndromes of thrombotic microangiopathy. N Engl J Med. 2014;371(7):654-666. doi:10.1056/NEJMra1312353

Wells PS, Ginsberg JS, Anderson DR, et al. Use of a clinical model for safe management of patients with suspected pulmonary embolism. Ann Intern Med. 1998;129(12):997-1005. doi:10.7326/0003-4819-129-12-199812150-00002

Wells PS, Hirsh J, Anderson DR, et al. Accuracy of clinical assessment of deep-vein thrombosis [published correction appears in Lancet 1995 Aug 19;346(8973):516]. Lancet. 1995;345(8961):1326-1330. doi:10.1016/s0140-6736(95)92535-x

Chapter 6:

Arnett DK, Blumenthal RS, Albert MA, et al. 2019 ACC/AHA Guideline on the Primary Prevention of Cardiovascular Disease: A Report of the American College of Cardiology/American Heart Association Task Force on Clinical Practice Guidelines [published correction appears in Circulation. 2019 Sep 10;140(11):e649-e650] [published correction appears in Circulation. 2020 Jan 28;141(4):e60] [published correction appears in Circulation. 2020 Apr 21;141(16):e774]. Circulation. 2019;140(11):e596-e646. doi:10.1161/CIR.0000000000000678

DEBAKEY ME, HENLY WS, COOLEY DA, MORRIS GC Jr, CRAWFORD ES, BEALL AC Jr. SURGICAL MANAGEMENT OF DISSECTING ANEURYSMS OF THE AORTA. J Thorac Cardiovasc Surg. 1965;49:130-149.

Ibanez B, James S, Agewall S, et al. 2017 ESC Guidelines for the management of acute myocardial infarction in patients presenting with ST-segment elevation: The Task Force for the management of acute myocardial infarction in patients presenting with ST-segment elevation of the European Society of Cardiology (ESC). Eur Heart J. 2018;39(2):119-177. doi:10.1093/eurheartj/ehx393

Isselbacher EM, Preventza O, Black JH 3rd, Augoustides JG, Beck AW, Bolen MA, Braverman AC, Bray BE, Brown-Zimmerman MM, Chen EP, Collins TJ, DeAnda A Jr, Fanola CL, Girardi LN, Hicks CW, Hui DS, Jones WS, Kalahasti V, Kim KM, Milewicz DM, Oderich GS, Ogbechie L, Promes SB, Ross EG, Schermerhorn ML, Times SS, Tseng EE, Wang GJ, Woo YJ. 2022 ACC/AHA guideline for the diagnosis and management of aortic disease: a report of the American Heart Association/American College of Cardiology Joint Committee on Clinical Practice Guidelines. Circulation. 2022;146:e334–e482. doi: 10.1161/CIR.0000000000001106

Levy D, Goyal A, Grigorova Y, Farci F, Le JK. Aortic Dissection. In: StatPearls. Treasure Island (FL): StatPearls Publishing; April 23, 2023.

Libby P. Inflammation in atherosclerosis. Nature. 2002;420(6917):868-874. doi:10.1038/nature01323

Knuuti J, Wijns W, Saraste A, et al. 2019 ESC Guidelines for the diagnosis and management of chronic coronary syndromes [published correction appears in Eur Heart J. 2020 Nov 21;41(44):4242]. Eur Heart J. 2020;41(3):407-477. doi:10.1093/eurheartj/ehz425

US Preventive Services Task Force, Owens DK, Davidson KW, et al. Risk Assessment, Genetic Counseling, and Genetic Testing for BRCA-Related Cancer: US Preventive Services Task Force Recommendation Statement [published correction appears in JAMA. 2019 Nov 12;322(18):1830]. JAMA. 2019;322(7):652-665. doi:10.1001/jama.2019.10987

Fujiyoshi T, Minatoya K, Ikeda Y, et al. Impact of connective tissue disease on the surgical outcomes of aortic dissection in patients with cystic medial necrosis. J Cardiothorac Surg. 2017;12(1):97. Published 2017 Nov 23. doi:10.1186/s13019-017-0663-8

Xie JX, Cury RC, Leipsic J, et al. The Coronary Artery Disease-Reporting and Data System (CAD-RADS): Prognostic and Clinical Implications Associated With Standardized Coronary Computed Tomography Angiography Reporting. JACC Cardiovasc Imaging. 2018;11(1):78-89. doi:10.1016/j.jcmg.2017.08.026

References

Chapter 7:

Global Initiative for Asthma. Global Strategy for Asthma Management and Prevention, 2022. Available from: www.ginasthma.org

Kumar RK, Antunes MJ, Beaton A, et al. Contemporary Diagnosis and Management of Rheumatic Heart Disease: Implications for Closing the Gap: A Scientific Statement From the American Heart Association [published correction appears in Circulation. 2021 Jun 8;143(23):e1025-e1026]. Circulation. 2020;142(20):e337-e357. doi:10.1161/CIR.0000000000000921

Ross DS, Burch HB, Cooper DS, et al. 2016 American Thyroid Association Guidelines for Diagnosis and Management of Hyperthyroidism and Other Causes of Thyrotoxicosis [published correction appears in Thyroid. 2017 Nov;27(11):1462]. Thyroid. 2016;26(10):1343-1421. doi:10.1089/thy.2016.0229

Chapter 8:

Bosman FT, Carneiro F, Hruban R H, Theise N. WHO classification of tumours of the digestive system, fourth edition. France: IARC; 2010

Nayar R Wilbur DC. The Bethesda System for Reporting Cervical Cytology: Definitions Criteria and Explanatory Notes. Third ed. Cham: Springer; 2015. doi:10.1007/978-3-319-11074-5

Chapter 9:

Brawer MK. Prostatic intraepithelial neoplasia: an overview. Rev Urol. 2005;7 Suppl 3(Suppl 3):S11-S18.

Chen N, Zhou Q. The evolving Gleason grading system. Chin J Cancer Res. 2016;28(1):58-64. doi:10.3978/j.issn.1000-9604.2016.02.04

Jancík S, Drábek J, Radzioch D, Hajdúch M. Clinical relevance of KRAS in human cancers. J Biomed Biotechnol. 2010;2010:150960. doi:10.1155/2010/150960

Wang H, Shen Q, Ye LH, Ye J. MED12 mutations in human diseases. Protein Cell. 2013 Sep;4(9) 643-646. doi:10.1007/s13238-013-3048-3. PMID: 23836153; PMCID: PMC4875528.

Chapter 10:

Gary C. Schoenwolf PhD, Steven B. Bleyl MD, PhD, Philip R. Brauer PhD and Philippa H. Francis-West PhD. Larsen's Human Embryology. Sixth Edition. Elsevier 2021. 3, 55-77

Larkin S, Ansorge O. Development And Microscopic Anatomy Of The Pituitary Gland. In: Feingold KR, Anawalt B, Blackman MR, et al., eds. Endotext. South Dartmouth (MA): MDText.com, Inc.; February 15, 2017.

Tani S, Chung UI, Ohba S, Hojo H. Understanding paraxial mesoderm development and sclerotome specification for skeletal repair. Exp Mol Med. 2020;52(8):1166-1177. doi:10.1038/s12276-020-0482-1

WHO Classification of Tumours Editorial Board. Soft tissue and bone tumours. Lyon (France): International Agency for Research on Cancer; 2020. (WHO classification of tumours series, 5th ed.; vol. 3). https://publications.iarc.fr/588.

GPSR Compliance

The European Union's (EU) General Product Safety Regulation (GPSR) is a set of rules that requires consumer products to be safe and our obligations to ensure this.

If you have any concerns about our products, you can contact us on ProductSafety@springernature.com

In case Publisher is established outside the EU, the EU authorized representative is:

Springer Nature Customer Service Center GmbH
Europaplatz 3
69115 Heidelberg, Germany

Batch number: 09709365

Printed by Printforce, the Netherlands